Health Assessment for Professional Nursing

A Developmental Approach

Health Assessment for Professional Nursing

Gloria J. Block, R.N., M.S.N., F.N.P., C.
Assistant Professor of Nursing
State University of New York at Binghamton

JoEllen Wilbur Nolan, R.N., M.S.N., F.N.P., C.
Assistant Professor of Nursing
University of Illinois
Chicago, Illinois

Mary K. Dempsey, R.N., M.S., F.N.P., C.
Assistant Professor of Nursing
State University of New York at Binghamton

with contributions by

Susan K. Pennington, R.N., M.S., M.P.H.
Nursing Director, University
    Health Services
University of Massachusetts
Amherst, Massachusetts

Toni Tripp-Reimer, R.N., Ph.D.
Associate Professor
College of Nursing
University of Iowa
Iowa City, Iowa

A Developmental Approach

APPLETON–CENTURY–CROFTS/New York

81 82 83 84 85 / 10 9 8 7 6 5 4 3 2 1

Prentice-Hall International, Inc., London
Prentice-Hall of Australia, Pty. Ltd., Sydney
Prentice-Hall of India Private Limited, New Delhi
Prentice-Hall of Japan, Inc., Tokyo
Prentice-Hall of Southeast Asia, (Pte.) Ltd., Singapore
Whitchall Books Ltd., Wellington, New Zealand

Library of Congress Cataloging in Publication Data

Block, Gloria J   1952–
    Health assessment for professional nursing.

    Bibliography: p.
    Includes index.
    1. Physical diagnosis.   2. Nursing.   I. Nolan,
JoEllen, 1946–   joint author.   II. Dempsey, Mary K.,
joint author.   III. Title.
RT48.B56   616.07′54   81-501
ISBN 0-8385-3660-3   AACR1

Text Design and Production: Judith F. Warm
Cover Design: Gretczko Advertising
Cover Photograph and Book Layout: Jean M. Sabato
Illustrations: Marion Eaton
Photography: Mary K. Dempsey

PRINTED IN THE UNITED STATES OF AMERICA

To . . .

Mom, Dad, Julie, and our Clara, and to those who are so special to me—with much love and a great big hug!

G.J.B.

My family.

J.W.N.

My family and friends for their love and support and to J.F.K. and T.J.
"Don't let it be forgot that for one brief shining moment it was known as Camelot"—It's not forgot!!

M.K.D.

Contents

2. The Physical Examination: An Introduction / 56

3. The Skin / 68

4. The Head, Face, and Neck / 90

5. The Eye / 106

9. The Cardiac and Peripheral Vascular System / 176

10. The Breast / 214

11. The Abdomen / 226

12. The Female Genitalia / 240

13. The Male Genitalia / 256

14. The Musculoskeletal System / 268

Foreword

With the advent of the nurse practitioner role in the mid-1960's health assessments by nurses took on marked improvement in quality and quantity by those who had had this training. By the mid-1970's several thousand nurses had become practitioners, and the trend had started to introduce aspects of this training into baccalaureate as well as masters programs. Today, health assessment has become part of the basic education of every nurse.

As rapidly as nurses take on new responsibilities for health assessment, the likelihood increases that better patient care will result. In every setting where nurses practice, definitive health assessment skills markedly improve the data base upon which their judgements are made in determining what to do, or not to do for the patient.

Nurses are becoming more and more prominent in many areas where careful health assessment is a critical part of the programming. Screening for a variety of health conditions, for example, is an important community service in which nurses have demonstrated competence, and health assessment is an integral part of preparing for primary care and primary nursing roles. This text provides the groundwork for these roles by integrating health assessment and health history within a clinical framework. This framework is then further extended to help the clinician consider potential problems based on the findings. This assessment prepares the learner for the next step, intervention, which can be introduced at a later time.

The authors are a talented group of nurses, who with a pioneering spirit, build from experience this guide to the expanded skills for professionals in nursing. The content is easily applied to units of learning that are intended to help the student apply basic science material to clinical assessment. The authors do not minimize the complexity of the human body, but have explained in a highly understandable form the specific applications of the sciences to the clinical assessment of the human being as a whole.

Several specific characteristics mark this book as an especially valuable resource. First, it integrates content across the age span in each chapter, giving the reader a comprehensive view of the important differences where relevant at the appropriate life stages. Second, the discussion includes many practical suggestions as to life-style and environmental factors to be taken into account in the history, in particular. These factors bring the usefulness of this resource into the real-life practice of nursing that assumes the assessment must include "where the *patient* is" as well as what the *clinician* needs to know. Further, the implication is clear that the patient is an active part of the process of health assessment. The sample interview questions are intended as guides for the nurse to facilitate elicitation of information from the patient.

A third characteristic of immediate help to anyone learning the material for the first time, as well as those who are reviewing the material, are the charts and tables so carefully developed. As the discussion expands the reader's understanding beyond these charts, the text develops an awareness of problems that may be present if deviations are found. In this way, while the emphasis is on the assessment of health, important deviations are brought out for consideration as the clinician begins to develop discrimination in using the health assessment skills. Further, each chapter includes a sample record of a history and physical to guide the student in written expression of the findings. One interesting inclusion in the health history is the section on patients' activities to maintain health. This information, together with the nurses' own findings, can form the basis for useful feedback to the patient in the general area of self-protective behavior.

The challenge to those studying this text is an exciting one. This material, together with guidance of experienced clinicians in clinical settings will make it possible for the learner to integrate health assessments into every situation in which patients are encountered. Having a detailed data base from which to select and to make judgements about the effectiveness of nursing care will result in greater satisfaction of the nurse and better quality of care for the patient. Undoubtedly, the health counselling given to patients will also improve as the understanding of the patient is more complete. Mastery of the content as presented in this is well worth the effort.

Judith A. Sullivan, R.N., Ed.D.
Clinical Chief for Community
    Health Nursing
Associate Professor of Nursing
    and Preventive, Rehabilitation,
    and Family Medicine
The University of Rochester
Medical Center
Rochester, New York

Preface

Nursing and nurses are growing—qualitatively! The role of the professional nurse is changing in all health care settings. Nurses are being called upon to make in-depth nursing assessments. In order to do this, they need tools at their disposal to validate their findings. A sound data base is needed by all nurses upon which to base assessments. The purpose of this book is to provide the professional nurse or the professional nursing student with the knowledge to elicit this important data.

Nurses have special qualities that often direct them into nursing. Generally they are excellent listeners and observers. Their basic education should and does nurture these characteristics. Nursing, however, as a discipline, determines its own scientific data base that has evolved far beyond listening and observing. Professional nurses are functioning more independently and making more autonomous decisions. Taking the patient's blood pressure was once the sole purview of the physician. Over the years the scope of nursing practice has expanded far beyond measuring blood pressures to the monitoring and use of complex sophisticated equipment. The nurse is expected not only to evaluate the patient's condition and response to increasingly complicated modes of treatment. This evaluation requires a greater knowledge of and responsibility for determining the state of health of the patient. Another word for the phrase "determining the state of health of the patient" is assessment. Assessment is the first phase of the nursing process. The level and depth of nursing assessment is expanding to meet the greater expectations of the nurse. Tools and techniques are being used to make more complex assessments. For example, the stethoscope once used for blood pressures and apical pulses is used now also to separate normal vesicular breath sounds from ronchii or normal heart sounds from murmurs.

The nursing history encompasses the health history. Eliciting the health history and performing a physical examination are today a part of nursing. Together they provide the data for the nursing assessment. It is a goal of this book to provide information for the professional nurse seeking to attain these skills.

It is the belief of the authors that they offer a unique approach to a health assessment text. Much thought went into this book before any writing was begun. The authors have had experience in teaching and practice. All three have taught health assessment to undergraduate and graduate nursing students as well as nurses in continuing education programs. All three practice as family nurse practitioners to maintain their role as providers in the nursing profession. All three were once students learning health assessment themselves. Because of this transition from student to educator and practitioner, the authors feel they have the expertise to present the right amount of knowledge in the most appropriate fashion. This book represents the culmination of their efforts.

A developmental framework with an integrated approach was selected as a design for the book. This has two benefits. First, health assessment can be discussed by each body system and each system can then be developed according to particular concerns and differences of each age group. Secondly, the book's structure can be easily utilized in an integrated curriculum model in a school of nursing. Thus, each system can be presented as it occurs in the sequence of the curriculum design. If the course is taught independently in a nursing curriculum, the framework works well, too.

The developmental framework was chosen by the authors as it offers the most adaptable design for their beliefs about patients and health. The patient is envisioned as a wholistic being composed of biopsychosocial needs. The nurse assumes "wholeness" and attempts to make assessments that include biopsychosocial facets. The person then is assessed within their life cycle as a whole person with integrated complex needs. The nurse assesses the relative health of the person. Thus, the patient receives the benefits of health assessment implemented with this philosophy as a guide.

For this book the term "health assessment" was selected for two reasons. Firstly, the authors believe that nurses do more than "illness assessment." The nurse who evaluates her patients wholistically looks at where they are situated on a continuum of health. It is as important to emphasize the patient's health as well as his illness. For this reason this book's emphasis is on "normal" health assessment with "abnormal" findings highlighted appropriately to the needs of the student learning this process. The goal of this book is not to make an expert diagnostician out of the reader, but to give her enough knowledge about health assessment to substantiate the actions she takes in her nursing decisions.

Secondly, the term health assessment was selected because it is more comprehensive than physical assessment or physical diagnosis, phrases commonly used in the past to describe this process. Health assessment features a wholistic approach. It not only includes the results of the physical examination, but also what the patient tells you about his wellness or illness. In other words, the term health assessment includes the process of history taking and physical examination.

The following statement is often professed to students on the first day of their health assessment course. "If you can learn to elicit a thorough and accurate history, you can be almost certain about what you will discover on the physical examination." The authors believe this statement to be entirely true. With that in mind we have selected to emphasize and reemphasize the history taking process throughout the book.

The first chapter is devoted exclusively to the health history. This chapter begins by reviewing some basic information about listening, questioning, and providing a supportive environment for the patient while collecting the data. This section not only discusses the principles of history taking, but also provides the student with suggestions for questioning the patient most effectively.

The components of the health history are then developed at length. The features of this chapter which give this book an extensive nursing emphasis are the psychosocial and nutritional sections. As nurses, we believe that developing these areas in the history is essential to evaluating the patient's overall health status. Therefore, within the chapter, the developmental, sexual, and nutritional histories are discussed according to every age and stage through the lifespan. Each section includes the necessary content that the student needs to be familiar with to explore specific areas with the patient.

In addition, each section provides examples of questions that can be used to elicit the data. The authors find this especially helpful for students who are struggling with how to ask the patient about his perception of his achievement of developmental tasks or feelings concerning his sexuality. It is not hard to convince students that this information is necessary to obtain, but they do seem to have a great deal of difficulty knowing how to elicit the data. Therefore, the emphasis is on the "how to's" of eliciting the data in these less tangible areas of the health history.

In addition to the chapter devoted to the Health History, there are short histories at the beginning of each chapter reviewing the body system being discussed. It is important for the student to understand that each system of the body when being evaluated has more than the physical findings which contribute to the final assessment of the condition of that system. For instance, when a stethescope is placed on a patient's chest and abnormal breath sounds are heard, and whether the patient has a previous diagnosis of congestive heart failure or has had an elevated temperature for three days, will channel the nurse's thinking about the nature of the problem. It is the combination of the history of the presenting complaint and the physical findings that lead the nurse to her assessment.

Each physical assessment chapter is organized in a similar fashion. There are four major sections: the historical review of the system being discussed, an overview of the necessary anatomy and physiology to assess the organs involved, the methods of physical examination used to evaluate the system and an example of how to record a chief complaint, history of present illness and physical findings of a problem commonly occurring in that system.

The repetitive format of each physical assessment chapter reinforces the necessity of a systematic approach to a physical examination. This is most important for the novice learning the process of health assessment.

Another unique feature of each chapter is the inclusion of transcultural aspects and physical features of various populations in the world. A nursing leader who is doctorally prepared in anthropology and sociology has incorporated this type of information throughout the book. All these very extensive discussions and highlighted areas throughout the book reflect the authors' wholistic approach to health assessment with its variations throughout the life cycle.

"Nursing means caring, comforting, counseling, teaching, guiding."* Caring and comforting are a great part of what this book is all about, for to take care of and give comfort to, a nurse must first listen, touch, and observe. Of all those whom the patient sees for health care, the nurse is likely to be the most consistent contact and the most available to evaluate the patient with tender compassionate interest.

Much has been written and continues to be written about the changing role of the professional nurse in the delivery of health care. The entire system is in a state of dynamic change at every

*Mauksch, Ingeborg. "The Future of Nursing." Presentation delivered in Binghamton, New York, May 1979.

level. These changes are especially apparent in legislative enactments, professional education, third-party payment demands, and the redistribution of responsibility among providers of health care. The role of the nurse has already changed a great deal. As the entire system changes, the function of the professional nurse will continue to develop. It is absolutely essential for the nurse to recognize how much the role of the professional nurse has already changed, if she is to be a full participant in the delivery of health care and especially if she is to be a creative contributor shaping still other changes which are bound to come.

The very fact that you, the nurse, have begun to read this book and study this subject, indicates that you acknowledge your awareness that the changes have indeed taken place and that you are making the professional decision to add to your learning and your skills, to the end that you will be doing all in your power to ready yourself for the professional demands of the nurses' role.

This knowledge can be incorporated into any area of nursing practice. Some nurses may find certain portions of the content more appropriate to their specialty. However, the book is written to meet the needs of the nurse in any health care setting. The nurse in a cardiac intensive care unit may become very proficient at listening to heart and breath sounds, but the very fact that she has the knowledge to evaluate psychosocial status or a skin rash reinforces the concept of wholistic nursing care.

The nurse practicing in a primary care setting will probably use this information for more generalized assessments as opposed to the nurse who has a highly specialized area of expertise. The authors wrote the book with the intention of meeting the needs of the professional nurse in any clinical setting.

Ideally, the book should be a valuable tool for nurses and nurses-to-be . . . and of equal worth to their teachers. This means that far more is envisioned than a "How To" teaching manual. The book, on the one hand should serve the already present desire of students to acquire new professional skills, without losing sight, on the other hand, of the importance of serving as a stimulus to the generation of ideas by the students themselves. The new nursing role calls for a greater degree of creativity and originality than was historically permitted.

The book, therefore, should be seen as opening doors for nurses in their expanding roles in the developing system of delivery of overall health care. "Expanding" is just the right word. The system is expanding. The nurses' roles are expanding. The book, too, should be designed for expansion . . . to keep pace with the dynamism of the nursing profession.

Nurses need to win the right to practice in settings which traditionally have provided little room for such nursing functions. To be successful, the book ought to help individual nurses learn to accept new responsibilities, to be comfortable where reliance is placed on their shoulders in unaccustomed professional areas, and finally, to be pioneers . . . that is, to show leadership in encouraging other professionals to accept them in wider roles.

The intention of this book is to give our nursing colleagues and nursing students the information they will need to be "astute assessors." Lacking this knowledge is like not having frosting on a layer cake. The cake might be adequate without it, but the frosting adds a flavor and richness that completes the taste. This book is for nurses who want to remain nurses!

Acknowledgments

Never in the course of Health Assessment have so few owed so much to so many . . .

We would like to thank:

Mary Ann Samsonik, our chief support, secretary, counselor, who typed every word of the manuscript in its several stages . . .

The Blocks, Katie and Paul Nolan, the Dempseys, the Wilburs, the Elinoffs, Denise Murray, Skip and Sharon Church, the Rymans, Margaret Tyson, Linda Rounds, Debby Dougherty, Danielle White, Phyllis Antos, the Haarsticks, Margaret Manley, Judy Kohl, the folks at 333 for all their TLC and understanding. . .

Victor Elinoff and Jonathan Harris who are anxious for this book to be done so they can get on with their lives!

Sharon Church, Victor, Cissy, Jed and Adam Elinoff, Gert and Mike Ryman, Alice and Jack Dempsey, Jamie Allen, Katie Nolan, Rosalyn Satterfied, Debbie Besen (MDT), Linda Rounds, Jon Harris, Dan Zatsick, Judy Nielsen, Nora Vallon, Jose Burgos, Casto Ramos, for their superb modeling . . .

Victor Elinoff, Jonathan Harris, and Dave Murrish for their technical consultation. . .

Gert Ryman, Paul Nolan, Sharon Church, Margaret Shea, Karen Herceg, and Liz Quilter for their proofreading. . .

Sue Rich and Herman Paikoff for their photographic consultation services. . .

Judy Sullivan for her support and Foreword. . .

Max Block, Jr. for his eloquent verbage P.R.N.!

Our students, especially Janis Riffanacht, Sue Frankowski, Michele Musto, Carol Kolarz, and Chris VanDelft. . .

Leslie Boyer, Judi Warm, Jean M. Sabato, Ray Lams, Gloria Moyer, and the rest of the staff at Appleton–Century–Crofts.

a personal note:

Health assessment, like so many key elements of health care, involves science, art, skill, technique, observation, logic, and most of all, caring. Success in the health assessment process depends on caring about people as well as caring for them. A nurse who truly masters this process will discover some unexpected "side effects". She will gain greater respect from health professionals with whom she works, and more appreciation from her patients. Adding this knowledge to her nursing practice will be a source of continuing professional pride and personal satisfaction.

One of the authors of this book was recently a patient in a teaching hospital which expects a high level of professionalism from its nurses. By coincidence, one of the author's former students was employed there. She felt she was succeeding while so many other new graduates were finding it difficult to meet the exacting demands of this institution. She was gracious enough to say, "The Health Assessment course put it all together for me."

It is hoped that authors' efforts to present an integrated approach to health assessment will help more nurses succeed in their complex and constantly expanding professional roles.

Max Block, Jr.

Health Assessment for Professional Nursing

A Developmental Approach

1

The
Health History

The information obtained for a patient assessment includes a health history, physical findings, and laboratory data. The history is the first and most important part of the data base. It serves as the foundation for the physical and laboratory data by directing the examiner toward the systems that should be examined. If a patient were to give a history of sore throat and rhinorrhea, the nurse would focus on (but not limit herself to) an examination of the ear and nasopharyngeal area. A detailed neurologic examination would be neither necessary nor appropriate. In addition to its influence on the course of the examination, the history gives meaning to the physical findings. Wheezing heard in the chest of an adult patient can be the result of a variety of causes. Knowledge of a 30-year history of heavy tobacco use might lead to the assessment: "Wheezes as a result of smoking." Without the support of historical data this wheezing would have been an isolated finding and the cause would have been difficult to determine. It is hard to overemphasize the importance of the history. It is fair to say that at least 80 percent of all diagnoses could be accurately made on the basis of history alone.

At this point it is important to distinguish between historical data and data obtained on physical examination and through laboratory tests. The pieces of information given by the patient while taking the history are called *symptoms*. These are *subjective* sensations which interfere with the patient's physical or mental comfort. *Signs* are *objective* evidence of a problem identified during the physical examination and from laboratory data. They are problems the examiner sees, feels, or hears with her* own senses. Pain, for example, is a symptom, while a mass is a sign. Symptoms are recorded in the history and signs are recorded in the physical.

*For the purposes of clarity, throughout the book the nurse (or examiner) will be referred to as "she" or "her" and the patient as "he" or "him."

This chapter will cover the complete health history, while following chapters will present the physical examination. Accompanying each chapter will be a brief example of subjective and objective data pertaining to the system being presented. This book will not address the use of laboratory data, with the exception of Chapter 12, The Female Genitalia.

THE HEALTH HISTORY

Traditionally, the patient's record contains a variety of histories. Under the premise that there is a body of knowledge specific to its field only, each professional group feels it necessary to gather its own information. This results in separate histories for nursing, medicine, nutrition, social service, etc. The main disadvantage of this system is that much of the data collected is redundant. The patient is subjected to many interviews consisting of repetitious questions. Because team members feel (perhaps with some justification) that information collected by other professionals does not meet their needs, they ignore it. This was often the case with the traditional nursing history, which was somewhat superficial and included such items as personal belongings brought with the patient to the hospital.

Nurses today are accountable for their actions. If a nurse is to arrive at an assessment, to determine the course of management or to make an appropriate referral, her decisions must be based on a body of professional knowledge combined with factual information about the patient under consideration. These data are then clearly documented.

The history is the primary source of patient information. It is a comprehensive record of the patient's present and past state of health. It reflects the patient as a complete entity both physically and psychosocially. Once the history is recorded, it gives any reader a clear picture of the patient and his problems. The availability of the history for use by all members of the health care team eliminates the need for repetitious interviews. Another professional may ask the patient to elaborate on a particular area, but then should not independently repeat material already collected. Thus time spent with the patient is used more efficiently, enhancing the interdisciplinary approach to health care.

Obtaining the History

The health history of a healthy or ill patient can be obtained at any point in his development. The source of information may be the patient, relatives, friends, old records, or any combination of these. Depending on the nature of the visit or severity of a problem, the history may take up to a half hour or even an hour to collect and an additional half hour to an hour to record. Ideally, all the information is collected at the time of the first patient encounter and ongoing data are obtained at subsequent visits. Realistically, time is often limited and portions of the history must be obtained over several patient contacts. The examiner should be sure to record in the notes the important facts to be elaborated on at the next meeting.

To ease the nurse's task, a predetermined format should be used to guide the interview. (See Worksheet for Patient History, p. 8.) This is merely a skeleton outline and not a check list or series of questions; the nurse's questions should be prompted by her knowledge of patient care. The structure keeps the interview efficient, and the nurse is better able to keep the patient on the topic at hand. This is not to say that flexibility is detrimental. If the patient jumps to the end of the outline, but the information is valuable, he should be allowed to discuss what is on his mind at that time. The gaps can be filled in later.

Taking occasional notes is necessary due to the volume of information obtained. Before beginning the interview, the examiner should inform the patient that she will be writing down some of the things he tells her. It is often reassuring to patients to know that their words are important enough to be recorded. The examiner should try to maintain eye contact, while writing and record just enough to later recall the data. It is important to remember that members of many ethnic groups may not wish to engage in direct eye contact. For example, some Appalachians, American Indians, and Orientals consider direct eye contact impolite and avert their eyes during an interview. This behavior should be respected and not misunderstood as disinterest or hishonesty.[1]

Approach to the History

The nurse's first contact with the patient is usually for the purpose of obtaining a health history. Ideally, this is time when the nurse establishes a trusting relationship that will facilitate the course of the patient's health care.

The patient can quickly detect whether the nurse is objective or judgmental and nonaccepting. There are several ways the nurse can help to make the patient feel comfortable and gain his trust. First, the interview should be conducted in a private environment. If this is impossible, the nurse should make sure that curtains are pulled and should talk only loud enough for the patient to hear. Second, the nurse should provide a relaxed setting. This is often accomplished by moving the interviewer's chair out from behind a desk, avoiding an authoritarian approach. Third, the nurse should make appropriate introductions, acknowledging all persons and their roles. If a young child has come with his parent, the nurse should be sure to recognize the child as well as the adult by name. She should tell the patient her name in the way she would like to be addressed in the future. Fourth, if possible, the nurse should take most of the health history prior to the physical exam, while the patient is still fully clothed. This gives the patient a sense of security. The nurse should avoid introducing certain questions once the physical exam has begun—the patient may become very anxious if he thinks a problem has been found. In most cases it is best to wait to ask these questions until after the examination is completed, although exceptions do occur and this approach may have to be modified. For example, some children are so frightened when they arrive for health care that it is best to take a brief history and quickly proceed to the physical examination. Once this is completed, the child may be sufficiently relaxed to give a detailed explanation of the problem.

There are several additional points to be aware of when approaching children, adolescents, and elderly adults for a health history.

Children. If the child is very young, the parent or guardian will give the information. Infants usually remain quietly in the parent's arms. An active toddler can be occupied with toys at this time. A school-age child, and occasionally a preschooler, is old enough to make a significant contribution to the history. The nurse should include the child in the questioning and allow him to speak without interruption (Fig. 1.1). The child can provide valuable information about himself, which is often very revealing to his parent. Sensitive areas regarding the child's problem are best discussed with the

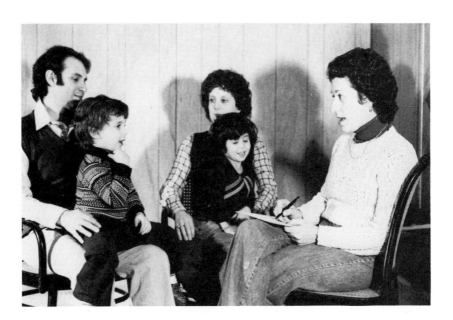

FIGURE 1.1. Interviewing the young family: the child shares his feelings.

parent in private. Because the school-age child may become concerned about what is transpiring in his absence, the nurse should talk with the parent when the child is occupied with, for example, laboratory work.

Adolescents. Children in early adolescence are beginning to assert their independence. Their parents, however, still want to be, and should be, involved in their children's care. The question of confidentiality can be awkward for the nurse. She must weigh the effect that talking with the parents will have on the youth's physical and mental well-being against the benefits of parental involvement. In order to retain trust, the nurse should discuss with the teenager which information will be shared with the parents and which will be kept confidential. By late adolescence the teenager's parents are much less frequently involved and questions of confidence rarely arise.

Elderly Adults. The elderly patient is sometimes the most difficult patient from whom to obtain a history. The list of prior illnesses and hospitalizations can seem overwhelming. In addition, recall can be vague about problems that occurred a long time ago or when there have been multiple hospitalizations for a chronic disease. The nurse should remain calm and allow for extra time if this is the first encounter with the patient. With time the nurse will learn to zero in on facts which are relevant to the patient's present state of well-being. The nurse should also be aware of sensory changes that come with age. For example, if there is a hearing impairment, the nurse should position herself in front of the patient so that he can see her speak.

Often the elderly patient feels uncomfortable discussing personal aspects of his life. This may be related to his having been raised in a less open era, and this uneasiness can be magnified if the nurse obtaining his history is young. The nurse should tread slowly into areas that are upsetting, always respecting the patient's privacy. She may need to wait until a firm relationship is established before probing sensitive areas.

The nurse should be aware of existing myths about aging. Some of the more common ones include tranquility, senility, unproductivity, and resistance to change. Elderly people have many of the concerns they had as young adults. Some of these, such as financial concerns, may be increased. It is not true that all elderly people are mentally confused, a condition which is referred to as senility. Nor does age mean that the person cannot be socially active or hold a job. Finally, resistance to change is probably related to lifelong personality traits rather than age. If the nurse ascribes to any of these myths she may structure her interview in such a way that she misses important pieces of information.

The Principles of History Taking

The principles of history taking include listening, questioning, observation, and integration.[2]

Listening. The interviewer should sit back and listen attentively as the patient tells his story (Fig. 1.2). A great deal of factual information can be obtained by letting the patient talk without interruption. This period of silence for the interviewer allows time to learn about

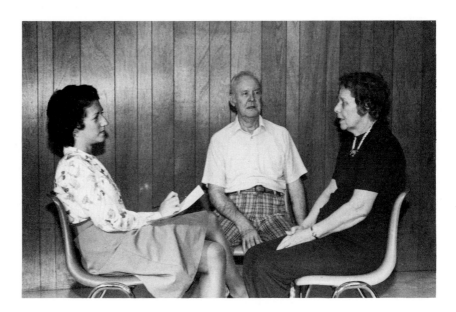

FIGURE 1.2. The art of attentive listening.

the patient's personality and emotional status and to assess his background, experience, and general level of intellectual functioning. It is important to evaluate these factors during the initial phases of the interview in order to be able to frame questions appropriately.

Questioning. After the patient has completed his story, the interviewer should ask specific questions to gain additional information. Some pertinent areas of the history may need clarification; other areas may have been omitted entirely. The nurse should resist the tendency to formulate the next question while the patient is still answering an earlier question. Valuable information may be lost by neglecting to give full attention to each response.

An open-ended approach should be used whenever possible—for example, "Tell me about your chest pain." This encourages verbalization, although some interviews can become rambling if too many open-ended questions are used. A more direct approach, involving primarily a "yes" or "no" response, can refocus and expedite the process. This tactic is also useful if the patient is having difficulty describing a problem, such as the intensity of his pain. In this case the interviewer might offer descriptive words, such as sharp, dull, throbbing, etc. When the interviewer offers descriptive words to the patient, offering choices rather than eliciting yes/no answers is helpful. The disadvantage in using direct questioning is that too many pointed inquiries tend to overwhelm the patient and put words in his mouth.

The nurse should avoid the use of leading questions, such as, "You don't have a history of emotional illness, do you?" This gives the patient an idea of the answer desired and, in an effort to please the interviewer, the patient often responds accordingly. The nurse's body movements, expression, and paralinguistics all indicate to the patient the expected response. The nurse should strive for neutrality in demeanor and try to eliminate personal idiosyncrasies, such as head nodding, while asking the questions.

Areas that may make the patient uncomfortable should be handled in a factual but not impersonal manner. If the interviewer conveys to the patient that she is comfortable with the information being obtained, the patient will usually respond honestly. Often patients are relieved when asked questions regarding personal matters which they may have been too embarrassed or afraid to introduce. However, the interviewer should not force sensitive issues the patient may not wish to discuss. These issues can be addressed later in the relationship, after trust has been established.

Observation.   The collection of objective data which later become part of the physical exam begins during the history. The patient should be observed during the interview for factors that may relate to his presenting problem. These include the patient's general appearance, demeanor, and stature and his attitudes toward himself, the interviewer, and his problems. Such information gives clues regarding the patient's sense of physical and mental well-being. If the patient is accompanied by someone else, as in the case of a child, their interactions should be observed. One can occasionally detect an emotional basis to a seemingly physical problem.

Integration.   It is helpful to periodically summarize the data that have been collected so far during the history. This clarifies the information and keeps the interview directly focused. The final summary is an integration of all the information gathered in the health history. If the task has been performed properly and completely, the nurse will have an accurate understanding of the patient and his problem.

Writing the History

The history should not be recorded during the interview. The nurse needs time to digest, sort, and integrate the information so that it can be put into a concise, coherent narrative. The same format used to guide the interview should be used to write it. It should be remembered that the history consists of the information gathered from the patient free of embellishment or reinterpretation by the interviewer. Interpretation should encompass all available information (history, physical, and laboratory data). Obviously, this is only possible at the end of the entire process.

OUTLINE FOR THE HEALTH HISTORY

A. Demographic data
B. Chief complaint (reason for visit)
C. History of present illness
   1. Usual state of health
   2. Chronologic story
      a. Sequence and chronology
      b. Frequency
      c. Location
      d. Character
      e. Quantity
      f. Setting
      g. Associated phenomena
      h. Aggravating and alleviating factors
   3. Relevant family history
   4. Disability assessment

D. Past history
    1. Childhood illnesses
    2. Immunizations
    3. Allergies
    4. Hospitalizations and serious illnesses
    5. Accidents
    6. Obstetric history
    7. Medications
    8. Habits
    9. Prenatal history*
    10. Labor and delivery history*
    11. Neonatal history*

*Recorded for a child under 4 years of age with congenital or developmental problems.

E. Family history
F. Review of systems
    1. General
    2. Skin
    3. Hair
    4. Nails
    5. Head
    6. Eyes
    7. Ears
    8. Nose
    9. Mouth
    10. Throat
    11. Breast
    12. Respiratory
        a. Child
        b. Adult
    13. Cardiovascular
    14. Gastrointestinal
    15. Genitourinary
        a. General
        b. Toddler
        c. School age
        d. Female menstrual history
        e. Male
            1. Adult
            2. Adolescent
    16. Back
    17. Extremities
    18. Neurologic
    19. Hematopoietic
    20. Endocrine
G. Nutritional history
H. Social data
    1. Family relationships and friendships
    2. Ethnic affiliation
    3. Occupational history
    4. Educational history
    5. Economic status
    6. Living circumstances
    7. Pattern of health care
I. Developmental history
J. Sexual history
K. Patient's activity to remain healthy

Demographic Data

There are some biographic facts that are necessary to the patient's record. This information is standard in all health facilities. The data to be collected for this section include:

1. Name
2. Address
3. Age
4. Sex
5. Marital status
6. Race
7. Religion
8. Usual source of medical care
9. Source and reliability of information

Chief Complaint (Reason for Visit)

The patient has arrived in the clinic office, signaled with his call bell in the hospital, or phoned the Public Health Department for a definite reason. The chief complaint (CC) is a brief statement of things that are troubling the patient and the duration of time the problem(s) has existed. Generally, it is the answer to the question, "What is troubling you?" or "What brought you to the clinic today?" or "Why did you come to the hospital?" Ideally the CC is the patient's first response to the nurse's question and is written in quotation marks. However, the patient may give a vague answer, such as, "I haven't felt well for the past week." It is important to be precise in exploring the patient's problem. A better CC would be, "I have felt weak and tired for the past week." Health-oriented terminology or disease entities should not be included in the CC. If a patient says his eyes are "yellow," his complaint should be recorded in his own words. It is not correct to record that the patient is complaining of "scleral jaundice." Using the name of a disease, such as "rheumatoid arthritis," tends to bias the subsequent readers of the record prior to adequate exploration of the problem. A better way of stating the CC would be, "Hands swollen and stiff for 10 days." In the case of a well client seeking a routine physical, there is no actual CC. The reason for the visit is recorded as, "Here for a physical examination, last complete exam two years ago." When a child comes to the clinic for an immunization, the CC is written, "Immunization needed. Second DPT two months ago." Brevity is important; elaboration of the CC is dealt with in the "history of the present illness."

The primary purpose of the chief complaint is to focus the nurse's attention on the reason for the patient's visit. It is easy to make assumptions as to the reason the patient is seeking care. For example, an elderly person who is being followed for elevated blood pressure may be more concerned about his constipation. The problem that is bothering the patient may seem trivial when compared to a problem that is more obvious to the health care provider. However, what the patient sees as a problem should be made a priority.

History of the Present Illness

The history of the present illness (HPI) is the narrative portion of the history. It gives the reader a clear idea of the patient's problem and how it affects his life. The HPI is a sequentially developed elaboration of the chief complaint. If it is written in a vague manner, it is meaningless and in some instances detrimental.

The HPI is divided into four sections: *usual health, chronologic story, relevant family history, and disability assessment.* The narrative is opened with a brief statement of the patient's usual long-term state of health. This gives the reader an idea of how the patient evaluates his health and indicates whether the problem is chronic or acute. The opening statement may read, "This patient considered himself in good health until yesterday, when . . ."

The *chronologic story* is the detailed section of the HPI. This is where the problem that brought the patient in is written down in the proper sequence of events. A great deal of time and investigative skill is needed to come up with meaningful data. There are general questions that help in the analysis of almost any symptom. These are referred to as the "eight areas of investigation" and should be learned thoroughly and used frequently. The eight areas of investigation include (1) sequence and chronology, (2) frequency, (3) location, (4) character of the complaint, (5) quantity, (6) setting, (7) associated phenomena, and (8) aggravating or alleviating factors.

Sequence and Chronology. When investigating the sequence and chronology, the nurse should determine when the symptoms first began. She should make it clear to the patient that she wants to know when the mildest symptoms were experienced and how long it took for them to reach a peak and subsequently to fade. She should also ask the patient if the onset of the problem was sudden or gradual. In the case of an episodic problem (such as an asthma attack) it is necessary to learn about the initial and later attacks. Whenever possible, specific dates should be used. Terms such as "two years ago" or "last week" are confusing to other readers of the record.

There are two approaches that can be taken when writing up the narrative. The nurse can record the most recent event first and then trace events backwards sequentially or she can start from the beginning, moving chronologically forward. Patients can usually give a clearer picture of the most recent episode of a problem. Regardless of the order used, it is important that the narrative be written according to a logical format.

Frequency. Frequency refers to how often the problem occurs. It is common for patients to be vague on the frequency of a problem. The interviewer should help the patient with direct questions, such as, "Does your headache occur more than once a month or more than once a week?" Another method of helping a patient to be more specific is to ask him to relate certain activities to the problem. This may help him recall the time frame more clearly.

Location. The location is where the distress is situated. Patients often use confusing terms when discussing the location of their problem. For example, a patient may say he has a "stomach ache" and really have prostatic pain. It is helpful to have the patient point with one finger to the exact location of his discomfort. Noting the exact location is beneficial when considering differential diagnoses. In the above example the examiner would focus his examination on the genitourinary organs and the epigastric area. When pain is reported, it is important to not only determine the location, but to pursue any radiation and determine whether the pain is on the surface or present in deeper organs of the body.

Character of the Complaint. When exploring the character of the complaint, the interviewer should try to get a description of the intensity of the discomfort. She should first try an open question—for example, "Could you tell me about the chest pain?" If this does not elicit the data needed, a "laundry list" type of questioning might be used, in which the patient is given a number of alternate adjectives or descriptive phrases to use. Some examples are: burning, sharp, dull, aching, gnawing, throbbing, shooting, viselike, and constricting. The terms mild, moderate, and severe can help to qualify the intensity. However, these words are very subjective and differences in interpretation do arise. A helpful way to find out the degree of the discomfort is to ask the patient if the pain interferes with his daily activities.

Character can also refer to the quality of the sputum, discharge, or stool. Sputum should be described in terms of thickness, color, and odor. When there is a discharge, the orifice from which it is coming is a key factor. The appearance of the discharge is recorded, as well as the color, thickness, and odor. The character of the stool describes the consistency (soft, firm, watery, etc.) and color.

Quantity. Quantity refers to the size of a lesion or the amount of discharge, mucus, blood, stool, or urine. The size of a lesion or mass is determined in centimeters or by comparing it to such common items as a nickel, a pea, or a walnut. Discharge is best measured in terms of teaspoons, tablespoons, and cups. If this is not possible, it can be estimated in terms of the number of pads or dressings saturated in a given period of time.

Setting. Setting most commonly refers to the activity the patient was involved in at the time his problem occurred. A pattern should quickly emerge. It may also be discovered that a problem is related to a season of the year or to a particularly stressful event. Questions like "Where were you or what were you doing when the problem occurred?" will be helpful in eliciting this information.

Associated Phenomena. Associated phenomena are symptoms that occur along with the chief complaint. These symptoms (or their absence) are additional aides in the assessment. With clinical experience and knowledge the nurse soon learns which systems of the body may be contributing to the CC. The nurse must inquire about each system involved in the complaint, looking for related symptoms. For example, if the patient is complaining of chest pain, the cardiac, respiratory, and gastrointestinal systems must be thoroughly reviewed. All positive and negative responses should be recorded. Those symptoms that do not occur with the chief complaint but could be related to it are referred to as *pertinent negatives.* If the nurse fails to record a pertinent negative response, subsequent readers will not be able to rule out that symptom as being related to the chief complaint. Pertinent negatives are recorded after the positive responses.

Aggravating or Alleviating Factors. Most patients are aware of the factors that aggravate their problems. Some of the factors that may contribute to a problem are emotional stress, fatigue, physical exertion, pregnancy, and use of certain drugs. Alleviating factors are those treatments the patient initiates or which have been prescribed to ease his distress. The success or failure of such treatments should be recorded. It may be discovered that the treatment utilized by the patient is harmful. The beginnings of a patient teaching plan are often formulated on the basis of this information.

Relevant Family History. The third section of the HPI concerns relevant family history. The patient is questioned about related problems of family members. For example, if the patient is having chest pain he is asked if there is any family history of heart disease. If there is a positive history the specific family member and his problem are recorded.

Disability Assessment. The last section of the HPI is the disability assessment. This is often a sensitive area because it explores the patient's feelings concerning the disruption of, or interference with daily life from his problem. The problem may result in strained family resources and relationships. For example, if the head of the household is ill, he may be unable to work. A child may be unable to attend school, resulting in his falling behind in his studies. With a long-term problem, relationships can become strained when all family energies are focused on the ill member. The disability assessment is important to the nurse in that it provides information regarding the patient's perspective of the severity of the problem.

Past History

The past history provides background for understanding the patient as a whole and his present illness. It is also a storehouse of information that may be relevant to management of the present illness. For example, if a patient comes to the clinic with right-lower quadrant pain and he has a past surgical history of an appendectomy, the possibility of appendicitis is ruled out.

Included in the past history are (1) childhood illnesses, (2) immunizations, (3) allergies, (4) hospitalizations and serious illnesses, (5) accidents and injuries, (6) obstetric history, (7) medications, and (8) habits.

Childhood Illnesses. The patient is asked if he has ever had chicken pox, mumps, rubella, rubeola, streptococcal infections, or scarlet fever. All patients are asked if they remember having had rheumatic fever. Most people cannot recall the dates of childhood illnesses. If they can, this is helpful information and should be recorded. If not, the approximate age at which they had the diseases should be recorded. The adult woman of childbearing age is asked when she had rubella. If there is a history of other significant childhood illness, dates, symptoms and signs, course of illness, treatment, and follow-up should be recorded.

Immunizations. The parent should be asked for the dates the child received the following immunizations: DPT; measles, mumps; rubella (MMR); and oral polio vaccine (OPV). The nurse should inquire about the occurrence of side effects. Also important are the dates and results of screening tests, such as the tuberculin skin test, the sickle cell test, and the G-6-PD (glucose-6-phosphate dehydrogenase deficiency). It is not necessary to obtain a complete immunization history from an adult, but the nurse should make sure that the necessary immunizations have been given and should note the date of the patient's last tetanus shot.

Allergies.   All patients should be asked about the presence of allergies to drugs (specifically penicillin), animals, insects, and environmental agents or irritants. It is not sufficient to record just the name of the offending allergen. The nurse should investigate exactly what type of reaction occurs and the treatment implemented. All types of untoward reactions to foods should also be discussed at this time. It is important to identify the offending food as well as the nature of the response, for this may be important in other areas of physical assessment. Thus, a true food allergy may present as an urticarial reaction to egg consumption. This response has different assessment implications than a response of hemolytic crisis when a person with Mediterranean G-6-PD deficiency consumes fava beans; or a response of bloating, flatulence, diarrhea, and cramping when a person with lactase deficiency consumes a threshold quantity of milk.

Hospitalizations and Serious Illnesses.   When asking about hospitalizations, the nurse should obtain exact information on the dates of hospitalization; the location or name of the hospital and the name of the attending physician; and the reason for the hospitalization, surgery performed, complications, and course of recovery. Obstetric hospitalizations are recorded under the obstetric history. The patient should be asked about past serious illnesses (which may not have required hospital admission), including dates, duration, severity, degree of recovery, and any sequelae. Some of the illnesses included in this category are high blood pressure, diabetes, pneumonia, pleurisy, tuberculosis, malaria, hepatitis, infectious mononucleosis, unexplained high fevers, and frequent colds and sore throats.

Accidents and Injuries.   The patient is asked about accidents and injuries that have been incurred, regardless of whether or not he was hospitalized. The interviewer should determine how the accident occurred, where it occurred, the type of injury and the treatment received, and what the sequelae were, if there were any. She should be alert to a pattern of injury. This is of particular importance when dealing with a child if abuse is suspected.

Obstetric History.   An obstetric history should be taken for all women, including those who are postmenopausal. The dates of birth, types of deliveries, weights of babies, lengths of gestations, and complications or illnesses during prenatal and postpartum periods are obtained. The obstetric history can provide a good reference point for learning about a woman's state of health during her young adult years.

Medications.   The patient is asked the names of prescribed medications he is taking currently or took for an extended period of time in the past. The nurse should also inquire about the use of over-the-counter medications. Patients may neglect to mention that they use vitamins, aspirin, nasal sprays, and laxatives that are obtained without a prescription. Because many patients, particularly those retaining strong ethnic ties, will prepare folk treatments themselves, patients should also be asked if they are using any home remedies or tonics. If they respond affirmatively, the method of preparation and administration as well as the frequency of use should be elicited. Many women do not consider the birth control pill a medication. A specific question about this is necessary. Although the patient may not be taking the pill currently, past use, side effects, and the reason for stopping use constitute important information and should be recorded. The dosage, routes of administration, frequency of administration, and reason for use should be noted for all medications.

Habits. The nurse should inquire about the use of illicit or recreational drugs; coffee, coke and tea; alcohol; and tobacco. When asking about illicit or recreational drugs, she should be sure to include drugs that were used extensively in the past. She should also ask about the frequency and duration of use and the good and bad effects.

Inquiry should be made into the amount of coffee or tea the patient drinks per day. It is interesting to ask about the use of sugar and cream in coffee and tea. This may account for a number of extra calories.

When asking about the patient's drinking habits, the interviewer should include types of alcohol, amount of alcohol consumed, pattern of drinking (morning or evening), drinking binges, and past treatment for alcoholism. It is sometimes difficult to assess the patient's consumption of alcohol. The nurse should obtain the exact number of bottles of beer or glasses of wine the patient drinks in a specified period of time. This lets the nurse, rather than the patient, decide whether the patient's drinking is occasional or not. This can be a sensitive area for both the nurse and the patient if a problem exists. Therefore, open-ended questions may be advisable, since they are less pointed and threatening.

In the case of cigarette use, the nurse should ask about the number of packs smoked per day, the type of cigarette, and the number of years the patient has been smoking. It is important to note the number of years the patient has been smoking rather than just his daily rate of consumption. Cigar and pipe smoking warrant obtaining the same information.

Habits specific to the child are covered in the developmental history. For a child under 4 years of age, additional information, including the prenatal history, labor and delivery history, and neonatal history, is essential to the data base.

Prenatal History. The gravity, parity, and number of abortions a mother has had may be important to the child's health. The mother should be asked when she first sought prenatal care for this child, how she felt physically and emotionally during pregnancy, the couple's feelings and acceptance of the pregnancy, and whether or not the baby was planned. All of these data may reveal very helpful information about the family's dynamics and health.

The nurse should explore for the presence of difficulties during the prenatal period. Some possible problems are diabetes, hypertension, unnecessary weight gain, poor nutrition, infections, rubella, vaginal bleeding, convulsions, and excessive stress. The use of alcohol, medications (amount and types), and tobacco during pregnancy should be recorded. The nurse should also note the length of gestation of the child.

Labor and Delivery History.   Difficulties during labor and delivery may indicate potential problems during childhood. The nurse should ask about the length and difficulty of labor, type of delivery, the presence of a significant other, and complications during the delivery. She should also inquire about problems specific to the child at the time of delivery. These include difficulty in breathing, seizures, jaundice, or low birthweight.

Neonatal History.   A good general question for establishing an idea of the newborn's health is, "Did your baby go home with you?" If the baby did leave the hospital with his parents, the nurse should inquire about the baby's first month of life. Helpful questions include: Were there any problems? Was the baby unusually fussy? How did the parents feel they adjusted to this new family member? What type of feeding was the baby on—breast or bottle? Was there any difficulty with feeding? Can the parents remember the frequency and give a description of bowel movements? How many times a day did the baby void? What were the baby's sleeping patterns?

If the baby remained in the hospital or was in a special nursery, the parents will probably recall special incubators or lights used. A detailed description of the prolonged hospitalization is necessary, if that was the case.

Family History

The purpose of the family history is to discover diseases of a hereditary nature, diseases that are communicable, and diseases that are environmental. Specific inquiry should be made regarding paternal and maternal grandparents, parents, siblings, spouse, and children. Their ages, general state of health, and health problems, if any, should be recorded. If any family members are deceased, the nurse should record the age at death and the cause (see pp. 48, 53). At the end, the patient should be asked if any other family members (aunts, uncles, or cousins) have the following diseases: cancer, tuberculosis, heart disease, hypertension, epilepsy, allergy, mental retardation, nervous or mental disease, and endocrine (diabetes) or other metabolic disorders. In the case of an adopted patient who is unaware of his blood relatives, it nevertheless may be beneficial to get a history of his adoptive family. The nurse notes on the record that the patient is adopted and has no access to his own family history.

Review of Systems

The review of systems (ROS) is a review of all complaints by body system, moving from head to foot. It is an evaluation of the past and present status of each system. The purpose of the review of systems is to act as a double check to prevent omission of data relevant to the present illness and to uncover other problems that might have been missed.

The review of systems is a list of symptoms that can be asked fairly quickly in a checklist manner. However, it is important to allow enough time for the patient to consider each symptom and to reply. The list of symptoms is fairly long and difficult to remember. It is therefore recommended that the nurse keep them on a reference card for easy access. Once she becomes practiced with the list, she will have it memorized. It is essential to record all negative as well as positive answers. If just the positives are written down the reader has no way to determine what other questions were asked. If there is a positive response, it should be explored via the eight areas of investigation utilized in the "history of present i'lness." When a response relates to the present illness it should be recorded under "present illness" and the following statement should be made in the ROS: "See HPI."

Nurses first learning the art of history taking often confuse the review of systems with a physical exam. This is evident when they record the history. The nurse will mistakenly write physical findings in the review of systems. It must be remembered that the review of systems contains subjective data given by the patient.

The systems to be reviewed include:

General: Height, weight, fatigue, weakness, night sweats.

Skin: Scaling, change in pigmentation, tendency towards bruising, lesions (i.e., birthmarks, moles), pruritis, rashes, dryness.

Hair: Amount, thickness, color, texture, alopecia.

Nails: Color changes, biting, clubbing, splitting.

Head: Problems with headache(s), falls resulting in unconsciousness, vertigo, syncope.

Eyes: Difficulty seeing, glasses (what for?), excessive tearing, pain, photophobia, diploplia, color blindness, cataracts, glaucoma, discharge, history of infections, date of last eye examination.

Ears: Discharge, tinnitus, history of infections, vertigo, pain.

Nose: Rhinorrhea, epistaxis, sinus problems, frequent colds, obstruction, loss of smell.

Mouth: Sore or bleeding gums; lesion on lips, tongue, or mucosa; excessive salivation; date of last dental exam; poor speech pattern; thumb sucking; hygiene practices; presence of dentures.

Throat: Soreness, hoarseness, frequent streptococcal or viral sore throats, difficulty swallowing, change in taste.

Neck: Swelling, stiffness, limitation of motion, thyroid disease, enlarged nodes.

Breasts: Adolescent pattern of development, discharge from nipples, masses, lesions, pain, pattern of self-examination of breasts.

Respiratory: Chest pain with breathing; cough; shortness of breath; night sweats; wheezing; frequent upper respiratory infections; history of emphysema, pneumonia, asthma, tuberculosis, bronchitis, or hemoptysis; date of last chest x-ray and results, if known; smoking habits.

Cardiovascular

Child: Fatigue, cyanosis, congenital heart disease, tiring with feeding, heart murmur.

Adult: Orthopnea, paroxysmal nocturnal dyspnea, edema, varicosities, chest pain, palpitations, claudication, history of heart murmur, hypertension, rheumatic fever, heart failure, heart attack (some questions regarding rheumatic fever and smoking habits may appear in more than one place; answers only need to be recorded once).

Gastrointestinal: Appetite, bowel patterns, changes in stools, diarrhea, constipation, abdominal pain, excessive flatulence, hemorrhoids, jaundice, dysphagia, changes in weight, tarry stools, anal itching, encopresis (child).

Genitourinary

General: Frequency, dribbling, pain, incontinence, pyuria, nocturia, urgency, color change of urine, hesitancy, history of venereal disease (type of treatment), history of urinary tract infection (type of infection).

Toddler: Toilet training.

School age: Bed wetting.

Female: Menstrual history; menarche, duration, regularity, amount, dysmenorrhea; date of last menstrual period, menorrhagia, metrorrhagia, vaginal discharge, vaginal itching, lesions, dyspareunia (see sexual history), history of vaginal infections (type and treatment).

Adolescent male: Nocturnal emissions.

Adult male: Lesions, impotence, prostate problems (symptoms and treatment), penile discharge, swelling, difficulty or stopping stream.

Back: Pain, stiffness, limited movement, history of injury or disease.

Extremities: Pain, swelling, redness, or deformities of joints; crepitation; varicose veins; gout, edema; limitation of movement; history of fractures, injuries, or disease.

Neurologic: Seizures, tremors, difficulty with balance, speech disorders, weakness, paralysis, limps, paresthesias, sleep disturbances, fainting, loss of memory, disorientation, mood swings, anxiety, depression, phobias.

Hematopoietic: History of anemia (type and treatment), spontaneous bleeding, blood dyscrasia, transfusions (reason for and reaction to).

Endocrine: Change in glove or shoe size, hirsutism, excessive sweating, polydypsia, polyphasia, history of goiter, heat or cold intolerance.

The nurse should be aware of the fact that if many of the questions are asked using this terminology she may obtain inaccurate information due to the patient's lack of understanding of the words. It is often necessary to change the wording according to the patient's age and level of understanding.

Nutritional History

The nutritional history is a vital part of the total picture of a person's health. The cliche, "A person is what he eats," is somewhat extreme, but does have some accuracy.

Our society tends to have problems with nutrition. As a whole we overeat; we eat the wrong types of foods; we cook in excess fat; we cover foods with extra calories and nonnutritional sauces; and we eat most of our calories at the wrong time of the day.

However, there is hope! More healthful nutritional practices are presently a trend. If we, as health care providers, reinforce the importance of good nutrition while it is in its "trend" state, maybe "the balanced diet" will become a way of life. Even the fast food restaurants, which have become so much a part of our lifestyle, are stressing items that are nutritionally beneficial. The push in this direction is strong, so let's not lose it!

Good nutrition is essential from birth to death. For this reason it is important to consider the nutritional history in a developmental framework. If specific questions are directed to the nutritional requirements of a particular age group, more accurate information will be obtained.

Before approaching the nutritional history developmentally, there are certain general areas to explore.

Eliciting a 24-hour diet history is a good way to gain some insight into a person's diet. The patient should be questioned about what he ate yesterday or the day before. It is also helpful to ask the patient if *he thinks* he eats a nutritionally balanced diet. Does he see himself as overweight or underweight, and how much? Have there been any recent weight gains or losses? This information provides the nurse with the *patient's perspective* of his nutritional status. Most people are aware of the quality of their diets. However, the patient should give his view and the nurse should not judge.

Other important general questions to ask are: Who does the cooking at home? Who does the grocery shopping? Does the patient eat out? How many times per week? What kinds of restaurants (i.e., fast foods, what types)? What financial concerns are there in terms of money spent on food? Are any family members on special diets? How does that affect the family's eating practices? And finally, it is advantageous to find out if there are any unusual weight problems in the family or any family history of obesity.

With ethnically distinct patients, food patterns are a particularly crucial area for assessment. An individual's culture defines what may be considered food. Within this range of culturally approved items, an individual diet depends on a host of economic, religious, psychologic, and personal preference factors. Because food traditions are among the last traditional ethnic customs to change, and because of the ethnic diversity in American society, the client's "foodways" may vary dramatically from those of the examiner. It is essential for the nurse to respect the food habits and preferences of all patients. It is important to investigate this area with culturally distinct patients, asking about methods of food preparation, meal ingredients, timing and frequency of meals, and foods considered harmful or beneficial to health.

Methods of *food preparation* merit special attention in the diet history. While some methods may remove nutrients (as in overcooking vegetables), other methods may increase available nutrients (soaking corn for tortillas in lime water adds calcium to the diet).

The *ingredients* used in cooking constitute another crucial area for diet assessment. Indochinese patients should be asked questions regarding the use of soy or MSG (monosodium glutamate) in addition to salt. Specific ingredients of ethnic foods should be elicited if the foods are not familiar to the examiner. For example, most nurses are familiar with lasagna, but not with pastitsio, a comparable Greek dish.

In addition to learning what is eaten and how it is prepared, it is important to determine the *timing and frequency of meals.* The examiner cannot assume that all persons eat three meals a day, with the largest meal in the evening. An often missed area of assessment concerns the timing of medications and treatments. Patients are often told to take a medication before or after meals, assuming a breakfast–lunch–dinner pattern. Variations in mealtime patterns should be noted in the record.

In obtaining a diet history, the nurse should also try to determine what the patient believes about *food and its relationship to health*. In many ethnic groups, infants and women during pregnancy and after delivery are placed on special diets, with some foods considered health-promoting and others considered dangerous. Many people, including the majority of those in Asian and Spanish-speaking groups, classify foods as *hot* or *cold* on the basis of inherent characteristics of the food, and not on their actual temperature. In this hot/cold system, foods are balanced for optimum health. In addition, if a person has a "cold" illness or condition, such as colic or earache, he should consume balancing or "hot" foods.

Assessing compliance with a prescribed therapeutic diet may pose difficulties for nurses unfamiliar with ethnic foods. To augment the examiner's skills, dietary exchange lists are available for some major ethnic groups.[3,4]

In addition to exploring these topical areas, Branch and Paxton suggest asking the following specific questions when assessing the diet of ethnic people of color:[5]

1. What times during the day do you usually eat?
2. Are there any circumstances that make you want to eat?
3. What takes your appetite away?
4. What foods do you like most?
5. What foods do you like least?
6. What foods are neutral?
7. What seasonings do you use regularly in preparing your foods?

After this information is obtained the nurse can further discuss the nutritional practices of the patient by considering his age. To make the *elicitation* of this easier, Chart 1.1 is available for reference. This chart is sectioned into various age groups. The questions included in the chart will help the nurse to gather a complete nutritional history.

CHART 1.1
Developmental approach to the Nutritional History

NEONATE (first 4 weeks)

Breast

1. How often?
2. How long on each breast?
3. Relief bottles? What formula? Type of nipple and bottle? How often?
4. H_2O intake? How much?
5. Supplements (i.e., foods, cereal)?
6. Mother's caloric intake, fluid intake drug usage, foods that bother her or infant?
7. Vitamins? Type?
8. Is feeding relationship pleasurable? Any problems? Concerns? How does father feel about breast feeding?

Bottle-fed

1. How often?
2. How much? Ounces? Times per day?
3. What type of formula (powder, concentrate, ready to feed)? Is evaporated milk used? Type of nipple? Type of bottle?
4. What dilution? How is formula prepared?
5. H_2O intake?
6. Who feeds the baby?
7. Is feeding relationship pleasurable? problems?
8. Who helps with feeding?
9. Supplements (i.e., foods, cereal)?
10. Vitamins? Type?

INFANCY (2 months–12 months)

Milk Intake

1. What kind?
   a. Formula (what kind)?
   b. Evaporated?

Intake of Solids and Other Supplements

1. When started?
   a. Cereal? How much? What type?
   b. Vegetables? How much? What type?

Milk Intake

c. Whole?

d. Two percent?

e. Skim?

2. How much? Ounces? Times per day?

3. When was breast feeding stopped?

4. When was formula feeding stopped?

5. When was other milk introduced?

6. Who feeds the infant?

7. Does the infant take a bottle to bed?

8. Does the infant drink from cup? Since when?

Intake of Solids and Other Supplements

c. Fruits? How much? What type?

d. Juice? How much? What type?

e. Meats? How much? What type?

f. Eggs? How much? Which part?

2. How are foods prepared? At home? Bought? Brand?

3. How far apart are new foods introduced?

4. What is a typical 24-hour diet?

5. Any allergies developed? With which foods? How manifested?

6. Likes and dislikes?

7. H_2O intake?

8. Fluoride in water?

9. Vitamins? Iron?

10. Who feeds the infant?

11. Does infant feed himself with fingers? What foods?

TODDLER (15 months–3 years)

1. Typical 24-hour diet (include amounts of food, fluid, and H_2O)?*

2. Milk intake (type, how much, cup used, etc.).

3. Who does the toddler eat with?

4. Does he feed himself?

5. Snacks? What types? How often?

6. Foods as rewards? Punishments?

7. Allergies? Which foods? How manifested?

8. Likes and dislikes?

9. Vitamins?

10. Parental concerns?

PRESCHOOL (3–5 years)

1. Independence in eating?

2. Willingness to try new foods?

3. See 1–8 under *Toddler*.

SCHOOL AGE (6–12 years)

1. Does child eat breakfast before school? What?

2. Does child eat school lunch? What does he eat? Does he take his own lunch? What does he take?

3. Attitude towards food?

4. See 1–8 under *Toddler*.

ADOLESCENT AND ADULT

1. Typical 24-hour diet?

2. Typical daily activities? Exercise?

3. Does patient eat at home? How often? With whom?

4. Does patient eat out? How often? With whom? What types of foods?

5. Snacks? What types? How often?

6. Fluids (types, amounts, H_2O)?

7. Likes and dislikes?

8. Allergies to foods? Which foods? How manifested?

9. Vitamins? Types? Amounts? How long taken?

10. Recent weight gain or loss?

11. Salt intake? How much (including that in canned foods, added salt to foods)?

12. Alcohol intake? What type? How often? How much?

13. Does patient feel knowledgeable about nutrition?

OLDER ADULT

1. Typical 24-hour diet or 3-day intake?

2. Interest in food?

(continued on p. 22)

CHART 1.1 (cont'd).

 3. Who cooks? How often?
 4. Who shops? How often? Does patient eat out? How often?
 5. How does food taste?†
 6. Salt intake? How much (including that in canned foods, added salt to foods)?
 7. Medications? What type? How much? How often? For how long?
 8. Vitamins? What type? How much? How often? For how long?
 9. Recent weight gain or loss?
10. Dentures? Condition and fit? Difficulty chewing?
11. Own teeth? Condition? Difficulty chewing?
12. Fluids (types, amounts, H_2O)?
13. Snacks? What types? How often?
14. Alcohol intake? What type? How often? How much?
15. Likes and dislikes?
16. Economic aspects?

*Sometimes a weekly diet history will give a better idea of the balance in the diet.
†Smoking may influence taste.

Social Data

Social data include family relationships and friendships, ethnic affiliations, occupational history, educational history, economic status, living circumstances, and pattern of health care. The nurse has traditionally given careful consideration to this area. However, when a nurse first becomes involved in taking the in-depth health history she sometimes neglects this area and concentrates on sections that are new to her. She must be reminded that she is to synthesize both the physical and social aspects of the patient history to make a meaningful assessment.

Family Relationships and Friendships

This can be a sensitive area and must be approached with care. Questions are directed toward assessing the quality and dynamics of the patient's significant relationships. The patient is asked how he gets along with family members and how he feels the other family members relate to him. He is asked such questions as, "Who do you feel close to in your family?" The nurse should determine whether anyone in the family is sick or has problems with behavior, school, work, drugs, or alcohol. If any of these problems are present, the nurse should ask how the patient feels they affect the rest of the family. The nurse should also ask if there are extended family members nearby to offer support in times of stress.

In our mobile society today there are many different types of relationships and "family" arrangements. For instance, the college student's "family" may be his roommates. A young man in the service may have a similar living arrangement and support system. Not all couples in love get married today. The relationship between these people should be considered as significant as a marriage if that is how the couple views their commitment to one another. Many people remain single today by choice and have other support systems to tap. The presence of these significant relationships should be explored.

The married patient should be questioned about the length of his marriage, previous marriages, duration of past marriages, the number of children from previous marriages, and how he feels about his relationship with his spouse.

Ethnic Affiliation

Cultural diversity accounts in large part for variations in family relationships, food preferences, religion, communication, and value patterns, as well as in health beliefs and behaviors. Ethnic affiliation differs from race, although both are important in health assessment. Ethnic identity concerns the cultural and social characteristics of a group of people. Racial identity has to do with biophysiologic differences among populations. Although there are certainly more biologic differences *within* a population than *among* populations, race is an important assessment variable because it indicates particular areas of attention. For example, persons of Mediterranean ancestry are routinely screened for glucose-6-phosphate dehydrogenase deficiency, blacks are commonly checked for sickle-cell anemia and hypertension, and Caucasians are the only group having a high rate of multiple sclerosis.

Ethnic affiliation may be determined by direct questioning as well as indirect assessment of such variables as language, manner of dress, and food preferences. While it is essential not to stereotype individuals, ethnic affiliation can serve as a clue in assisting the nurse in understanding client customs or beliefs. Sensitivity to ethnic differences is an important element in the delivery of quality health care. This variable should not be ignored because of a misguided notion that all people are the same.

Occupational History

The occupational history should include all jobs the patient has held. The type of work, where employed, when employed, and for how long should be noted, along with any jobs that may have involved an environmental hazard with a potential for future disease or accident.

The patient should be asked if he has ever been required to change jobs because of illness and how he feels about that. The nurse should not neglect to obtain a job history for housewives. If a woman has no work experience outside the home she may be at risk for adjustment problems when the children leave home or she loses her spouse.

Educational History

The interviewer asks the parent of a grade school child how the student learns in relation to children of the same age and in relation to members of the same family. The parent is asked if the child has ever had to repeat a grade or has ever been told he has a learning disability. The child is asked if he likes school and how well he feels he is doing. The nurse also asks the child if he likes to learn and what his favorite subject is. Inquiry is also made as to how the child relates to his teachers and peers at school.

The nurse should determine whether the high school student is satisfied with his academic performance and what he plans to do after high school. The student should be asked how he relates to his teachers and peers at school, too.

The nurse should record the highest level of education attained by adult patients and determine whether the patient feels this education is adequate. Inquiry is also made about past difficulties with learning in school. These difficulties can influence plans for patient education.

Economic Status

Inquiry into the family's economic status is another sensitive area. The nurse should determine whether the patient feels the family income is sufficient to meet the family's basic needs. The patient should be asked how he is paying for his medical care. This includes the type of medical and hospitalization coverage he holds. Last of all, the nurse should ask if the patient's illness has affected his savings.

Living Circumstances

In this section the adequacy of the home and surrounding community is assessed. This can be done by questioning the patient and his family. However, the information is best obtained by making a home visit. The nurse should ask about the type of home (i.e., apartment, single family) and whether it meets the present needs of the family. Do family members have enough privacy? The nurse should determine whether the location provides easy access to shopping, schools, churches, and parks. She should assess the safety of the neighborhood and home, and find out if the home is near any industrial sites that may present an environmental hazard.

The safety of the home should be explored in detail if there are young children or elderly people living there. For young children it is important to discuss placement of poisonous substances (such as cleaning solutions), home repair equipment, and medications. The tragedies that occur annually because of neglect in this area are devastating. Thus, the covering of electric sockets is necessary for the infant or toddler, who is busy moving around the house.

Accidents in the home are also common for the elderly client. Are there loose rugs or mats around? Are the stairs getting harder to maneuver without help? Is there a safety rail and bath mat in the bath tub? Is there adequate light to find the bathroom at night? All this information may prove crucial in preventing an accident and is the basis for good preventative teaching.

Patterns of Health Care

Interesting information is obtained by inquiring into the patient's pattern of health care. In an age of specialization, many patients refer themselves to specialists. The patient may have a variety of health care providers meeting specific needs. However, there may be no one who is treating the individual holistically. This can also result in duplication of services. The nurse should record all other health resources that are currently used and that were utilized in the past, including periodic visits to dentists, eye doctors, etc. If folk practitioners, such as herbalists, curanderas, or granny midwives, are also treating the patient, the nurse should obtain information concerning the nature of and reasons for treatment.

Inquiry should be made into the sources of health care received by other members of the family. The children may see a pediatrician and the mother a gynecologist, and the father may have no care provider.

The patient's general attitude toward the health care system should be obtained. The patient should be asked if he feels the care he is receiving is adequate. Any bad experiences with health care providers, either personal or involving family members or friends, should be recorded. The nurse should explore factors that may have interfered with the family's ability to procure medical care when needed (i.e., no transportation, little money, no baby sitter).

Developmental History The developmental history is elicited to collect information regarding a person's accomplishment of developmental tasks within a particular stage of the life cycle. To gather this information, the nurse needs to know what stage the person is in by noting his age. Erikson's developmental framework is a universally accepted method of assessing a person in a particular stage.

Chart 1.2 is constructed to help the health care provider gather data to evaluate whether or not a person has accomplished the tasks within each stage. This chart provides *examples* of questions used to elicit the appropriate material.

Some of the information will be collected in other areas of the health history (i.e., neurologic history, sexual history). There is no need to repeat this information in two places. It is important, though, to record all pertinent data regarding the accomplishment of the developmental tasks somewhere within the total health history.

CHART 1.2

Developmental Tasks	*Examples of Questions to Elicit Data*
AGE: BIRTH–12 MONTHS DEVELOPMENTAL STAGE: INFANCY DEVELOPMENTAL CRISIS: TRUST VS. MISTRUST	
1. Adjusts physiologically to his physical environment after birth.	(Address questions to parents.) Did you take your baby home with you when you went home from the hospital? Were there any problems after birth? Do you remember the Apgar score? How is the baby sleeping? How is he eating? Does he seem fussy? Does anything in particular bother him?
2. Totally depends on others, but establishes a separateness.	How is your baby special? What seem to be his own unique habits and responses? How does he let you know when he needs you?
3. Becomes a social being, can differentiate between people and objects and strange and familiar.	How does your baby know and respond to you? Your faces? Your voices? Some of your habits? Does he smile? After 6 months: Does he recognize his own environment (i.e., room, toys)? Does he seem to be afraid of strangers?
4. Develops need for affection and returns affection to others.	How does your baby respond to hugging and kissing? Does he seem to "love" back (i.e., hugging, kissing, reaching out to be picked up)?
5. Begins to interpret expectations of others.	How can you tell when he detects displeasure? How does he respond to "no"?
6. Makes strides developmentally.	(See Denver Developmental section pp. 337–8 for questions appropriate to age)
7. Explores world around him.	Depending on age: Does he follow objects with his eyes? Does he reach out for things? Does he try to move to what is intriguing him?
8. Develops a communication system.	How does he let you know when he wants something? Is he happy? Is he sad?
AGE: 15 MONTHS–3 YEARS DEVELOPMENTAL STAGE: TODDLER DEVELOPMENTAL CRISIS: AUTONOMY VS. SHAME AND DOUBT	
1. Begins to adjust to daily routines.	What does the toddler do all day? What are his activities? His resting patterns? Does he sleep through the night? Does he have a planned bedtime and bath time? Are parents consistent with maintaining structure in the schedule?

Developmental Tasks	Examples of Questions to Elicit Data
2. Develops good nutritional practices.	What times does he eat? Snack? Does he eat table food? What? What utensils does he use? Who does he sit with at mealtimes? (See nutritional history for further detail.)
3. Begins to demonstrate the basics of toilet training.	Earlier stages: Does he indicate when his diapers are dirty? How does he tell you that he has to "go potty?" Does he have a bowel movement when placed on the toilet? Later stages: Does he begin to indicate signs of nighttime control?
4. Develops physical skills appropriate to his age and stages.	What gross-motor, fine-motor, language, and personal–social skills does he demonstrate? (See Denver Developmental section pp. 337–8 for further detail.)
5. Begins to participate as a family member.	What does he enjoy doing with the family? How does he get along with members? Who is he close to? How does he demonstrate affection? How does he play with his brothers and sisters? How does he want to help mommy and daddy?
6. Begins to communicate with people outside his immediate family circle.	How does he play with other children, other adults? How does he communicate with people other than his family?
7. Shows signs of autonomous behavior.	How does he express his needs, wants, likes, and dislikes? What does he do for himself?

AGE: 3–5 YEARS
DEVELOPMENTAL STAGE: PRESCHOOL
DEVELOPMENTAL CRISIS: INITIATIVE VS. GUILT

Developmental Tasks	Examples of Questions to Elicit Data
1. Adjusts to daily routines of good nutritional habits, physical activity, and appropriate amounts of rest.	What does the preschooler do all day? What are his activities? Eating practices? Who does he sit with at mealtimes? What time does he eat? Snack? Rest? When does he nap? For how long? How many hours of sleep does he get at night?
2. Develops physical skills appropriate to his age and stage.	What gross-motor, fine-motor, language, and personal–social skills is he capable of? (See Denver Developmental section for further detail).
3. Participates actively as a family member.	What does he enjoy doing with the family? How does he get along with members? How does he show affection? Who is he close to in the family? What responsibilities does he assume as a family member (household chores, picking up toys)? What are the feelings between siblings?
4. Becomes toilet-trained.	Is he bowel and bladder trained? Since when? Any enuresis or encopresis? Day or night? What problems did he have?
5. Tries to monitor impulsive actions and reactions.	Does he laugh and cry at seemingly appropriate times?* What does "no" mean to him (7)? How does he show anger? How do parents deal with anger or temper tantrums?
6. Responds to expectations of others.	How is discipline handled? Is praise given, too? How does he respond to praise, direction, discipline?
7. Develops appropriate emotional expression for various experiences.	Does he seem like a happy child? Is he unusually afraid (5)? What does he do to show happiness, sadness, affection?
8. Learns to communicate effectively with more and more people.	Does he talk? What does he say or talk about? How are his sentences formed—two words, three words, complete? (See Denver Developmental section—language skills.) Does he listen to you as well as others? How is his attention span? Does his social circle go beyond the immediate family? How does he act around strangers?

Developmental Tasks	Examples of Questions to Elicit Data
9. Begins to handle potentially dangerous situations.	What does he do if he is confronted by a barking dog? What does he understand about poisons, electrical outlets, hot stoves, etc.? What safety signals does he understand?
10. Is developing autonomy.	What things does he want to do for himself (i.e., dress, bathe)? How does he differentiate between and explore the concepts of boy and girl? What typical "little boy" ("little girl") things does he do?
11. Begins to understand life's meaning ethically, religiously and philosophically?	What seems to be important to him? What does he understand about religion, the church, or God (if this is a family value)?

AGE: JUVENILE PERIOD, 6–9 YEARS
      PREADOLESCENCE, 10–12 YEARS (ONSET OF PUBERTY)
DEVELOPMENTAL STAGE: SCHOOL AGE
DEVELOPMENTAL CRISIS: INDUSTRY VS. INFERIORITY

1. Becomes an active and cooperative family member, at the same time decreasing dependency on family for total love and support.	(These questions are directed to the child.) What do you do to be helpful as a family member (i.e., chores)? What does the family do together? Do you have friends outside the family? Who is your best friend?
2. Develops physical characteristics and skills to join in activities in school and with peers.	What kinds of things do you like to do with your friends (i.e., games, hiking, riding)? Do you like sports, running games, etc.?
3. Begins to show active problem-solving, especially relating to activities of daily living (ADL) and role for this age.	What do you do when you have a problem with a friend? If you come home from school and no one is home yet, what do you do? What happens when you disagree ·vith your brother or sister?
4. Begins "realistic" communication with parents, siblings, teachers, etc.	What do you and your family talk over together? When you plan a family project, does everyone talk it over? When you have a problem, who do you talk to? When you don't agree with your parents (i.e., at bedtime, going somewhere with a friend), what usually happens?
5. Begins to understand the definition of friend and to learn about give and take with family and peers.	How do you feel about sharing (1, 2, 4)?
6. Begins to learn how to handle money in both saving and spending aspects.	What do you do with your own money? How do you get it? What chores do you do around the house? Do you get an allowance? How do you save money?
7. Handles strong and impulsive feelings.	When you are very happy, how do you show it? When you get very mad, how do you show it? When you are sad, what do you do?
8. Acknowledges body changes and understands some concepts of masculinity and femininity.	What do you notice that is different about your body? How do you feel about that (see sexual history)?
9. Relates to aspects of society beyond self—religious (if it is a family or personal value) and community participation.	What kinds of groups or clubs do you belong to? (Girl Scouts, Boy Scouts) What activities does the group participate in? Community programs? Charity projects? How do you feel about going to church? Sunday school? What about religion is special to you?
10. Thinks of self as healthy and engages in healthy activity.	Do you like yourself (1, 2, 4, 8, 9)? Do you feel healthy? How could you be more healthy?

AGE: EARLY, 12–14 YEARS (FEMALE)
          14–16 YEARS (MALE)
     MIDDLE, 15–18 YEARS (FEMALE)
          16–20 YEARS (MALE)
    LATE, 20–25 YEARS
DEVELOPMENTAL STAGE: ADOLESCENCE
DEVELOPMENTAL CRISIS: IDENTITY FORMATION VS. IDENTITY DIFFUSION

1. Acknowledgement and acceptance of physical changes in body and body image.	(These questions are directed to the adolescent.) How do you see your body changing? How do you feel about it?

Developmental Tasks	Examples of Questions to Elicit Data
2. Attains male or female role.	In today's world, what do you think it means to be a man (woman) (1)? How do you see yourself as a man (woman)?
3. Understands body function and utilization.	What do you understand about reproduction, love-making, birth control, etc.? Where did you get this knowledge? What further questions do you have (1)? (See sexual history—adolescent.) If you have decided to be sexually active, what are your beliefs about and practice of birth control?
4. Has peer relationships of both sexes.	Do you have friends that you enjoy? Male and female? What kinds of activities do you and your friends participate in? Do you have a best friend?
5. Seeks more of a peer relationship with parents, changing from dependence to supportive.	How would you describe your relationship with your parents? What kinds of issues do you agree about? Disagree about? Do you feel they listen to your reasoning? How do you help them to understand you?
6. Begins to make decisions regarding future career, etc. (occupation).	What kind of work would you like to do? Do you have a job now? What will you do when you finish high school? Do you "wish-dream?" What about?
7. Develops a relationship on a deep personal level with future commitment in mind (although this is not the central focus of this task at this age).	Do you date? Do you have a boyfriend (girlfriend)? If so, what kinds of things do you enjoy talking over and doing together? What issues do you disagree about? How do you resolve the discussion when you disagree?
8. Considers role as citizen and contributions that can be made to community life.	What projects do you get involved in that benefit others? Do you belong to a club of any sort? What kind?
9. Develops a set of values, ideals, and ethical standards that contributes to a philosophy of life.	What in life is important to you? What are your personal goals? How do religion and/or spiritual beliefs fit into your life?
10. Promotes good health.	What do you do to be happy and healthy? What sports do you engage in? What do you do if you get sick or need information regarding your health?

AGE: 25–45 YEARS
DEVELOPMENTAL STAGE: YOUNG ADULT
DEVELOPMENTAL CRISIS: INTIMACY VS. SELF-ISOLATION

1. Stabilizes self-image.	How do you feel about yourself as a person? How do you feel about the direction your life is taking?
2. Establishes personhood away from parent's home and financial support.	Where do you live? Do you live alone? Are you satisfied with where and with whom you live?
3. Selects a job or career which supports a strong self-image, financial independence, and satisfaction.	What career choice have you made? How did you choose your occupation? Are you satisfied with that decision? What direction is your career taking? Does your income meet your basic needs?
4. Is having (or has had) an intimate relationship which is more than infatuation or just for the purpose of self-gratification.	Are you involved in an intimate relationship (have you been at some point)? How does (did) this relationship enrich your life? What do (did) you find particularly satisfying in this relationship?
5. Makes and maintains a home.	How does your home meet your needs (i.e., comfort, life space) (2)?
6. Has a meaningful social life.	Do you have friends that you enjoy? What activities do you participate in together? How do you seek out an interesting life outside your work?
7. Determines desires for having a family.	Do you see yourself becoming a parent? How do you think parenthood will fit into your life and personal goals?
8. Participates in social, civic, and community roles.	Are you involved in any community activities (i.e.,

Developmental Tasks	Examples of Questions to Elicit Data
	PTA, school board, community organizations)? How do you contribute to this (these) groups?
9. Maintains an optimal level of wellness.	What is your daily diet? What physical exercise do you do? How do you relax? How much rest do you need? Do you get it? From whom do you obtain your health care?
10. Formulates philosophy of life. Continues to develop values and ethical standards that contribute to this philosophy.	What gives your life meaning? What in life is important to you? What are your personal goals in life? How do religion and/or spiritual beliefs fit into your life?

AGE: 45–65 YEARS
DEVELOPMENTAL STAGE: MIDDLE AGE
DEVELOPMENTAL CRISIS: GENERATIVITY VS. SELF-ABSORPTION AND STAGNATION

Developmental Tasks	Examples of Questions to Elicit Data
1. Acknowledges and accepts the physical and emotional changes of the middle years.	What physical changes do you see happening to you? What emotional changes are you aware of? How do you feel about these changes?
2. Works on marriage (or significant relationship) and its growth by developing new joint activities and goals with spouse as well as building on existing love and friendship (including sexual relationship). If need be, they together reassess feelings and commitment and build on that or restructure the relationship in a way appropriate to both members.	How do you feel about your marriage (or significant relationship)? How do you spend your time together? How do you feel about the communication in the relationship? What do you like best and least about being married? How do you see your spouse: as a friend, lover?
3. Fosters independence of grown children.	Are your children still home? Where do they live? How do you feel about your relationship with them? How do they fit into your lives? How do you encourage independence in your children?
4. Finds satisfaction and accepts new responsibilities in work. May be peak time in career.	How do you feel about your work? What do you see yourself doing in later years? How do you feel about retirement?
5. Considers plans for retirement.	How will you keep busy after you retire (4)? How will you maintain economic stability during these years?
6. Creates a comfortable living environment.	Do you feel that your home offers a safe and comfortable environment? How do you maintain your home to your satisfaction?
7. Assists aging parent(s) in finding satisfactory living accommodations and lifestyle for their later years.	Where are your parents living? Are they healthy and independent? How do you see yourself helping them in the future?
8. Maintains and/or enhances civil and social responsibilities.	How do you contribute to your community and/or charity organizations?
9. Develops friendships with new and old friends of both sexes and assorted ages.	Do you have a social life that you enjoy? What activities do you and friends participate in together? Do you find rewards in friendships with people of all ages, and both sexes?
10. Spends liesure time satisfactorily.	What do you do to relax? What do you do in your free time (9)?
11. Practices preventative health care and maintains stability with existing chronic disease, if possible.	What is your daily diet? In what physical exercise do you participate? How much rest do you require (10)? Do you get it? From whom and for what do you obtain health care? Are you satisfied with this (these) resource(s)?
12. Continues to build on existing philosophy of life, if pleased with it, or changes as needed.	What gives your life meaning? What in life was, is, and will be important to you? How do religion and/or spiritual beliefs fit into your life? What are your future goals and plans?

Developmental Tasks	*Examples of Questions to Elicit Data*

AGE: 65 AND OVER (QUESTIONABLE; MAY BE 70 AND OVER)
DEVELOPMENTAL STAGE: LATER MATURITY
DEVELOPMENTAL CRISIS: EGO INTEGRITY VS. DESPAIR

1. Makes decisions concerning how and where to live for the rest of his life.	Where do you live? Does your family live nearby? How and where would you choose to live for the rest of your life?
2. Provides self with safe and pleasant living environment within economic means.	Where and how do you see yourself situated if illness or a loss of independence becomes a problem (1)? Whom do you call in an emergency? Do you think your home is safe (i.e., throw rugs, stairs)?
3. Continues close, warm, loving relationship with spouse and helps her (him) to adjust to life in these years.	Do you enjoy the companionship of your spouse? How do you spend your day? What sort of things do you do together?
4. Acclimates himself to retirement income and augments this if desirable and possible.	Does your income meet your needs? In what areas is most of your income spent?
5. Promotes for himself and spouse the highest level of wellness possible. Seeks care and complies with and practices prevention wherever possible.	How do you feel physically and emotionally? What type of diet do you follow? What exercise do you get? How do you see your body changing? How do you feel about its changes? For what and from whom do you seek health care? Do you have Medicare? What other agencies do you use? Do you go for follow-up visits at recommended times (2)?
6. Maintains close relationships with children, grandchildren, and other relatives and friends.	How often do you correspond and visit with your family? Do they live nearby? How often are you able to visit and communicate with friends and relatives?
7. Maintains old interests and develops new ones with both activities and people.	Are you lonely? How do you spend your day? Are you active in any clubs, groups, etc.?
8. Copes with and hopefully accepts illness or death of spouse, aging relatives, and friends.	(Questions will vary according to the recency of deaths. For the most part, open-ended questions like "How are you feeling since your (husband) wife died?" will open communication.)
9. Continues to uphold his philosophy of life and feeling of self-worth.	How do you see that your life has meaning, to you and to others? How do religion and/or spiritual beliefs fit into your life?
10. Develops his philosophy of life so that death is accepted as a part of life.	Have you thought about death? How do you feel about dying? Do you feel you have your affairs in order to your satisfaction (i.e., wills, finances)?

*Questions may fit in with other categories. Numbers in parentheses refer to the developmental task and its corresponding questions.

Sexual History

The discussion of the sexual history is based on the premise that man is a holistic being and his sexuality is part of that holism. If we as nurses believe that statement, then the sexual history is as important as any other component of the total health history. Worthy of consideration, too, is the fact that many physical ailments are a result of or are incorporated with psychosocial stresses. This relationship is reciprocal—stresses can precipitate a sexual dysfunction or, similarly, a sexual dysfunction can produce biopsychosocial responses.

Until recently, elicitation of the sexual history as an integral part of the health history was given little attention. There is one recurrent reason why nurses and other health providers deemphasized their role in this process—namely their own discomfort. These feelings inhibit them in broaching the subject with a client.

Four key factors contribute to this discomfort: (1) the acceptance of self as a sexual being, (2) the acceptance of other definitions of sexuality, (3) a lack of knowledge about human sexuality, and (4) a lack of self-confidence as a professional in this area.

Regardless of how a person defines his sexuality, it is of the utmost importance that he be comfortable with this aspect of his life. To be comfortable does not necessarily mean that this person is sexually active (engaging in intercourse). It does mean that he is comfortable with however he chooses to define his sexuality.

Accepting another person's sexual beliefs can be very difficult. If a person tells the nurse that he is a homosexual or bisexual and that poses a conflict for her in terms of her own values, then she must recognize these feelings and attempt to elicit information without imposing her values. Her responsibility as a health care provider is to offer the patient the highest quality of care that she is capable of giving. In this instance that may mean that she identifies and accepts her feelings and refers this patient to someone who is comfortable dealing with people who define their sexuality in that way. That is a mature and honest way of dealing with such feelings. The nurse should not consider herself inadequate because she refers the patient to another provider.

A knowledge base about the physiologic, cultural, and developmental aspects of human sexuality is essential if the nurse expects to be effective. It is not enough for the nurse to be able to answer questions that a patient may have. The nurse as a teacher and counselor must assess the patient's developmental level, health or illness status, and his unique characteristics as a human being. She is then in a position to provide anticipatory guidance as he needs it.

The first three of the four factors mentioned earlier in this discussion contribute greatly to self-confidence. If a nurse accepts her own sexuality and the sexuality of others and has a strong knowledge base on the subject, then her level of self-confidence in this role will improve markedly. If she can convey an attitude of self-assuredness and trust, the patient will most likely respond to her with frankness and honesty.

The approach to the sexual history that the nurse selects will be based on two considerations: (1) the patient's level of illness or wellness, and (2) the patient's developmental stage. It goes beyond the scope of this text to discuss the sexual problems of the physically ill. However, one must remember that history taking is a process and its general principles should be equally applicable regardless of whether the nurse is eliciting such information from a person who is sick or from one who is well. The primary goal of taking a sexual history is for the nurse to gain knowledge about the patient's feelings and/or concerns about his sexuality so that teaching, counseling, and support may be given to the patient when necessary.

The sexual history usually flows rather easily from the genitourinary history in the review of systems. Asking a woman about her menstrual pattern, etc., facilitates the discussion of her sexuality. For the male, the dialogue can continue from questions pertaining to urinary symptoms, etc.

The patient's developmental stage will help the nurse decide on an approach to elicit appropriate and pertinent information. The questions asked of a school-age child will obviously differ from those asked of an older person. Therefore, the best way for the nurse to develop an approach is by starting with an assessment of the developmental stage.

School Age. The child in these years is very curious and asks a lot of questions. The "rule of thumb" is to be honest and straightforward when responding. The nurse should *not* make assumptions about what the child knows or does not know. In addition, it is important to consider the parent's feelings about what and where their child learns about the "facts of life." It should be remembered, too, that when a child asks a sex-related question, one should clarify what the child wants to know. The following questions are *examples* of how a nurse might elicit a sexual history from the school-age child.

1. What do you know about having babies?
   a. From whom and where did you learn this information (school, friends, etc.)?
   b. When you have questions about having babies, etc., whom do you ask?
2. What do you notice about your body changing? How does that make you feel?
3. What do you know about having "periods?"
4. What other questions do you have?

This information will provide a beginning data base regarding the child's perceptions and knowledge about pregnancy and puberty. The nurse can then decide whether the child is adequately informed. If he is not, she must make some decisions about what to say to the parents. This can be a sensitive area, especially if the parents do not feel secure discussing sex with their children. In any case, the nurse must see that the child has access to appropriate information, so that any major physical changes in the child do not frighten or repulse him.

Adolescence. The physical and emotional changes that a teenager undergoes affect his sexual identity. Each adolescent responds differently to these changes. Some will be more embarrassed than others. Some will try to defy the existence of these changes. Others will explore all facets of their development. A teenager's attitudes and acceptance of these changes may reflect how he feels about himself as a person. The accomplishment of the developmental tasks will depend in great measure on the adult support and guidance available to him during this period. Peer relationships will also influence risk-taking and testing. The nurse should be prepared to listen objectively and offer support and factual information. Directness is very important, as is mutual understanding of the terms used in the dialogue. Privacy and confidentiality are fundamental to the trust that develops in this relationship.

Assessing the youth's maturity and development is helpful so that the nurse does not ask inappropriate questions. Once assured that the patient can answer the questions appropriate for school-age children, she may then gather information more directly by asking the questions for adolescents.

It is not unlikely that the teenager will have had a sexual experience at some time. It may have been heterosexual, bisexual, or homosexual. The nurse should be prepared to respond as she would to any other information the patient reveals. However, without making any assumptions, the nurse must find out whether the adolescent is sexually active or not. Once she determines this, she can guide the conversation accordingly.

There are several methods of approaching the question, "Are you sexually active?" Sometimes a general statement to open the dialogue is helpful; such as, "Some teenagers have decided to be sexually active. How do you feel about that?" (Be sure to use terminology familiar to the patient.) From the patient's response there will probably be some cues that the nurse can pick up and use for further exploration by saying, "How does that fit into your life?" If it is determined that the patient is sexually active, then birth control and satisfaction with any relationship should be discussed. The following questions are *examples* that may be helpful to the nurse:

1. Birth control
   a. What birth control method(s) are you using?
   b. What do you like or dislike about it (them)?
   c. What other methods are you familiar with? What do you know about (them)?
   d. What other method(s) have you used in the past?
      (1) What did you like or dislike about it (them)?
      (2) What problems did you have with it (them)?
   e. What other method would you like to consider?
      (1) What do you know about how it works?
      (2) Why do you feel that method would be good for you?
   f. If pregnancy were to occur, how would you feel? How does this affect your sexual pleasure and/or relationship?
2. Satisfaction with the sexual relationship
   a. "How do you feel about the sexual relationship? Do you talk over your feelings, pleasures, and displeasures with your partner(s)?
   b. For women
      (1) Do you have pain with intercourse? Dryness?
         (a) At what point during intercourse does this occur? With entry? With deep thrusting?
         (b) Do some positions cause the symptom(s) more than others? Which position(s)?
      (2) Do you have orgasms? (Be prepared to describe the term!) How often?
         (a) Do you notice that they occur more easily when you are relaxed, rested, and feeling good about yourself and the relationship?
         (b) Do you notice that they occur more easily if you have more time, privacy, and/or foreplay?"
   c. For men
      (1) Do you have any problems with having or maintaining an erection? If yes:
      (a) How often?
      (b) Do you notice that fatigue, stress, and how you are feeling about yourself and the relationship affect this?
      (2) Do you have problems with ejaculation? (Be prepared to describe the term!)
      (a) What happens?
      (b) How often?
      (c) Do you notice that fatigue, stress, and how you are feeling about yourself and the relationship affect this?

If the teenager is not sexually active, it is important to ascertain whether he anticipates becoming active in the near future. The nurse should discuss the patient's feelings about his not being sexually active yet. There may be some peer pressure either to alter or maintain his present state. How does the patient handle that pressure? This is a good time in the interview for the nurse to provide anticipatory guidance regarding responsibility for birth control, including information about various methods and about facilities that provide birth control services. The nurse's confidentiality as well as availability as a resource person must be emphasized to the patient.

Young Adult. Within this developmental stage one of two situations is likely to exist. The patient may or may not be married.

For the single patient many of the same approaches that are used with the unmarried adolescent may be employed to elicit the sexual history. A general comment can be used to open communication, such as "Many single people decide that being sexually active fits into their lifestyle. How do you feel about that?" As with the teenager, it is necessary to establish whether or not the patient is sexually active and what his feelings are about his choice. If the patient is engaging in intercourse, the same questions that are used with the sexually-active teenager may be used. If the patient is not active, the basic approach used with the nonactive adolescent may be helpful to the nurse.

When the patient is married, discussing how he feels about his relationship with his wife may flow easily into his sharing how he feels about their sexual relationship. Care should be taken not to make any assumptions regarding marital fidelity or the lack of that commitment. Open-ended questions such as, "How would you describe your sex life?" or "How are things for you sexually?" will prevent falling into an embarrassing trap.

When children are born into a marriage, a couple's energy dissipates in new directions. This is a common time for sexual tension to occur. The patient should have an opportunity to express his feelings about the changes that occur in a growing family. Again a general statement might open communication, such as, "Many couples notice that when they have children their own relationship changes significantly. What have you noticed that's different in your relationship since the birth of your child(ren)?" After the patient has shared his feelings about this, the nurse should further explore the patient's overall satisfaction with his sexual life. (See questions regarding satisfaction with sexual relationships.)

The desire to have children can affect the purposes of lovemaking. If there is a difficulty with conception, lovemaking can become task-oriented. Here again, the nurse should give the patient an opportunity to identify this aspect of the relationship and share his feelings about it. As the quality of the sexual relationship is discussed the presence of this task orientation often becomes clear.

In this developmental stage career goals or job related stresses are often a major focus of the patient's life. Many times, working towards achieving these goals or resolving the stresses takes a great deal of physical and emotional energy. The result of these efforts and the time commitment involved may cause unusual fatigue and strain, thus affecting the patient's libido and sexual abilities. Unusual financial concern may also have the same affect. It is important to explore this with the patient. A general statement such as the following may facilitate conversation: "Some people notice that when they are under severe job or financial pressure there is a change in their sexual abilities or desires. Have you noticed this happening to you?" If yes, "What have you noticed that is different? How do you feel about that?" These kinds of life stresses are not necessarily unique to any particular developmental stage and should be considered whenever the possibilities exist.

Middle Age. Many changes occur during this developmental period. The nurse can incorporate the tasks of this stage and the likelihood of change occurring in order to provide anticipatory guidance. Whether a person is single, married, widowed, or divorced, general inquiry about how he feels about his sexuality is appropriate. However, in this age group there are some key areas that might affect the patient's feelings, desires, and self-image.

For the female the most obvious physiologic change that is likely to occur is menopause. This can have a positive or negative effect or even no effect at all. For some women, freedom from a fear of becoming pregnant makes menopause a great relief. For others, no longer having the ability to become pregnant may seem like a great loss. Before making any assumptions, the nurse should explore how the patient feels about the changes taking place in her body (a discussion of what she notices happening will probably precede this in the menstrual history). Once her feelings have been discussed and the fact that she remains sexually active has been established, it is important to share with her that some women notice dryness and/or pain with intercourse during or after menopause because of physiologic changes in the vagina. Such symptoms are a common problem, and can often be treated effectively with lubricating creams, if the physiologic change is the primary reason for the problem. The nurse should find out whether or not there are situational or self-image crises. If there are emotional stresses superimposed on the physiologic changes, then these feelings should be explored as well.

Physiologically, the male at this stage has changes, too. Attainment of an erection takes longer, sustainment time decreases, and ejaculatory force lessens.[6] These changes are likely to happen gradually throughout the aging process. The nurse should explore with the patient his fears and feelings about these occurrences.

The nurse should be alert to common life stresses during these years. The patient may be at the height of his career, or he may be trying to keep his job safe from the "younger fellow in the department." There may be a problem with physical illness that keeps him from doing his job. He may have major expenses in terms of educating his children or helping his retired parents financially. In any event, the impact of these types of stresses can affect his sexual desires and abilities. The nurse must be able to elicit information to help the patient identify the presence of these problems. She can then follow with a discussion of how he feels about his sexual life. (It is important not to make assumptions or inferences about the existence of one or more than one partner.)

After exploring these areas with the patient it is important to discuss his feelings about the quality of the existing relationship(s). Such questions as the following are helpful in eliciting information on these feelings: How would you rate your marriage sexually? How would your wife rate it? What would you do to make it better? What would your wife do to make it better? These questions can be asked of any patient married or not. Anticipatory guidance regarding normal developmental struggles may help the patient avoid long-term concerns which can cause sexual problems.

Late Maturity. Elderly people are as sexual as those in any other group. They may have different needs or desires, but physically many can still enjoy a very fulfilling sex life. A general statement that can be used to open the dialogue is: "Many older people enjoy a close physical relationship with a loved one. How do you feel about that?" Then a question regarding how the patient feels about that portion of his life should be asked. It is especially helpful to ask the patient if he has discomforts or problems. At this stage chronic illness often exists and can interrupt a person's sex life abruptly or insidiously. The astute nurse may be very valuable to such a patient. For instance, when a patient has arthritis, a certain time of day or certain positions used for intercourse may again make possible a sexual relationship he thought could no longer be. The same types of questions mentioned earlier regarding satisfaction with the sexual relationship can then be used. The "rating" questions are open-ended and give an opportunity for the patient to share his actual perception of that portion of his life.

Sensitivity on the nurse's part is important, too. Some patients may prefer not to share this information or may need a long-established relationship before they can do so. The nurse must decipher the patient's verbal and nonverbal cues. She must try to ascertain what the patient is really trying to tell her. In addition, the nurse must be aware of traditions and long-standing cultural beliefs. This will add to her ability to provide anticipatory guidance in these situations because her knowledge base will be broader.

A most important fact to remember is that there is no *one* way to elicit this information. Every nurse must find a method that is comfortable for her and for her patients. The text above gives the nurse a few *suggestions* to start. It is expected that she will develop her own style as she gains self-confidence in the art of taking a sexual history.

There are other aspects of sexuality and sexual practices that go beyond the scope of this text, such as masturbation and oral–genital sex. Exploration of these practices may be necessary to further understand the patient. The principles of gathering data in these other areas are consistent with what is described throughout the sexual history. The nurse should be confident in her approach and have a good knowledge base on the subject matter. If her questioning is open-ended and clear to the patient, she should have no trouble collecting this information. It should be remembered that all people are sexual beings and that the nurse who gives the patient the opportunity to share his feelings and/or concerns in this area is providing holistic care.

The Patient's Activities to Maintain Health

This category of information has four purposes. First, it provides the nurse with knowledge regarding the patient's perception of his approach to maintaining an optimal level of wellness, both physical and emotional. Second, the patient has an opportunity to share with the nurse his own ideas (or lack thereof) of what he does to maintain his health. Third, these data give the nurse an idea of the patient's leisure activities which contribute to his health. Fourth, it alerts a patient to the fact that he has responsibilities for his health.

Eliciting information regarding the patient's hobbies (cooking, stamp collecting, etc.), recreational interests (fishing, camping, etc.), and physical activity (jogging, swimming, etc.) will give the nurse further insight into the patient's lifestyle.

REFERENCES

1. Tripp–Reimer, T., & Friedl, M. Appalachians: A neglected minority. *Nursing Clinics of North America*, 1977, *12*, 41–54.
2. Prior, J., & Silberstein, J. *Physical diagnosis: The history of the patient* (4th ed.). St. Louis: Mosby, 1973, p. 5.
3. Biermann, J. *The diabetes question and answer book.* Los Angeles: Sherbourne, 1974.
4. Whitaker, J. *Guidelines for primary health care in rural Alaska.* Washington: DHEW (No. 017–026–00049–6), 1976.
5. Branch, M., & Paxton, P. *Providing safe nursing care for ethnic people of color.* New York: Appleton–Century–Crofts, 1976, p. 177.
6. Masters, W., & Johnson, V. *Human sexual response.* Boston: Little, Brown, 1966, pp. 233–236.
7. Duvall, E. *Family development* (4th ed.). Philadelphia: Lippincott, 1971.
8. Erikson, E. H. *Childhood and society* (2nd ed.). New York: Norton, 1963.
9. Murray, R. & Zentner, J. *Nursing assessment and health promotion through the lifespan* (2nd ed.). Englewood Cliffs, N.J.: Prentice–Hall, 1979.

BIBLIOGRAPHY

Froelich, R. & Bishop, M. *Medical interviewing* (2nd ed.). St. Louis: Mosby, 1972.
Mahoney, E., Verdisco, L., & Shortridge, L. *How to collect and record a health history.* Philadelphia: Lippincott, 1976.
Patient assessment: Taking a patient's history. *American Journal of Nursing*, 1974, *74*, 293–324.

WORKSHEET FOR PATIENT HISTORY

NAME _____

ADDRESS _____

AGE_____ SEX_____ MARITAL STATUS_____

RACE _____ RELIGION_____

OCCUPATION_____

USUAL SOURCE OF MEDICAL CARE_____

SOURCE AND RELIABILITY OF INFORMATION _____

CHIEF COMPLAINT:

PRESENT ILLNESS:

PAST HISTORY:

    Childhood Illnesses:

    Immunizations:

    Allergies:

    Hospitalizations and Serious Illnesses:

    Accidents:

    Obstetrics History:

    Medications:

    Habits:

*Recorded for a child under 4 years of age or with congenital or developmental problems.

    Prenatal History:*

    Labor and Delivery History:*

    Neonatal History:*

REVIEW OF SYSTEMS:

    General:

    Skin:

    Hair:

Nails:

Head:

Eyes:

Ears:

Nose and Sinuses:

Oral Cavity:

Neck:

Nodes:

Breast:

Respiratory:

Cardiovascular:

Gastrointestinal:

Genitourinary:

Menstrual History:

Back:

Extremities:

Neurologic:

Hematopoietic:

Endocrine:

FAMILY HISTORY:

NUTRITIONAL HISTORY:

SOCIAL DATA:
Family Relationships and Friendships:

Ethnic Affiliation:

Occupational History:

Educational History:

Economic Status:

Living Circumstances:

Pattern of Health Care:

DEVELOPMENTAL HISTORY:

SEXUAL HISTORY:

PATIENT'S ACTIVITY TO REMAIN HEALTHY:

**EXAMPLE OF A
HEALTH HISTORY (A)**

NAME _____K. J._____

ADDRESS _____

AGE _1 month_ SEX ___F___ MARITAL STATUS __S___

RACE _Caucasian_ RELIGION _Protestant_____

OCCUPATION _Not applicable_____

USUAL SOURCE OF MEDICAL CARE_HMO_____

SOURCE AND RELIABILITY OF INFORMATION_Mother,_____
who appears articulate and reliable_____

CHIEF COMPLAINT: "She's due for her 4-week check-up, but I think she looks thin."

PRESENT ILLNESS: Mother says the baby has been "healthy" and "doing well" since birth.

The baby came home from the hospital with her mother 2 days postpartum. She was born after an uncomplicated spontaneous vaginal delivery (see Labor and Delivery History). She cried immediately. Her weight was 8 lbs. 6 oz.; length 21″. She had a stool shortly after birth and the mother thinks she urinated at the time.

Mother states baby could not suck breast for the first 24 hours. Sterile water and 1 supplemental bottle given. Second day, baby was able to nurse 5 minutes on each breast with use of nipple shield. Continued like this for 3 more days. Mother "frustrated and ready to give up." Developed "clogged nipples and ducts." The next few days baby "struggled with grasping the breast, but eventually was able to nurse 10 minutes on each breast." Until 2 weeks ago, nursed 6 times/day. Mother now gives pacifier after baby nurses 20 minutes (10 minutes/side), to "satisfy sucking."

The last 2 weeks things much improved. Continues to nurse 4 to 5 times per day. Both mother and baby "satisfied." Presently no supplements. Baby does not like H_2O. She urinates "6 to 9 times per day." Has "squirty, soup-like" yellow stool every day or every other day. Moderate to large amount ("fills diaper").

Sleeps for 4 to 6 hour periods. Does not cry often if not hungry or wet. Mother states her husband is "very supportive and helpful. He's thrilled to death with the baby. He knows the first few weeks are a big adjustment and tries to remind me of that."

In general, mother feels things are going "as smoothly as possible now." She's concerned about the baby being "too thin because of our problem in the beginning, and she just looks small to me."

PAST HISTORY:

Childhood Illnesses: None yet.

Immunizations: None yet.

Allergies: None known to foods, clothes, soaps.

Hospitalizations and Serious Illnesses: None yet.

Accidents: None yet.

Obstetrics History: Not applicable.

Medications: None since birth.

Habits: Not applicable.

Prenatal History: Mother had no health problems during pregnancy. Considered herself in "excellent" health. "We were anxious to become parents and the timing could not have been better." Tried to eat balanced diet with right amount of vegetables, meat, fruit. Gained 25 lbs. Had "low blood count." M.D. prescribed $FeSO_4$ tablets t.i.d. No toxemia, diabetes, heart disease, or depression during pregnancy. Felt life at "4 months." Baby carried to term. Duration of pregnancy 40 weeks.

Labor and Delivery History: Modified LeBoyer birth. Father present throughout. Mother feels labor was "easy." Ten hour duration. Delivered vaginally. No forceps. Pudendal block used. "Very effective." Baby cried instantly. Weighed 8 lb. 6 oz. Then given to father so he could hold and give bath. After bath, mother, dad, and baby spent 2 hours together in recovery room. "Apgar 9."

Neonatal: (See HPI.) No respiratory distress, jaundice, seizures, paralysis, congenital anomalies, or blood group incompatibility.

REVIEW OF SYSTEMS:
General: "Pink and healthy." (See HPI.)

Skin and Mucous Membranes: No rashes, no diaper irritation, moles, birthmarks. "Black and blue" bruise on frontal area of scalp from birth—disappeared at 2 weeks.

Hair: "Light peach fuzz on head."

Nails: Seem to grow fast. Must trim 2 ×/wk.

Head: No lump, lesions. "Soft spot" in top of head; it seems to "pulsate" sometimes. Baby has no hair yet, "fuzzy light hair" covers scalp.

Eyes: No discharge, redness. Can cry real tears. Looks at mobile in crib. Squints in bright light.

Ears: No discharge, redness, lesions. Seems to listen to music box in mobile. Responds with a startle to loud noises.

Nose and Sinuses: No discharge, no bleeding.

Oral Cavity: No drooling, lesions, teeth. Can purse lips to suck.

Neck: "Floppy." No masses or stiffness.

Nodes: No masses noted in cervical, axillary, epitrochlear, or inguinal areas.

Breast: Had "small breast buds" when born. Resolved at 2 weeks. No discharge then. No masses, discharge now.

Respiratory: No cough, breathing difficulties, wheezing, or history of respiratory illness.

Cardiovascular: "Can feel her heart beating when I hold her against me." No cyanosis, peripheral edema, or varicosities.

Gastrointestinal: "Nurses well." Burps 2 to 3 times during feedings. No apparent colic or abdominal cramping. No constipation, diarrhea. (See HPI.)

Genitourinary: Voids yellow, not strong-smelling liquid 6 to 8 times per day. No vaginal discharge.

Menstrual History: Not applicable.

Extremities: Fingers and toes symmetrical bilaterally. Legs "long and thin." Feet and hands warm to touch. No apparent redness, edema, stiffness, or deformity.

Back: No noticeable curvature of spine. Able to lift head from bed when lying on abdomen. Cannot hold head up without support.

Neurologic: No seizures, paralysis, tics, tremors, projectile vomiting; no difficulty sucking. Cries when hungry or wet. (See Developmental.)

Hematopoietic: No known anemia, need for "purple light" after birth. No bleeding or bruising tendencies. Mom and dad's blood types both A positive.

Endocrine: No apparent heat or cold intolerances. No hair on body.

FAMILY HISTORY:

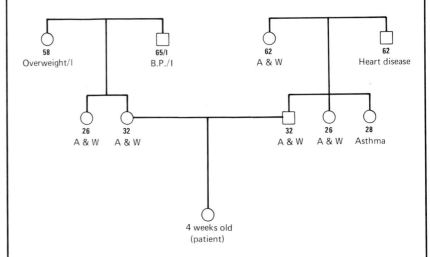

○ = female; □ = male; no family history of cancer, epilepsy, stroke, tuberculosis, diabetes, mental illness, mental retardation, or kidney disease.

NUTRITIONAL HISTORY: Breast feeding. No supplements. (See HPI.)

SOCIAL DATA:
Family Relationships: "We hope she is as pleased with us as we are with her." Grandparents on both sides live nearby and visit often. They like to baby-sit. No siblings.

Ethnic Affiliation: Irish-German descent.

Occupational History: Not applicable.

Educational History: Not applicable.

Economic status: Parents both work. Income meets needs. No extras right now. Mother plans to return to part-time in 3 months. Working on baby-sitting arrangements.

Living Circumstances: Family lives in 3-bedroom ranch house in suburb. All conveniences: gas heat, city water, air conditioning, etc. Baby has own room. In cradle at present. Will move to her crib when she gets bigger.

Pattern of Health Care: Family practice M.D. and nurse practitioner team. Parents very satisfied with availability, teaching, and care by the team.

DEVELOPMENTAL HISTORY: Mother notices that when she strokes baby's cheek she begins to suck; there is no difficulty sucking; when finger is inserted in baby's hand, she grasps finger; if loud noise, baby is startled; when she is held in a standing position and her feet touch a flat surface she "tries to step;" she lifts her head up when laying on abdomen, but cannot hold it straight yet (for vision and hearing see Review of Systems)

SEXUAL HISTORY: Not applicable.

PATIENT'S ACTIVITY TO REMAIN HEALTHY: Not applicable.

EXAMPLE OF A HEALTH HISTORY (B)

NAME ___L. R._____

ADDRESS ___Harvey University, Boston, MA_____

AGE ___21___ SEX ___F___ MARITAL STATUS ___S___

RACE ___Caucasian___ RELIGION ___Baptist_____

OCCUPATION ___Student; part-time nurse's aide (home care of elderly)_____

USUAL SOURCE OF MEDICAL CARE ___Family physician___

SOURCE AND RELIABILITY OF INFORMATION ___Patient, who appears reliable.___

REASON FOR VISIT: "I need a physical. I haven't had a good one in 3 years."

PRESENT HEALTH: This 21-year-old female considers herself to be in "excellent" health. States she has never been seriously ill or hospitalized and has never had surgery. Patient states she was diagnosed with "anemia" by a blood test at her "doctor's office" in 1975. She was treated with $FeSO_4$ gr. V. q.d. × 1 month. Rechecked at that time. Blood test revealed "anemia gone." No further treatment. In the summer of 1979 began to feel weak and tired. Went to M.D. He did a "CBC" and it showed that she "was mildly anemic." He gave the same "iron pills" to take 3 times a day for 1 month. "I haven't been back since I stopped the pills, I feel so much better."

Patient feels she has no major concerns or stresses at the moment. She is graduating from nursing school this spring and is anxious to "go to work" for a few years. She states she "likes herself as a person," although there are times when "we don't feel as good about ourselves as other times." She feels that her friends and family respect her, as she does them. She exercises daily (since 3 months ago jogs 1 mile) and tries to eat a balanced diet with "extra red meat and leafy vegetables."

PAST HISTORY:

Childhood Illnesses: Mumps, German measles (rubella), rubeola, chicken pox under 10 years of age. No strep throats or scarlet fever. (See Chest and Respiratory section.)

Immunizations: Had usual immunizations—doesn't remember which ones or when. Had tetanus booster this past summer (1980).

Allergies: No allergies to foods, medications, or environmental factors.

Hospitalizations and Serious Illnesses: None.

Accidents: None.

Obstetrics History: Gravida ÷ 0, para ÷ 0, abortions ÷ 0.

Medications: ASA gr. × approx. 1 time per month for headache; Mycolog cream; Nystatin cream q.h.s. (see Skin section).

Habits: Does not smoke cigarettes or "grass." Drinks 1 or 2 glasses of wine on weekends; 1 or 2 cups of coffee or tea per day. No soda.

REVIEW OF SYSTEMS:

General: Height 5'4". Usual minimum–maximum weight 120–125 lbs. No recent weight gains or losses. Denies fatigue, malaise, or weakness.

Skin: Winter 1976 had "rash" consisting of "little dry, flat, brown spots" covering area from axilla to waist in midaxillary lines (R and L). Went to M.D. because of itching. Doesn't remember diagnosis. Prescribed Mycolog cream during day, Nystatin at night. Continued with medications for 3 months until rash subsided completely. Last month noticed same type rash about 6" to 8" underneath axilla, at midaxillary line. Did not visit M.D. Starting using Mycolog and Nystatin again. No associated pruritis or scaling of this area. Rash improved slowly. No further rashes, spreading, or itching. No lesions, color changes, tendency toward bruising.

Hair: No alopecia or brittleness; thick, blond, shoulder-length hair. Washes daily, no use of dyes.

Nails: No splitting, peeling, cracking, or biting.

Head: No pain, dizziness, vertigo, or history of injury or loss of consciousness. No history of headache.

Eyes: Wears corrective lenses for distance vision. Last eye exam 1 year ago. No recent change in visual acuity, pain, infection, watering or itching eyes, diplopia, glaucoma, cataracts, blurred vision.

Ears: Denies hearing loss, discharge, pain, irritation, or tinnitus. Impacted cerumen in both ears during Jr. High School. Visited physician, irrigation without further occurrence of this condition.

Nose and Sinuses: No sinus pain, congestion, postnasal drip, impairment in olfaction, discharge, sinus infection, sneezing. Infrequent cold, 1 ×/year, lasting a few days. No meds for cold.

Oral Cavity: No problems with teeth. Sees dentist yearly. Few cavities. None in years. No bleeding or swelling of gums, lips, mouth, or tongue. Rare sore throat, 1 ×/year. No meds.

Neck: Denies pain, stiffness, limitation of motion, swelling, or history of goiter.

Nodes: No node enlargement or tenderness in cervical, axillary, or epitrochlear areas.

Breast: No masses, pain, tenderness, or discharge. Does self breast exam every month 7 days after menses in lying down position. Learned about it in nursing magazine and nursing class.

Chest and Respiratory: No past diagnosis of respiratory disease, cough, dyspnea, hemoptysis. Denies wheezing or history of asthma. Pneumonia age 4—visited physician. No hospitalization. Doesn't remember meds. During early childhood years, yearly occurrence of bronchitis. Seen by physician each time. No hospitalizations. No recurrence since 11 years old. No TB, asthma, emphysema. Denies orthopnea and night sweats. Last chest x-ray Summer 1979 for employment purposes. Tinné test done at same time—negative.

Cardiovascular: No precordial pain, palpitations, cyanosis, edema, or varicose veins. Denies Hx [history] of heart murmur, heart disease, high blood pressure, or rheumatic fever. Rheumatic fever in family—sister. No complications. (See Family History.)

Gastrointestinal: No abdominal pain or disease. Appetite "too good, sometimes." Belching after eating for a few hours. "Think it is a nervous habit." No food intolerances or M.D. care for this. No associated pain. No dysphagia, nausea, vomiting, diarrhea, constipation, hemorrhoids, hematemesis, jaundice. Bowel movement q.d. or q.o.d.—moderate amount firm, brown stool.

Genitourinary: Denies history of bladder or kidney infection, hematuria, urgency, stones, frequency, dysuria, nocturia, incontinence, polyuria, or venereal disease.

Menstrual History: Menarche 12 years. First 1½ years of menstrual cycle 19 to 21 days. Since has had 26 to 28 day cycle. Duration 4 to 5 days. First 2 days uses tampons × 7; days 3 to 5, decreased flow, uses 3 to 4 (tampons). No cramping, slight bloating, mood change (irritable first couple days), and breast tenderness. Denies dysmenorrhea, menorrhagia, infection, or pruritis. No history of pelvic exam with Pap—has had no problems, "never got around to go for an exam."

Back: No past problems. Denies pain, stiffness, limitation of ROM, postural problems.

Extremities: No history of disease. No coldness, deformities, discoloration, varicosities, crepitation, pain, history of phlebitis. Denies muscle weakness, pain. No joint swelling, stiffness, redness, limited ROM, or history of fracture. No history of arthritis.

Neurologic: One episode of fainting in 1975. "Blacked out" for 10 to 15 seconds. Got up in the night to go to the bathroom and "passed out." Went to M.D.. No diagnosis offered or studies done. No repeat incident. Denies loss of consciousness, change in sleep patterns, weakness, tic, tremor, numbness, tingling, speech disorder, paralysis, anxiety, phobias, mood change, difficulty with balance, seizures, aphasia, change in memory, disorientation, and hallucination. Denies pain and paresthesia.

Hematopoietic: See HPI. No bleeding tendencies, transfusions, blood diseases. Does not know blood group or type.

Endocrine: No change in eating patterns; no unusual growth patterns, thyroid problems, heat or cold intolerance, polyuria, polydypsia, polyphagia. No change in glove or shoe size or hirsutism.

FAMILY HISTORY:

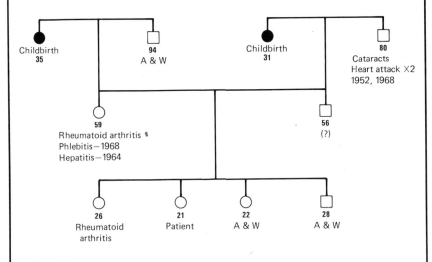

○ = female; □ = male; ●, ■ = deceased; denies family history of cancer, diabetes, tuberculosis, epilepsy, mental retardation, mental illness, kidney disease, or asthma.

NUTRITIONAL HISTORY: Tries to include basic four food groups daily. Likes most foods except for an occasional vegetable. Eats out with friends at fast food places 2 or 3 times per week.

A.M.: Eats breakfast q.o.d. or so (does not always have time). Grapefruit; cereal with milk, no sugar; coffee with cream

Lunch: Sandwich (2 slices bread with 2 slices lunch meat); 1 piece fruit; 1 can soda

Dinner: 1 portion meat or fish (2 slices); 1 vegetable (1 cup frozen); 1 dish of salad with dressing (2 tbsp.); 1 glass milk (8 oz.)

Snacks: Popcorn, chips approximately q.o.d.

SOCIAL DATA:

Family Relationships and Friendships Feels positive about relationship with mother and brother and sisters. Feels they relate well, talk over problems, are close to one another. Enjoys being with family. Father and mother divorced for 18 years. Doesn't remember father. "He doesn't come around or keep in touch. I'm not angry anymore, but I'd like to know him." Presently lives with four housemates. "We're all good friends." Rarely disagree. "I'll really miss them next year."

Occupational History: Attends baccalaureate nursing program full-time. Work-study in office on campus 10 hrs/wk. Takes care of elderly woman 6 hrs/day on weekends. Feels satisfied with job and school. Wishes she had more leisure time.

Educational History: Senior undergraduate nursing student.

Economic Status: Income satisfactory. Putting herself through school. Receives adequate financial aid. Just has to pay for rent, food, and personal articles. "Everything is O.K. with the finances."

Living Circumstances: Lives with four others in apartment. Own bedroom, two bathrooms, large living room, and kitchen with appliances.

Pattern of Health Care: No routine health maintenance, except for dentist and eye doctor. Only sees physician when ill. Doesn't want to spend money to see physician when well.

DEVELOPMENTAL HISTORY: Patient considers herself an adult, having "moved out of the adolescent stage." States she knows the direction she would like her life to take. She plans to work in nursing for a while and eventually return to school to get a Master's in her area of specialty, which is undetermined at this time. She hopes to marry and have a family, although she has not met anyone yet who "fits the bill." The things in life that are most important to her are her friends, family, and work.

SEXUAL HISTORY: No sexual intercourse up to present time. "I want the relationship to be special." Not necessarily "saving myself for marriage; just haven't met the right man."

Desires a mutually loving relationship in which intercourse would be enjoyable. Knows about birth control methods. Does a lot of reading on the subject. "I'd like to try a diaphragm when the time comes."

PATIENT'S ACTIVITY TO REMAIN HEALTHY: Enjoys music, going out with friends to movies and parties. Also enjoys walking in forests and reading novels. She feels "good health comes from good food, rest, and a sensible approach to life."

EXAMPLE OF A HEALTH HISTORY (C)

NAME ___N. M._____

ADDRESS _____

AGE ___71___ SEX ___M___ MARITAL STATUS ___M___

RACE ___Caucasian___ RELIGION ___Catholic___

OCCUPATION ___Civil engineer at consulting firm—full-time___

___since retirement 7 years ago.___

USUAL SOURCE OF MEDICAL CARE ___General practitioner,___ ophthalmologist.

SOURCE AND RELIABILITY OF INFORMATION ___Patient,___ who appears both articulate and reliable.

CHIEF COMPLAINT: "Chronic shortness of breath since childhood which has become gradually worse over the past year."

PRESENT ILLNESS: This 72-year-old man has considered himself to be in good health. He does not feel dyspneic at the moment. As a child, he noticed he would become dyspneic following running sooner than his peers. During grade school and high school he had frequent absences due to bronchitis and asthma for which he was treated at home. During college he was well, but became short of breath with exertion, such as running or pushing a car. In (approximately) 1957, he had a lung capacity test done in Rochester, Minnesota, and was told he had 50 percent lung capacity. In 1969, the test was repeated and again he was told he had 50 percent lung capacity due to emphysema. There is no pain with inspiration, no coughing, no wheezing, no night sweats. Shortness of breath is only associated with exertion, such as lifting a moderately heavy box, walking fast, or playing golf on a hot day. He notices that less exertion causes shortness of breath than was required 1 year ago. When shortness of breath occurs, he ceases activity and it improves in 3 or 4 minutes. His work involves no real physical activity. He has an attack of "asthma" with wheezing 2 or 3 times a year. He uses "a squirt or 2" of Primatene Mist, which relieves symptoms. The asthma can be brought on by humid weather, cold weather, vapors from fried cooking, horses, cats, or excess dust. He does not consider his life stressful at present and also does not feel that anxiety ever precipitated an episode. He has never been formally tested for allergies. No interference with sleep.

For 20 years he smoked 2 to 2½ packs of cigarettes a day without inhaling. He stopped in 1954. He then smoked 2 cigars a day and stopped in 1969. He noticed no change in shortness of breath after he ceased smoking. He drinks 1 beer a day. Other than 2 uncomplicated surgical procedures (see section on Hospitalizations and Serious Illnesses), he has never been ill. His father had asthma and one of his sons has a history of asthma. He does not consider this disease life-threatening, just a "nuisance" which interferes with his golf game on occasion. Last chest x-ray 1973. Does not recall any "unusual comments from the doctor regarding the findings."

PAST HISTORY:

Childhood Illnesses: Chickenpox–under 10 years; "hard" measles–under 10 years; no history of German measles, mumps, strep throat, or scarlet fever. Bronchitis at least twice a year during grade school and high school.

Immunizations: Last remembers being immunized before college. Last tetanus shot 12/70.

Allergies: Vapors of fried cooking, animal hair, wheat (see HPI), caviar; none known to medications.

Hospitalizations and Serious Illnesses: 1943 hernia repair, no complications, Peoria, Illinois. 1945 bilateral vein ligation, no complications, Peoria, Illinois. In February, 1973, bronchoscopy at Wesley Hospital by Dr. Buckingham. At routine physical in January, 1973, "whistling" was heard on right frontal chest. It persisted following one month of cough medicine. "Laminar" chest x-rays were negative. Bronchoscopy negative.

Accidents: None.

Medications: Primatene Mist 2 to 3 times per year.

Habits: Not smoking presently, beer (1 × day), no other drug usage; 2 cups decaffeinated coffee per day; does not drink soda.

REVIEW OF SYSTEMS:

General: Height 6', Weight 180 lbs. Considers himself a "good weight." No recent gains or losses. Denies fatigue or weakness. Feels good, generally.

Skin: White flat elevations on chest and back present for 10 years. February, 1973 had some removed—none malignant. Have reappeared in greater number. Mild itching of skin on legs in the winter; treated with hand lotion. No rashes, lesions, tendency to bruising.

Hair: Gray, balding on frontal aspect, no dandruff.

Nails: No splitting, cracking, or biting.

Head: No headache, dizziness, or trauma. Occasional pain in anterior to right auricular area, enough to wake him at night. A sharp pain relieved after hot water bottle applied for ½ hour. Occurs approximately once a month for three-four years. Not associated with activity or weather. No treatment sought.

Eyes: Glasses for reading for 15 years. Sees ophthalmologist yearly for tonometry test. Was told his pressure is normally high. No diploplia, pain, history of infections, spots, photophobia, excessive lacrimation. No problems with night vision.

Ears: For past year, humming in both ears when he wakes mornings. Goes away when he gets up. No discharge, vertigo, earaches, or history of infections.

Nose and Sinuses: Mild epistaxis with colds when he blows his nose. No sinus pain, obstruction, discharge, post nasal drip, frequent colds, trauma, sneezing, or loss of smell.

Oral Cavity: No problems with teeth. No recent extractions, no soreness or bleeding of lips, gums, mouth, or tongue. Few sore throats, no disturbance of taste, no hoarseness. Sees dentist yearly.

Neck: No pain or limitation of motion, swelling, or history of goiter.

Nodes: No tenderness of cervical, axillary, or epitrochlear areas. Mild swelling in inguinal area first noticed by M.D. in 1969. No change—remains swollen. Was told it is like a varicose vein. No discomfort.

Breast: No pain, lumps, discharge.

Respiratory: See HPI.

Cardiovascular: No palpitation; dyspnea with exertion. Edema of both ankles 1971 to 1972, at end of day. He began wearing socks with loose tops and edema has not been present since 1973. No chest pain, orthopnea, paroxysmal nocturnal dyspnea, cyanosis, history of heart disease, murmur, rheumatic fever, palpitations, ↑ B.P., cramps, or varicose veins at present. (See Hospitalizations and Serious Illnesses section.)

Gastrointestinal: No history of abdominal pain or disease; no disturbance in appetite; no indigestion or food intolerances; no nausea, vomiting, belching, flatulence, or jaundice; no change in bowel habits or use of laxatives; has one formed brown stool daily. No diarrhea, constipation, use of laxatives, or hemorrhoids.

Genitourinary: No frequency, nocturia, polyuria, hesitancy, hematuria, or kidney stones; no history of UTI or V.D.

Back: No back stiffness, limitation of motion, or injury.

Extremities: No pain, swelling, redness, deformities of joints, crepitation, gout, limitation of movement, or history of fracture, injuries, or disease.

Neurologic: No speech disorder or change in sleep pattern; no tremors or weakness; no convulsions, loss of consciousness, strokes, mental illness, numbness, limps, paralysis, disorientation, mood swings, anxiety, depression, or phobias.

Hematopoietic: In 1957, was told he was anemic, asked to have test rerun as he did not believe diagnosis and then refused test. Took medication (iron) for 1 year. No tiredness. No bleeding tendencies or other blood diseases or transfusions.

Endocrine: No change in eating patterns. No unusual growth problems, thyroid problems, heat or cold intolerance, polyuria, polydypsia, polyphagia. No change in glove or shoe size or hirsutism.

FAMILY HISTORY:

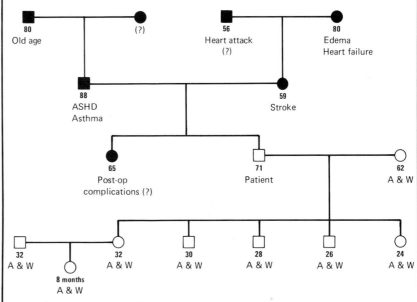

O = female; □ = male; ●, ■ = deceased; no family history of cancer, diabetes, tuberculosis, epilepsy, mental illness, mental retardation, or kidney disease.

NUTRITIONAL HISTORY: Wife does all cooking and shopping. Tries to include "meat and vegetables" in diet daily. Dines out for dinner one time per month with wife and friends.

Enjoys "all" foods, especially desserts. Two meals per day. Lunch—sandwich, fruit; dinner—meat, vegetables, potato, salad, dessert, and a glass of milk; 1 glass of beer in the evening.

Diet Yesterday: A.M.—1 cup of coffee; lunch—ham sandwich (2 pieces of white bread with mayonnaise and 3 slices of ham), 1 apple; snack—1 cup of coffee; dinner—2 slices pot roast with gravy, 1 cup (or so) peas, 1 baked potato, 1 lettuce salad with dressing, 1 piece of apple pie with ice cream, 1 glass of milk; P.M. snack—1 glass of beer.

SOCIAL DATA:

Family Relationships and Friendships: Client feels "positive" about relationship with his family. He and his wife like one another both as people and as spouses: "There are 35 years of affection in our marriage." They talk over problems together and share decisions. His children are grown and he feels close to them. His first granddaughter was born 3 months ago and this gives him "a great thrill."

Ethnic Affiliation: Irish.

Occupational History: Worked for 40 years at L&R Railroad as a chief bridge engineer. Was required to retire in February, 1973 at 65 years of age. Started work full-time at consulting engineering firm the next week. Hopes to work until 75 years old and longer if his health remains good.

Educational History: Obtained B.S. and M.S. in Engineering at Fulton University.

Economic Status: Very happy that he found good employment following retirement. He is involved with different areas in his field which he has found challenging. Receiving retirement benefits. Feels economically secure at present. Helping children through graduate school as best he can.

Living Circumstances: Lives in two-bedroom home in a suburb of upstate New York. Has lived in this house for 23 years. He lives there with his wife. This home has gas heat, running water, etc. It is well insulated. There are no loose rugs, mats, etc. The house is easy to manage and he and his wife hope to live there until "our health gives out."

Pattern of Health Care: Sees his M.D. as needed and "every couple of years for a physical." Has eyes checked yearly and also goes to the dentist annually. Doesn't have much faith in physicians. When he questions diagnosis or treatment, responses make him question their reliability. Has a complete record of all medical reports, bills, etc., since the early 1960s.

DEVELOPMENTAL HISTORY:
Client and his wife feel financially secure for the future. They have arrangements with their children for their future residence, health needs, and other relevant concerns. He has strong religious beliefs

which "give me courage when thinking of dying." Some of his children live nearby and they visit often. He is proud of his children and their accomplishments. He sees his life's goals as being fulfilled and still "learns new things about himself" every day.

SEXUAL HISTORY: Believes strongly in marital fidelity and feels he and his wife share very positive feelings about the sexual portion of their marriage.

PATIENT'S ACTIVITY TO REMAIN HEALTHY: Patient enjoys taking walks with his wife in the neighborhood when the weather permits. He relaxes by reading books in his field. Another favorite pastime is visiting with his family and granddaughter. He feels rest is essential to his "well-being" and retires by 10:00 P.M. every night.

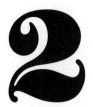

The Physical Examination: An Introduction

Ideally, the trusting relationship and rapport between the nurse and the patient have been established during the elicitation of the history. The existence of this kind of relationship will decrease the stress the patient may have in anticipation of what is about to be done *to him*. An additional way to facilitate the physical examination is for the nurse to be meticulous about explaining to the patient what will be done and the reason a particular test is performed. For most people a physical exam is not painful, unless there is something wrong. In many instances, only the area or system involved in the ailment will cause pain during the exam. A patient will be much more relaxed and cooperative if he is assured that he will be told when to expect any discomfort and is given a description of what to expect.

Achieving this trust with children is sometimes more difficult. However, *honesty* is essential. In the long run, the child will benefit from straightforwardness. Some children may have terrible fears and cry from the beginning of the history to the end of the physical. If a child is so terrified that he has to be restrained in order to be examined, evaluating the necessity of the examination is appropriate. In general, most children, if reassured that it is alright to cry when something hurts, and that they will be told in advance, begin to separate the unpleasantness from the more reasonable portions of the exam and cooperate beautifully. It should be remembered, too, that much of this can be made into a game.

Working in an organized and systematic fashion and having all the equipment that will be needed ready and available is another method of making any physical examination as pleasant as possible. The more systematic and organized the provider is, the more cooperative and relaxed the patient will be. The patient's participation is essential at various times throughout the exam. He will be asked to sit up, lie down, and stand. If the patient is not asked to do each of these several times, he will be less fatigued. As many of the "sit up" assessments as possible should be done before the "stand up" tests are started. Equally important to remember is the fact that the readiness of the equipment will contribute to the expediency of the exam. Time will be saved and organization will be maintained if the nurse does not have to hunt for equipment either inside or outside the examination room.

The patient should also be undressed appropriately. If a thorough history has been elicited, then the nurse should have a good idea about what she will be examining. A patient in the hospital will most likely be undressed already. An outpatient will have to undress. (Ideally, the patient is able to remain clothed during the elicitation of the history. This does not always work out because of the way a facility may be organized, but it certainly helps to preserve the patient's dignity.) For a chief complaint that only involves certain systems, the patient may only have to get partially undressed. Proper covering should be provided, regardless. If a complete physical is being done, all clothes will have to be removed. A gown and sheet (to drape over the patient's lap) should be made available to the patient. Some people, both children and adults, may feel more comfortable leaving their underwear on until the genitalia are examined. This is up to the nurse and the patient. However, it should be remembered that preserving the patient's dignity is an important part of the nurse–patient relationship, and a small consideration like this may contribute significantly to the patient's trust and relaxation.

Two other aspects to consider before starting the exam are the room temperature and the lighting. The temperature should be high enough so that the patient is not chilled during the exam. The light available should be sufficient to see clearly for overall as well as for close inspection.

A last thought to keep in mind relates to the patient's own needs. Every person is unique and has individual concerns. As nurses, we identify as one of our strengths the ability to incorporate those individual concerns into our nursing practice.

THE FOUR TECHNIQUES OF PHYSICAL EXAMINATION

There are four techniques in physical examination: *inspection, palpation, percussion,* and *auscultation.* Unless otherwise specified, they are implemented in this order. Occasionally, the sense of smell is used. This technique is used to help describe the character of things like mouth odors and discharges. Precisely where this is used will be discussed within pertinent chapters.

Inspection

Inspection is the observation portion of the exam. It is probably the most revealing technique, yet the most underused. There is no fancy equipment for this. The quality of the inspection depends on the observer's astuteness as well as the willingness to invest the time to do a thorough job.

When a person is looked at as a "whole" (as opposed to looking at a particular portion of his body), notations should be made regarding posture, gait, stance, anomalies, motor activity, affect, and mood (specifications of each are discussed in related chapters). When focusing in on a specific area or lesion, other information can be collected concerning color, edema, discharge, texture of the surface, etc.

The most frequent mistake made during inspection is consistently rushing through it. This is primarily true because it is hard to take time just to stop and look at a patient without reaching for a piece of equipment or laying on hands. Needless to say, good lighting and exposure of the area(s) which are being inspected are a must.

Palpation

Palpation means to feel. One can feel heat, cold, vibrations, moisture, or masses. Palpation is also used to elicit tenderness. Superficial or light palpation detects palpable findings on the skin surface or the area immediately below. Deep palpation is used to confirm superficial findings, feel deep organs, and elicit deep pain. Some systems do not require palpation. These are described within each chapter.

Percussion

Percussion is used to detect air, fluid, or solid mass in an underlying area. The skin's surface is struck with a specific gesture of the examiner's hand which sets the organs below into motion.[1] The result of this causes a vibration known as a *percussion note.* These notes vary in quality according to the density of the underlying structures (see Chap. 8 for further discussion of the percussion notes).

Auscultation

To auscultate means to hear. For the purpose of physical examination the terms listening and auscultating are separated. There is little that can be auscultated without a stethoscope. Voices and sounds in the air are listened to. Heart sounds, bowel sounds, and bruits are auscultated.

EQUIPMENT

The discussion thus far indicates the need for a patient who is appropriately undressed and a room that provides good lighting, warmth, and privacy. In addition to the eyes, nose, and hands of the examiner, other special equipment will be needed:

1. A diagnostic set which includes an otoscope, ophthalmoscope, and various-sized speculum tips
2. A Snellen chart—the illiterate "E" chart, the picture chart, and the alphabet chart
3. A penlight
4. A nasal speculum
5. Tongue blades
6. A tuning fork (either 256, 512, or 1024 cycles/second)
7. A wrist watch with a second hand
8. A stethoscope with a diaphragm and bell
9. A sphygmomanometer
10. A reflex hammer
11. A safety pin
12. Cotton
13. A cloth tape measure with centimeter calibrations
14. A scale with a device that measures height
15. Alcohol swabs
16. Gloves (sterile and unsterile)
17. Lubricant
18. Vaginal speculums
19. Hemocult test slides
20. A microscope and slides

THE GENERAL REVIEW

Before eliciting the review of each specific system in the history or performing the physical (objective) exam, some *general information* is collected.

In the history portion, this category, called *general*, begins the "review of systems" (see p. 17). The information obtained includes the patient's perception of his height and weight, any recent weight gains or losses, and any problem with fatigue or weakness.

As concerns the physical exam, this section includes the measured height and weight, a notation on general appearance and any obvious signs of distress, and the vital signs.

The General Subjective Review

It is important to ask the patient what he weighs and how tall he is. This gives the nurse an idea of how the patient perceives his height and weight. If the information the patient gives differs greatly from the measurements obtained, this is a clue to a possible problem in how the patient views himself. It is helpful when recording the patient's stated weight in the *subjective* review of systems to put quotation marks around the figure, so that it is not confused with the *objective* measurement.

This question provides a good opening to ask about any recent weight gains or losses. If a positive response is given, further data are needed. The patient should be asked how much weight was lost or gained and over what period of time this occurred. He should be questioned further as to whether this type of weight change has ever occurred before, when it took place, and what the patient's physical condition and stresses were at the time. The nurse should ask him if the change was a desired one and whether it is still desired. Any changes in the patient's life may precipitate this pattern, and he may be very aware of this tendency. This should be confirmed, if possible. Further elaboration can be included in the nutritional review.

The last area to discuss in this portion of the history is any notice of fatigue or weakness. Again, a positive answer always requires an elaboration of the circumstances and events. This area is often particularly difficult to discuss because it is hard to get the patient to be specific. However, a good way to begin is by asking the patient what he means by "fatigue" or "weakness." To some, fatigue may be the result of lack of sleep. To others, all the sleep in the world does not alleviate the feeling. After a detailed history of a patient's sleep pattern has been discussed, a look at the psychosocial stresses he is under at the time may prove helpful.

If weakness is a concern, there are many possibilities. Once the patient has tried to define exactly what he means by this sensation, taking him through the *eight areas of investigation* may offer some clues to the source of the problem. With a complaint like this, a complete health history should be elicited.

The General Objective Review

Height and Weight. An accurate recording of the height and weight can be made on a scale that can measure both. The patient should have on street clothes or only the clothing necessary so as not to "expose" him. No shoes should be worn. Every scale weighs differently, so if accuracy is essential, then an effort should be made to use the same scale each time. (Fig. 2.1 and Charts 2.1 and 2.2. It is important to note that most standardized growth charts are based on Caucasian standards. Although standardized growth charts for culturally diverse patients have not yet been produced, recent research allows us to make some very gross generalizations. The International Biological Programme has determined that children of predominantly African descent tend to be taller and heavier at all ages than children of European descent, even at somewhat lower economic levels. Individuals of Asiatic descent tend to be less tall at all ages than individuals of European or African descent. Body shape and proportions also differ according to population group. A number of investigators have concurred with Barr et al. in stating that "race-specific standards are required before growth achievements in infants and children can be properly evaluated."[2-4] Figures 2.2 (a-f) give examples of differences between population groups of children found in two studies.[2,3]).

Appearance. Note signs of physical age, size, stature, gait, obvious motor dysfunction, deformities, affect, speech, mood, alertness, hygiene, and dress (appropriate to weather).

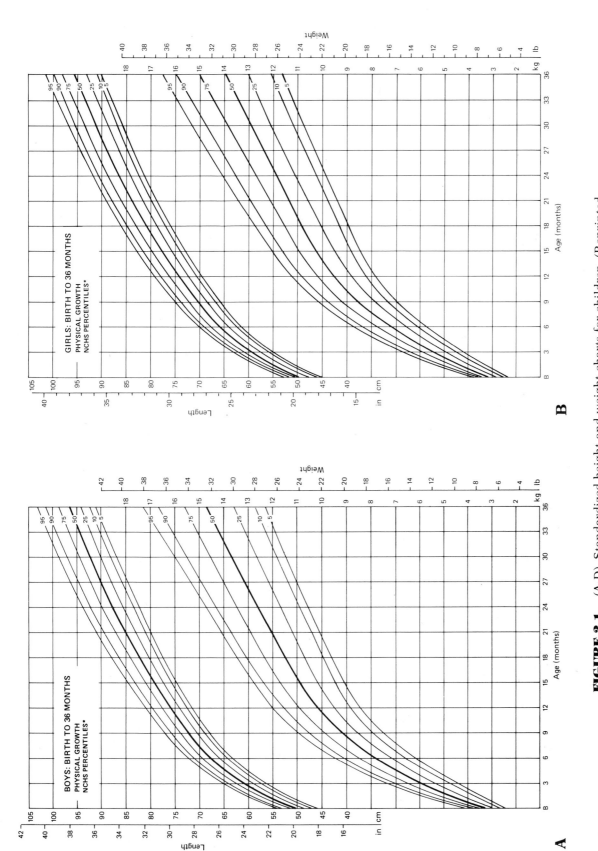

FIGURE 2.1. (A-D). Standardized height and weight charts for children. (Reprinted with permission from Ross Laboratories, Columbus, Ohio, C. 1976. Adapted from National Center for Health Statistics: NCHS Growth Charts, 1976. Monthly Vital Statistics Report. Vol. 25, No. 3, Supp. (HRA) 76–1120. Health Rescources Administration, Rockville, Md., June, 1976. Data from The Fels Research Institute.)

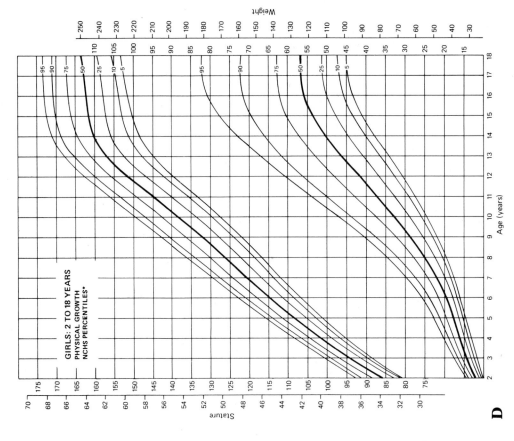

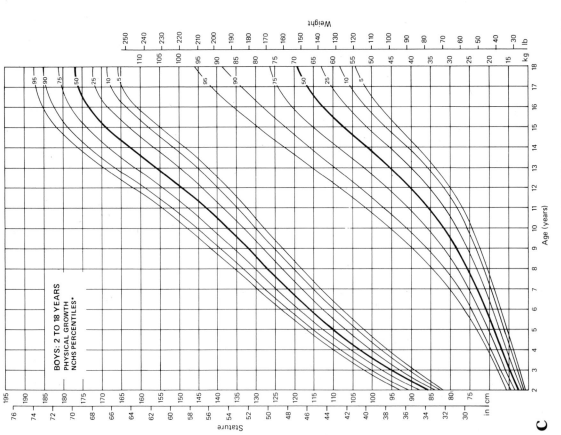

FIGURE 2.1. Standardized height and weight chart for children (continued).

CHART 2.1.

Desirable Body Weights: Men

Height with Shoes on		Weight in lbs., as Ordinarily Dressed, Including Shoes and Suit		
FEET	INCHES	SMALL FRAME	MEDIUM FRAME	LARGE FRAME
5	2	112–120	118–129	126–141
5	3	115–123	121–133	129–144
5	4	118–126	124–136	132–148
5	5	121–129	127–139	135–152
5	6	124–133	130–143	138–156
5	7	128–137	134–147	142–161
5	8	132–141	138–152	147–166
5	9	136–145	142–156	151–170
5	10	140–150	146–160	155–174
5	11	144–154	150–165	159–179
6	0	148–158	154–170	164–184
6	1	152–162	158–175	168–189
6	2	156–167	162–180	173–194
6	3	160–171	167–185	178–199
6	4	164–175	172–190	182–204

Courtesy of Metropolitan Life Insurance Company Statistical Bureau

CHART 2.2.

Desirable Body Weights: Women

Height with Shoes on; 2 in. Heels		Weight in lbs., as Ordinarily Dressed, Including Shoes and Dress		
FEET	INCHES	SMALL FRAME	MEDIUM FRAME	LARGE FRAME
4	10	92–98	96–107	104–119
4	11	94–101	98–110	106–122
5	0	96–104	101–113	109–125
5	1	99–107	104–116	112–128
5	2	102–110	107–119	115–131
5	3	105–113	110–122	118–134
5	4	108–116	113–126	121–138
5	5	111–119	116–130	125–142
5	6	114–123	120–135	129–146
5	7	118–127	124–139	133–150
5	8	122–131	128–143	137–154
5	9	126–135	132–147	141–158
5	10	130–140	136–151	145–163
5	11	134–144	140–155	149–168
6	0	138–148	144–159	153–173

Courtesy of Metropolitan Life Insurance Company Statistical Bureau

Signs of Distress. Note any signs of pain, anxiety, depression, or inappropriateness.

Vital Signs. The following should be measured and recorded.

Temperature. Until a child is old enough to hold his lips closed around a thermometer (usually at about 5 to 6 years of age), a rectal

FIGURE 2.2. (A–F). (A) Selected centile estimates for weight by age for young white and black boys. (B) Selected centile estimates for weight by ages for young white and black girls. (From Robson, J. K., Larkin, F. A., Bursick, J.H., Perri, K.P. Growth Standards for Infants and Children: A Cross-Sectional Study. *Pediatrics* 56 (6): 1017–18, December, 1975, Copyright by American Academy of Pediatrics 1975).

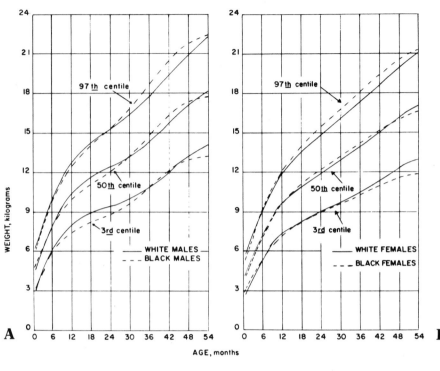

FIGURE 2.2. (C) Selected centile estimates for height by age for young white and black boys. (D) Selected centile estimates for height by age for young white and black girls. (From Robson, J. K., Larkin, F. A., Bursick, J.H., Perri, K.P. Growth Standards for Infants and Children: A Cross-Sectional Study. *Pediatrics* 56 (6): 1017–18, December, 1975, Copyright by American Academy of Pediatrics, 1975).

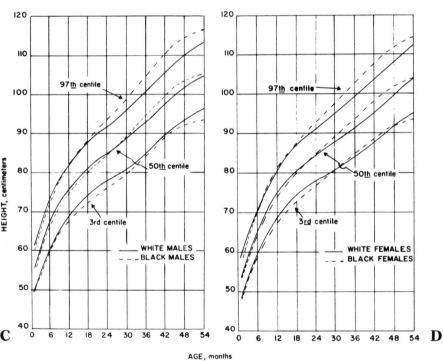

temperature is indicated. If a parent is nearby, the child's stress may be decreased if the parent is permitted to take the temperature. In addition, this gives the nurse an opportunity to observe the parent, and if any teaching is necessary, it can be done at that time. Any illness that prevents any patient from closing his lips around the thermometer also requires taking a rectal or axillary temperature. A rectal recording provides far more accuracy than an axillary measurement. Some geriatric patients may have difficulty with oral thermometers, too. Again, if accuracy is necessary, a rectal temperature is indicated.

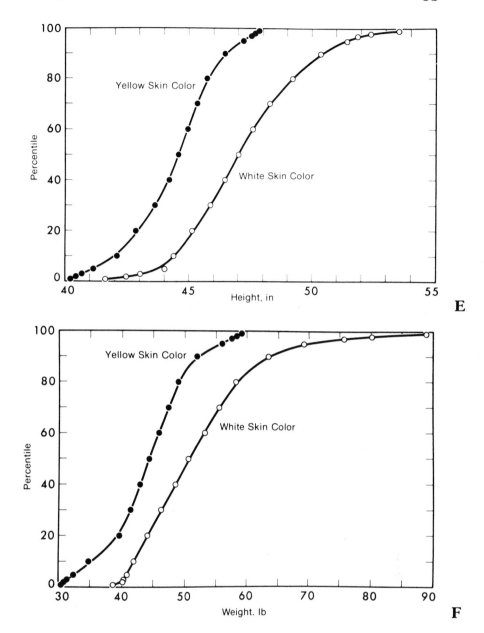

E

F

FIGURE 2.2. (E) Percentiles of height compared in 6 year-old boys white and yellow skin color. (F) Percentiles of weight compared in 6 year-old boys of white and yellow skin color. (From Barr, G.D., Allen, C.M., & Shinefield, H.R. *American Journal of Diseases of Children, 124,* December, 1972 pp. 871–2, Copyright 1972, American Medical Association.)

The average body temperature is 98.6° F (37° C). There are various ranges of acceptable normal temperatures. Some individuals have a normal temperature of 97° F, others 99° F. The important consideration is that whatever is average for that person when he is well should be considered his normal body temperature. Remember that rectal temperatures may run as much as a whole degree higher than oral temperatures.

Pulse. For a routine pulse check, a radial pulse will do. Further discussion of appropriate rates and other pulses can be found in Chapter 9.

Respiration. Respirations are counted and recorded. A discussion of abnormalities and acceptable rates can be found in Chapter 8.

Blood Pressure. Adults can have their blood pressure taken in various settings: doctors' offices, clinics, dentists' offices, hospitals, shopping malls, etc. Because elevated blood pressures are such a common problem, health facilities have begun taking blood pressures on children, too. All adults should have their blood pressure checked routinely. Children over 3 years old (who are healthy) should also be checked annually. Further discussion of technique and acceptable normal ranges can be found in Chapter 9.

The following chapters of the book deal with the assessment of individual systems. For all practical purposes, it is always best to "start at the top and work down." Some systems will be examined at the same time as others. For instance, the cranial nerves (described in Chapter 15, The Neurologic Examination) are usually evaluated while examining the head, ears, eyes, nose, throat, and neck. Everyone must develop her own system. The most important aspects are thoroughness, organization, and consideration of the patient's needs and abilities.

REFERENCES

1. DeGowin, E. & DeGowin, R. *Bedside diagnostic examination.* New York: Macmillan, p. 36.
2. Barr, G., Allen, C. & Shinefeld, H. Height and weight of 7500 children of three skin colors. *American Journal of Disease in Children,* 1972, *124,* 866–872.
3. Eveleth, P. & Tanner, J. *Worldwide variation in human growth.* Cambridge: Cambridge University Press, 1976.
4. Robson, J. K., Larkin, F. A., Bursick, J. & Perri, K. Growth standards for infants and children: A cross-sectional study. *Pediatrics,* 1975, *56,* 1017–1018.

3

The Skin

The skin is the body's external protection. It is the first line of defense. The integumentary system holds the "inside" in and keeps the "outside" out!

Another primary role of the skin concerns body temperature regulation. The anatomic structure houses the mechanisms for heat dissipation (the sweat glands) and heat storage (subcutaneous tissue). Finally, the skin is the sensory organ for temperature, pain, and touch.

HISTORY

The main focuses of the integumentary system are the skin, the hair, and the nails. The review of this ystem includes general questions regarding any problems in these areas. The nurse should explore with the patient any tendency towards any of these symptoms:

1. Skin: Dryness, itching, rashes, bruising; existence (either now or in the past) of lesions, moles or lumps; any problem with excess or lack of perspiration.
2. Hair: Any loss or excess, change of growth patterns, texture (described as dry, brittle, coarse, fine), scaliness of scalp; also note use of dyes or chemical treatments.
3. Nails: Biting, splitting, change in appearance (pitting, ridging), markings under nailbeds, or thickening (especially common in toenails).

Remember that if a patient gives a positive response to any of these symptoms, it is important to explore further. A description of the data that are collected when a rash exists illustrates this point. The chronologic story includes answers to the following questions (note that the duration of the problem is recorded in the chief complaint).

1. Location: Where is it? Is it spreading? If so, where is it spreading to and how (i.e. in a linear or circular pattern)?
2. Frequency: Have you had it before? If so, how often?
3. Sequence and chronology: If it has occurred before, describe a typical course of the problem. When did it occur? Was it treated successfully? How was it treated? When did it return again? In terms of the present episode, is it getting progressively worse? Does it heal in one place and appear in another?
4. Quantity: How far does it extend? Is it in more than one place? Where else? Are there several lesions or just one?
5. Quality: Describe the rash. What color is it? Is it raised or flat? Fluid-filled? Crusty? Oozing? If so, describe the discharge. Is there an odor? Does the involved area feel tender or warm to the touch? Are the borders regular or irregular in shape (Figs. 3.1 and 3.2)?
6. Setting: Where does the patient work or go to school? Does anyone there have a similar complaint? Any recent travel? Camping? Involvement in any new activities?
7. Associated phenomena: Itching? (Is it worse at night?) Is there a fever? Nausea? Vomiting? Diarrhea? Sore throat? Cold? Stiff neck? Any different or unusual foods or restaurants? New soap, perfumes, lotions, or detergent? New

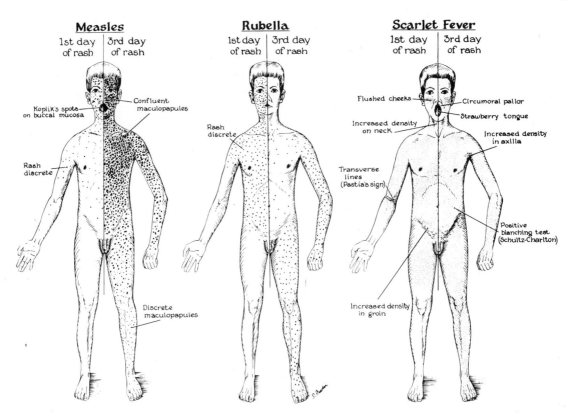

FIGURE 3.1. Signs of communicable diseases. (From McMilan, J. Stockman, J., III, & Osk, F. *The whole pediatrician catalogue* (Vol. 2). Philadelphia: Saunders, 1979, pp. 163–164).

clothing or bed linens? Any allergic history or tendencies? Taking any medications? Recent treatment with any medication? What type? Under any stress other than usual?

8. Aggravating factors: What makes it worse? Scratching, medications, lotions or soaps, bathing, jewelry or clothing?

9. Alleviating factors: What makes it better? Home treatments, baths, showers, medications, or lotions?

Certain skin changes, both normal and abnormal, are more common in some age groups than others. For instance, in the newborn, a benign condition called *milia* is a common occurrence (Chart 3.1). Birthmarks may also appear at this time. As the baby gets older and begins to eat solids, allergic reactions to some foods may occur. The most typical response manifests as a generalized skin rash. Diaper rash is another frequent concern during the early years of life.

In the school-age child many of the skin disorders that occur are of a *contact* or *atopic* (allergic) etiology. This is also the age group in which communicable diseases are likely to appear (Chart 3.2). Adolescence is the time for acne. Some people do not develop acne until the young adult years, but that is less common.

Skin conditions that are likely to exist during the adult years are: psoriasis, eczema, neurodermatitis, folliculitis, and skin cancer (Chart 3.3). In addition, there are some normal physiologic changes which occur during adulthood. A gradual loss of hair on the scalp (especially in the male) will begin. Women may notice a decrease in

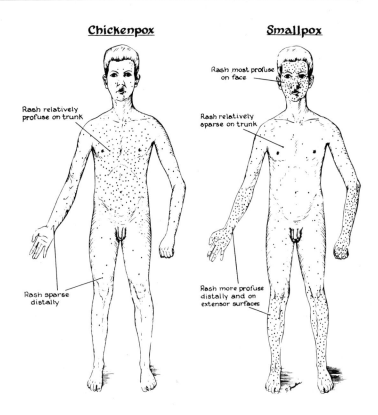

FIGURE 3.2. Signs of communicable diseases. (From McMilan, J., Stockman, J., III, & Osk, F. *The whole pediatrician catalogue* (Vol. 2). Philadelphia: Saunders, 1979, pp. 163–164).

the firmness of the body's subcutaneous tissue. This is especially true of breast tissue and the upper arm.

The older patient may notice an overall wrinkling of the skin which is due to the decreased elasticity of the skin turgor itself. In this age group the consistency and quality of body hair as well as the hair on the head will change. Hair covering the extremities will decrease in amount and become straighter. This is true of axillary and pubic hair, too. In addition to the normal changes associated with aging, some systemic diseases may affect the integumentary system. For instance, the patient with venous insufficiency and diabetes often has poor peripheral circulation, resulting in thinning of the skin and edema of the legs, eventually leading to a venous stasis ulcer.

CHART 3.1.

Examples of Common Skin Conditions of Infancy

Name	Age	Etiology	Appearance
Erythema toxicum neonatorum	First 3 days of life	Unknown	Pinpoint red macules on cheeks, trunk
Physiologic jaundice	3rd–4th day of life	↑ Number of RBC hemolyzing after birth	Yellowing of skin and mucous membranes, sclera
Milia	Neonate–infancy	Collected area of epithelial cysts	Tiny white spots on cheeks, forehead, and nose
Mongolian spot	Birthmark, may fade gradually	Clusters of melanocytes in dermis	Blue-black markings, often on buttocks or lower back

CHART 3.2.

Common Infectious Diseases with Dermatologic Manifestations

Name	Incubation Period	Subjective	Objective
Rubeola (hard measles)	10–12 days	Rash preceded by fever, cough, cold, lethargy, photosensitivity, some itching with rash	Koplick spots,* watery eyes, maculopapular rash—first on face, then behind ears and down trunk and extremities
Rubella (German measles)	14–21 days	May be no symptoms preceding the rash, with the exception of the classic enlargement and tenderness of lymph nodes; mild to moderate itching may accompany rash; no fever	Enlargement of post-auricular, occipital, and posterior cervical nodes; maculopapular rash begins on face and moves to trunk, clears by about third day; afebrile
Exanthema subitum (roseola infantum)	7–17 days	Sudden high fever 3–4 days prior to rash eruption	Few objective signs at this time—possibly slight cold, inflamed pharynx; fever drops and maculopapular rash appears, first on trunk and then on arms and neck; rash usually lasts 24 hours
Erythema infectiosum (fifth disease)	7–28 days (average 16)	None until rash appears and then complaints are present of rash and some itching	Bright red cheeks and the eruption of maculo-papular rash on trunk and extremities—rash may last 2–39 days (average 11)
Varicella (chicken pox)	13–21 days	Symptoms 24 hours before rash; slight fever, lethargy, anorexia	Red papules which become clear vessicles on red base; vessicles break and get scabby; rash erupts over 4-day period, begins on face and then goes to trunk and extremities
Scarlatina (scarlet fever)†	1–2 days	Sore throat, vomiting, malaise, headache, ↑ temperature	Very red pharynx, probably exudative; strawberry, red tongue; cervical adenopathy; maculopapular red rash, first on skin folds and then on trunk and extremities; rash appears on 1st–2nd day of illness and peels by 3rd–7th day, desquamates

*Koplick spots are white spots on the buccal mucosa which precede the appearance of the rash by about 48 hours.
†Scarlatina is the only bacterial communicable disease listed; all of the others are viral.

CHART 3.3.

Common Skin Conditions

Category/Name	Definition	Etiology	Clinical Features
Allergic dermatitis			
Contact	Reaction to external substances which are primary irritants	Contact allergens—i.e., shampoos, soap, clothing, jewelry, lotions, chemicals	Redness → vesicle formation → rupture of vesicle → crusting and scaling of area contacted by irritant
Eczema (atopic dermatitis)	Chronic, recurrent dermatitis	Skin as a target organ of allergic response of chronic or subacute outcome—i.e., milk	Infancy—red, weeping, irritated rash; adult—red, weeping → scaling → hyperpigmentation
Diaper rash	Local irritation with prolonged exposure to urine and stool, over-cleansing	Contact allergen; soap, diaper material	Erythema, oozing vesicles; in diaper area, abdomen, gluteal folds, genitalia, and inner aspects of thighs
Drug rash (dermatitis medicamentosa)	Allergic response to ingestion of drug	Drug allergen	Depends on drug; generally erythematous, macular, or maculopapular rash; vesicles or wheals may form; rashes all over; sudden onset and itching are noted
Urticaria (hives)	A local edematous response of the skin, often to an allergen; may be acute or chronic	Unknown; allergens frequently are food, drugs, inhalants.	Pink-white wheal which may become bullous; redness around borders; may occur anywhere on the body; much itching
Infectious dermatitis **Bacterial**			
Folliculitis	Infection in the hair follicle	Exposure to staphylococci	Superficial inflammation; single or multiple pustules at hair follicles, usually buttocks, face, scalp, posterior neck
Furuncle	Deeper inflammation than in folliculitis; one follicle	Exposure to staphylococci	Larger, red, painful, hard pustules which will often drain; posterior neck, buttocks
Carbuncle	Deeper inflammation than folliculitis; more than one follicle	Exposure to staphylococci	Larger, red, painful, hard pustules which will often drain; posterior neck, buttocks
Abscess	Often starts as a folliculitis and develops into a collection of purulent material deep in the skin	Exposure to staphylococci	Deep in the skin; hard, red, tender mass in which purulent material exists but not evident on skin's surface

(continued on pp. 74–5)

Category/Name	Definition	Etiology	Clinical Features
Impetigo	Very contagious superficial pyoderma; may be associated with poor hygiene	Exposure to staphylococci; B-hemolytic streptococci	Begins with red macules and these become serous vesicles surrounded by erythematous ring; vesicles rupture, leaving yellow, crusty area surrounded by erythematous ring; most often found on face, arms, and legs
Cellulitis	Bacterial infection of dermis and subcutaneous tissue	Exposure to staphylococci; B-hemolytic streptococci; H-influenzae	Tender, erythematous, raised, warm area, well marginated; may be associated with lymphangitis
Syphilis	A venereal disease	*Treponema pallidum*	Painless, moist ulceration with raised, firm edge
Primary	Initial lesion is a chancre at site of contact.	*Treponema pallidum*	Painless, moist ulceration with raised, firm edge
Secondary	Appears 6 weeks to 6 months after chancre	*Treponema pallidum*	Scaling papular rash found on soles of feet and palms of hands; generalized macular rash of trunk; mucous patches of oral and vaginal mucosa; flat wart-like white lesions in groin and axilla (condylomata lata)
Viral Herpes simplex I (cold sore, fever blister)	A viral syndrome which causes vesicles to occur on the skin and mucous membranes	Viral; often follows sun exposure, stress, fatigue, trauma, other viral syndromes	Groups of small vesicular lesions which erupt and crust within 48 hours
Herpes simplex II (herpes genitalis)	A viral syndrome causing painful vesicular lesions on the genitalia; associated with history of malaise, fever; may be sexually transmitted	Viral; suggestive relationship with cancer of the cervix	Primary occurrence most severe; vesicular eruption on labia, perineum vestibula, or cervix; much pain; recurrent episodes less painful, milder
Herpes zoster	Viral syndrome	Same virus that causes varicella (herpes virus varicellae)	History of chicken pox in childhood; unilateral area involved which follows pattern of dermatone; usually face, trunk, lower extremities; painful vesicular eruptions accompanied by erythema

Category/Name	Definition	Etiology	Clinical Features
Warts	Viral tumors of the skin	Viral	See specific type
Common wart			Papillary eruption, from pinhead to pea size; may have gray or brown surface; most often on hands
Filliform			Flesh-tone finger-like projections that occur on eyelids, face, neck
Plantar			More painful; flatter than the common wart; surrounded by thickened skin; often mistaken for calloused area; commonly on foot
Venereal (condylomata acuminata)			Cauliflower-white skin, tag-like lesions; multiple, may be found in genitalia, perineum, vestibule, or cervix; itching discharge may accompany
Fungal			
Moniliasis	A fungal infection caused by *Candida albicans*	Increased candida in body, often following antibiotic treatment or while on oral contraceptives; may be active in diabetes, obesity	See specific type
Thrush	Moniliasis in the mouth	See moniliasis etiology	Thick, white, curd-like patches on pharynx or oral mucosa; removal causes bleeding
Vaginal moniliasis	Moniliasis of the female genitalia	See moniliasis etiology	Thick, white, nonodorous discharge, white curds in vestibule and on cervix, much itching
Moniliasis of onychia paronychia	Monilial involvement of the nail and surrounding skin	See moniliasis etiology	Tender edematous of the skin around nail's ridge, become thickened and discolored
Moniliasis intertrigo and crural areas	A form of moniliasis; common in warm weather, affecting the skin folds and external genitalia	See moniliasis etiology	Bright red macules with satellite areas; vesicles and pustules interspersed throughout; occurs mostly in skin folds, under breasts, axilla, and groin; typical diaper rash in infants; will spare scrotum and penis in adult male

(continued on pp. 76–7)

Category/Name	Definition	Etiology	Clinical Features
Tinea versicolor	Superficial fungus infection	Exposure to fungal agent *Malassezia furfur*	Flat, itchy, yellow, pink, tan patchy areas on shoulder and upper chest and back; some scaling possible
Tinea	Ringworm; a fungal infection (further defined according to body part)	See description of specific body part	See description of specific body part
Capitis	A fungal infection/ringworm of the scalp, found mostly in children	*Microsporum audouini or M. canis*	Broken hairs and patchy hair loss; inflammation of the areas; some scaling possible; common in occipital region
Corporis	Fungal infection/ringworm of the body	*Microsporum audouini or M. canis*	Red, scaly, macular, papular, vesicular areas; eventual lichenification erythematous ring surrounding lesion; much itching; occurs on face, neck, trunk, and hands
Pedis (athlete's foot)	Fungal infection/ringworm of the foot	*Trichophyton mentagrophytes or T. rubrum*	Fissuring, scaling between the toes, some maceration, much itching; fourth web common; may spread to sole of foot, causing scaling, vesicles, erythema
Onychosis	Fungal infection/ringworm of the nails	*Trichophyton rubrum, or T. mentagrophytes*	Particularly in toenails; nail gets white or yellow at borders, infection moves in, and nails get very thick; nail splits (often due to *Candida albicans*)
Infestations			
Pediculosis	Lice infestation of the body	Exposure to lice	
Pediculosis corporis (body lice)	A body louse that lays eggs near clothing seams	Exposure to lice	Pinpoint small, red, macular lesions; scratch marks obvious, as itching is severe; papules and secondary infection may develop (comes in contact with body only to eat; hard to find lice on body)
Pediculosis capitis (head lice)		Exposure to lice	Not easily seen; nits if present appear as little white specks attached to hair; typical in children; itching and scratching very prevalent; eventually weeping, crusty areas develop on scalp

Category/Name	Definition	Etiology	Clinical Features
Pediculosis Pubis (pubic lice)		Exposure to lice, often sexually transmitted	Reasonably easy to see; Looks like gray flecks attached to pubic hair; head often buried in hair follicle; ova attach to hair
Scabies	Infestation of an itch mite in the epidermis; highly contagious	Exposure to itch mites; *Sarcoptes scabies*	Severe itching—worse at night; white-gray winding, linear pattern at the end of which there is a gray-black dot; papules and pustules and vesicles may accompany; most likely to occur on the flexor surface of the wrist, finger webs, axillary areas, nipples, waistline, lower abdomen, genitalia (for pruritic rashes always think scabies!)
Tumors			
Malignancies			
Basal cell	Tumor of the skin that arises from epidermis	Malproduction of basal cell; may be highly related to ultraviolet light exposure	History of outdoor occupation or activities; small, smooth-surfaced, well circumscribed areas that may have indentation in the center of the lesion; ulceration may follow; likely to occur on areas exposed to sun
Melanoma	Highly cancerous and lethal tumors of the skin and mucous membranes; malignancy of the melanocytes	Unknown	Smooth, isolated, non hairy; pigmented lesions; may be irregularly shaped; darkening and increase in size may occur. May erupt anywhere.
Squamous cell	Tumor of the epidermis which in its early form is potentially malignant	Exact cause unknown; high probability that there is a relationship to ultraviolet rays and light skin color	May be preceded by keratoses, leukoplakia; nodular area eventually forming crusty ulceration, commonly on lower lip, tongue, ears, neck, dorsum of hands
Benign			
Seborrheic keratosis	Common tumor of older adult	Unknown	Yellow/brown, roughened surface; slightly elevated, about 1 cm; usually on upper torso
Sebaceous cysts	Blockage of sebaceous gland duct	Same as definition	Usually less than 3 cms; well defined, round, firm mass attached to skin; may be inflamed

(continued on p. 78)

Category/Name	Definition	Etiology	Clinical Features
Pigmented nevi	Tumors containing nevus cells	Stimulated growth of nevus cells	Colored or noncolored; raised or flat; associated with hair growth or non-growth; of varying size, shape, and texture
Miscellaneous dermatitis			
Acne	Inflammatory response of sebaceous glands	↑ Oil production; secondary to hormonal stimulation	Blackheads, papules, cysts; typically on face, back, chest (any, some, or all)
Psoriasis	Chronic skin condition in childhood which lasts through life, often associated with arthritis; exacerbation and remissions continuous	Unknown: genetic transmission; possibly environment- or stress-related	Thick, white, scaly patches surrounded by erythema; when scales picked off, may bleed; commonly on elbows, knees, feet; much itching, often only in scalp
Neurodermatitis	Allergy-like dermatitis; emotional stress acting as a contributing feature; may be contained in one area	See allergic dermatitis; emotional stress; chronic local irritation from neurotic scratching	See allergic dermatis; may be in one area if repeated scratching takes place there; hyperpigmentation
Seborrhea dermatitis	Biochemical imbalance of sebaceous glands	↑ Oil production of sebaceous glands	Greasy scales on scalp, face, eyebrows, naso-labial folds; may spread to body, chest, abdomen, and skin folds; If so, scales are usually salmon colored

ANATOMY

There are three layers of the skin: *the epidermis, the dermis,* and *the subcutaneous layer* (Fig. 3.3).

Epidermis

This is the outermost covering and is considered a protective barrier. There are two components of the epidermis: the *horny layer* and the *inner layer*. The horny layer is made up of *keratinocytes*. This is a protein also found in the hair and nails. The horny layer sloughs off continuously and is replenished by new cells. The inner layer contains *melanocytes*, which produce a brown-black pigment called eumelanin and a yellow-red pigment called pheomelanin. In the absence of pathology, skin color depends on the relative proportions of the two melanin compounds and on hemoglobin, the red pigment of red blood cells.[1]

The *epidermal appendages* are the *hair, nails, apocrine glands, eccrine glands,* and *sebaceous glands*. All are indirectly related to this layer of the skin. The hair and nails are of no particular physiologic value to man. However, in most societies people emphasize them for cosmetic purposes.

There are two types of sweat glands: apocrine and eccrine. They respond to physiologic and emotional stimuli. Apocrine glands are located throughout the dermis and subcutaneous layers (Fig. 3.3). They are found in the axilla, breasts, and genitalia of both men and

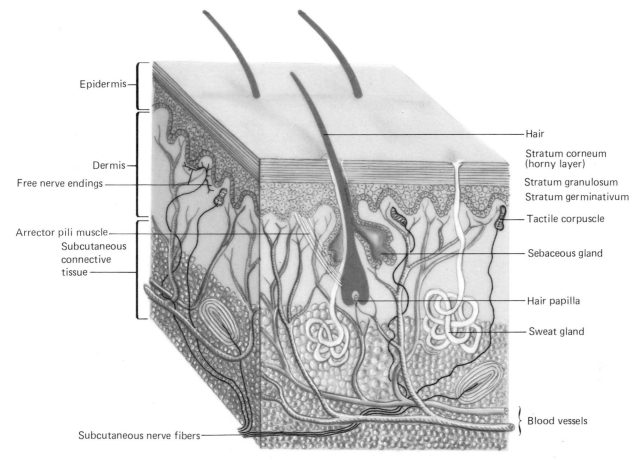

Epidermis

Dermis

Free nerve endings

Arrector pili muscle
Subcutaneous connective tissue

Subcutaneous nerve fibers

Hair

Stratum corneum (horny layer)

Stratum granulosum
Stratum germinativum

Tactile corpuscle

Sebaceous gland

Hair papilla

Sweat gland

Blood vessels

FIGURE 3.3 Structure of the skin. (From Heagarty, M., Glass, G., King, H., & Manly, M. *Child health: Basics for primary care.* New York: Appleton–Century–Crofts, 1980, p. 108).

women and do not begin to function until puberty. The secretion from these glands, called "apocrine sweat," empties into the hair follicles and then onto the skin. Apocrine secretions are thick and milky and are comprised of many organic components. The bacterial action causing the breaking down of these organic components can create distinctive body odors.

The eccrine glands are the most prevalent sweat glands in the integument (Fig. 3.3). They are located throughout the body and are the mechanism of heat dissipation. Both water and salt are secreted by the eccrine glands.

Eccrine "sweat" is basically clear and thin. It has few organic components and is odorless.[2]

Sebaceous glands are also located throughout the body, with the exception of the palms of the hands and soles of the feet (Fig. 3.3). They are most copious on the forehead, scalp, face, and chin. These glands secrete assorted lipids which are collectively called *sebum*. Sebum is a lubricator of the skin surface.

Dermis

This layer also acts as a protective barrier. It has many blood vessels and nerves that supply the nutritional needs of the skin. The dermis contains *collagen* and *elastin*, which hold the epidermis in place. In an emergency the epidermis can be a storage center for the body's fluid and electrolytes.

Subcutaneous Layer   This is where the body stores its fat. There are also nerves, sweat glands, and blood vessels in this layer. The subcutaneous tissue acts as the insulation for the body.

PHYSICAL ASSESSMENT

Examining the skin is often erroneously looked upon as the least significant portion of the physical. The skin can tell the examiner so much! Not only can it be a fair indicator of illness or wellness, but the skin can reveal signs of anxiety and aging. While the condition of the skin can also be a good indicator of general hygiene, the normally sloughing horny layer of highly pigmented patients may appear to be "dirt" to the inexperienced examiner.

No fancy equipment is needed for this exam except the examiner's hands and eyes and, in some instances, the nose. Good lighting and full exposure of the area being evaluated are essential. A magnifying glass and a small flashlight may also be of help. The two methods of examination used are inspection and palpation.

Skin

Inspection. The skin is inspected for color, lesions, obvious moisture (or lack thereof), edema, and vascular changes. (Obvious changes in turgor and texture are discussed more thoroughly in the section on palpation.)

Color. Skin color varies from body part to body part and from person to person. An individual's genetic composition is the most dominant factor in his overall coloring. In general, skin tones can range from shades of ivory to deep brown. Different hues of pink, green, and orange are usually apparent and vary among individuals. If a person spends a good portion of his life outside, the exposed areas are likely to be more pigmented than the rest of the body. Vasodilation of the superficial vessels occurs in fevers, sunburns, or blushing and can alter the skin color temporarily. A common characteristic during sexual arousal is a generalized flush over the body, and in a woman the labia will change color markedly. The most common changes in skin color are described in (Chart 3.4).

Assessing skin color changes may be more difficult in darkly pigmented individuals. With pallor, dark skin loses the normal underlying red tones, so that patients with brown skin may appear yellow-brown and the patient with black skin may appear ashen gray, particularly around the mouth and on the buccal mucosa. Cyanosis is best detected at the sites of least pigmentation: lips, nail beds, palpebral conjuctiva, palms, and soles. In highly pigmented individuals, just as in lightly pigmented ones, the sclera exhibits yellow pigmentation with jaundice. However, because dark-skinned individuals may normally have yellow subconjuctival fatty deposits, inspection of the hard palate should also be made if jaundice is suspected (See Chap. 4). Skin color changes which appear red in lighter-skinned individuals may also be missed in darkly pigmented individuals. In blacks, the characteristic red flush of fever may be visible at the tip of the ears. Inflammation and rashes may best be detected by palpation in combination with patients' verbal reports.[3-5]

Lesions. There are many varied causes of lesions. Normal, inconsequential markings are usually freckles *(lentigos)*, some

CHART 3.4.

Common Changes in Skin Color

Color/Response	Conditions or Cause	Typical Location
Yellow-orange		
Jaundice	↑ Total serum billirubin (above 2–3 mg/100 ml)	Generalized; sclera, mucous membranes
Carotene (carotenemia)	↑ Serum carotene usually due to excessive intake of carotene-related vegetables (i.e., carrots); typical in infants; pathologic in such conditions as hypothyroidism and diabetes	Palms, soles, around mouth
Bluing		
Cyanosis	↑ Deoxygenated hemoglobin (unsaturated hemoglobin)	Nail beds, lips, mucous membranes, skin
Petechiae (1–3 mm) Ecchymosis (larger petechiae)	Bleeding outside the vessels due to the trauma or systemic disease	Anywhere on body
Pallor	↓ Hemoglobin due to anemia, shock, fatigue, startling emotional upset	Generalized, conjunctiva
Albinism	Transmitted metabolic defect of melanocytes, causing lack of pigment	Hair, body, eyes
Vitiligo	Lack of pigment in patchy areas due to an autoimmune or neurogenic etiology	Patchy spots on body
Red		
Erythema	↑ Oxygenated blood to a particular area or all over body as in infection	Local area infected
	↑ Alcoholic intake	Face, cheeks
	Exposure to cold	Areas exposed
	Trauma	Local area involved
Tan-brown	↑ Melanin, as in pregnancy or with oral contraceptives	Face, areola, nipples, linea nigra
	Sun tan	Exposed areas to sun
	Hyperthyroidism, Addison's disease	Diffuse, prevalent in genitalia, areola, recent scars, knees, elbows
Café-au-lait spots (sharply delineated tan-brown patches)	Nonpathologic	One or two small spots on body
	Albright's syndrome, von Recklinghausen's disease (neurofibromatosis)	Spots which vary in size scattered over body

birthmarks, and some aging spots. Primary lesions are an initial response to some stimulus on the skin (*macule, papule,* etc.) (Fig. 3.4, Chart 3.5). Secondary lesions may occur as an alteration in a primary lesion (*keloid, scales, fissures,* etc.) (Fig. 3.4 and Chart 3.6).

These skin changes can exist in groupings or as isolated lesions. The three most common classifications for groupings are *linear, clustered,* and *circular.* A lesion should always be described according to its location, distribution, color, type, size, discharge (including description), and grouping. In darkly pigmented individuals, lesions may be difficult to identify by inspection and may necessitate identification by palpation, observation of patients' scratching, or patients' verbal reports. However, in only moderately pigmented

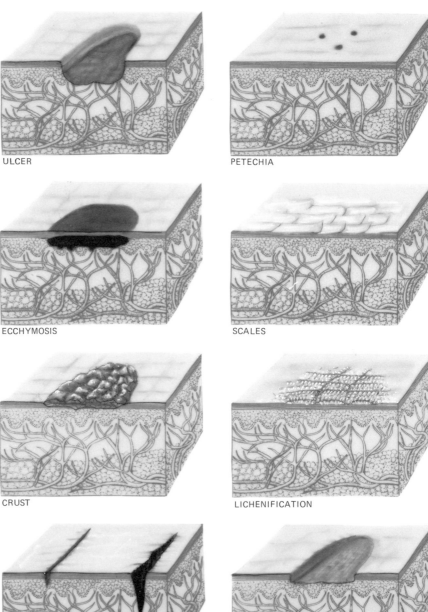

FIGURE 3.4. Skin lesions. (From Heagarty, M., Glass, G., King, H., & Manly, M. *Child health: Basics for primary care.* New York: Appleton–Century–Crofts, 1980, pp. 108–109).

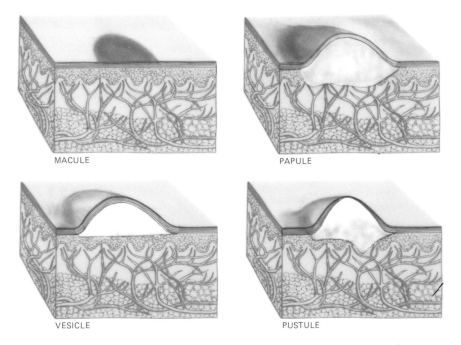

MACULE

PAPULE

VESICLE

PUSTULE

FIGURE 3.4 (Continued).

skin, a macular rash may be more recognizable if the skin is gently stretched between the thumb and finger (as for administration of an injection). This maneuver decreases the normal red tone and thus brightens the macules. In addition, some generalized rashes can be seen in the mouth, especially on the palate (See Chap. 7).[3]

Moisture. Perspiration is the most obvious moisture seen on the body. The face, axilla, and skin folds are the likely places for it to occur. Dehydration is detected by noting the moisture on the mucous membranes. For instance, in mild dehydration, the mucosa of the oral cavity is likely to look dry. In a more serious stage, the lips may be cracking and look parched and other mucosa of the body

CHART 3.5.

Primary Lesions

Name	Size	Description
Macule	↓ 1 cm	Flat, circumscribed alteration of skin color (freckle)
Papule	↓ 1 cm	Solid, raised area (pimple)
Patch	↑ 1 cm	Flat, discolored area (Mongolian spot)
Nodule	↓ 1 cm	Solid mass in dermal or subcutaneous layer (wart)
Tumor	↑ 1 cm	Solid mass, may extend through subcutaneous layer
Cyst	Varies	Encapsulated, fluid-filled mass, may extend into dermis and epidermis
Wheal	Varies	Erythematous, smooth, irregularly shaped, flat-topped
Vesicle	↓ 1 cm	Fluid-filled area below skin surface (varicella)
Bulla	↑ 1 cm	Like vesicle, but larger (blister)
Pustule	Varies	Similar to vesicle and bulla, but pus-filled (acne)

CHART 3.6.

Secondary Lesions

Name	Size	Description
Erosion	Varies	Rubbing away of epidermis (abrasion)
Crust	Varies	Dried serum, pus, blood (scab)
Scar	Varies	Healed injury
Keloid	Varies	Overgrowth of scar that extends at least into dermis; fibrous
Scales	Varies	Flakes of skin, especially epidermis (psoriasis)
Lichenification	Varies	Thickening of all layers—an area that is repeatedly exposed to trauma or disease (eczema)
Hyperkeratosis	Varies	Extreme lichenification (callous)
Fissure	Varies	Linear furrowing in the epidermis and dermis, may go further (lip-splitting, especially in cold weather)
Ulcer	Varies	Loss of epidermis and portion of dermis (decubiti)

may look very dry. Darkly pigmented blacks often have dry skin under normal conditions, not necessarily indicating dehydration. Black skin tends normally to be dry and may appear "ashy" or flaky. Many patients use Vaseline-like compounds as moisturizers.

Edema. Obvious areas of swelling are inspected and palpated. An edematous area is described in terms of location, shape, tenderness, mobility, consistency, and color. Edema masks the intensity of skin color because the distance between the skin surface and the pigmented and vascular layers is increased. This increase in distance causes darkly pigmented skin to become lighter. Changes in color indicating pathology, such as pallor of cyanosis, may be obscured.

Vascular Alterations. There are normal and abnormal vascular changes. *Petechiae, ecchymosis, telangiectasis, venous stars,* and *spider angiomas* are usually abnormal (Chart 3.7). *Cherry angiomas* and other hemangiomas present at birth may be normal findings. In any case, the recorded description includes noting location, distribution, color, size, amount, and the presence of pulsations. In highly pigmented individuals, these vascular changes may be difficult to detect. However, ecchymosis resulting from a systemic disorder can usually be detected on the buccal mucosa. Petechiae can be most easily identified on the bulbar and palpebral conjunctiva as well as on the buccal mucosa (see Chaps. 4 and 5).[3,5,6]

Palpation. Inspection and palpation of the integumentary system go "hand in hand". Some features noticed in inspection can be examined by palpation, too. Palpation is used to detect moisture, temperature, texture, and turgor.

Moisture. The moisture seen on inspection should be felt. What appears to be thin and watery may be thick and oily. Fluid oozing

CHART 3.7.

Vascular Markings Throughout the Life Span

Name	Age	Physiologic Cause	Description
Hemangiomas	Birth or old age	Vascular lesions	See specific type.
Nevus flammeus infantile	Present at birth, fades by 2 years	Vascular lesion	Small, superficial, flat, irregularly shaped, pink patches over eyelids, especially around nose and forehead
Port wine stain	Present at birth, may fade gradually	Vascular lesion	Larger nevus may be dark pink to red; often on scalp; if on central face there may be associated neurologic disease
Strawberry	Develops from birth and enlarges through 6 months, may start to resolve by 2 years	Vascular lesion	Raised red lesion, may occur anywhere
Cavernous (mature hemangioma)	May be present at birth and not change in size; does not fade usually	Vascular lesion	Red-blue, spongy, irregularly shaped mass
Cherry angioma (senile hemangioma)	Develops in aging persons	Vascular lesion	Small, nodular, red; most frequently on trunk; may blanch with external pressure
Spider angioma	Any age	Can be normal vascular lesion or pathologic indicator (liver disease, pregnancy, ↑ estrogen)	Small, star-like, with a solid circular area in the middle; may pulsate when pressure applied; often below waist
Telangiectasia	Middle age	Sun exposure, polythemia, alcoholism	Large or small generalized areas of venous or capillary dilatation, appear as erythematous linear markings
Venous star	Varies	Vascular force on vein	Various sizes, small, blue, star-like; found near veins, often on legs

from a lesion should be described by its color, amount, thickness, and odor.

Temperature. One of the most traditional ways to detect an elevated temperature is by laying the back of one's hand on the patient's forehead or neck. If there is a fever, a warm or hot sensation can be felt. The examiner must not have cold hands or the results of this gross estimation will be useless. Isolated areas that have been traumatized or are infected or sunburned may feel warm, too. The opposite physiologic occurrence (reduced blood flow) causes a cooler feeling of the skin and may be evidenced in peripheral arteriosclerosis, Raynaud's disease or syndrome, shock, or any circulatory disturbance of significance.

Texture. Skin texture varies on different parts of the body. Normal descriptions include thick, thin, rough, smooth, etc. A sculptress's hands may be rough and the skin may even be lichenified from contact with harsh materials, whereas the rest of her body will probably be much smoother. People with an overactive thyroid (hyperthyroidism) may notice their skin becoming smoother and softer. Those with an underactive thyroid (hypothyroidism) may have dryer, flaking skin. In both thyroid conditions, the skin changes will be generalized, rather than localized. In darkly pigmented individuals, palpation of skin texture may be the best method of detecting a rash. Roach contends that with a little practice, papular rashes can usually be identified by palpating gently with fingertips. However in the case of a macular rash, the nurse may have to rely on the patient's complaints of itching or on evidence of scratching.[3]

Turgor. Skin *turgor* is a term used to describe the skin's elasticity. In advanced dehydration, large amounts of weight loss or stretching, or even in normal aging, elasticity of the skin will lessen. To test skin turgor, one gently pinches an area of skin (usually the abdomen, if not too flaccid, or the skin over the radius at the wrist), noting how quickly the skin returns to place. If the elasticity is decreased, the skin will recede very slowly or stand by itself. If the turgor is normal, it will go right back into place.

Epidermal Appendages

Fingernails and Toenails. The nails and hair are inspected and palpated. The nails are inspected for color, shape, biting, unusual curvature, thickness, and markings in the nail beds themselves. In light-skinned patients, healthy nails appear reasonably smooth, convex, and pink over the nailbeds. While pigmentation of the nails is unusual in normal Caucasians, it is not uncommon among blacks, who may normally have brown or black pigmentation along the edge of the nail or in a pattern of longitudinal streaks.[7]

The nurse should next push on two or more of the nails and look for blanching and the immediate return of the pink color to the nail bed. If the pinkness does not return promptly, she should consider the possibility of a circulatory insufficiency or an anemia. In highly pigmented individuals, the rate of return of the nail bed color may be a more useful indicator than the actual color of the nail. The nails themselves do not change much throughout life unless abnormalities develop (Chart 3.8 and Fig. 3.5).

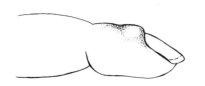

FIGURE 3.5. Clubbing of the fingers.

CHART 3.8.

Abnormalities of the Nail beds

Name	Description
Clubbing	This is the result of advanced heart or lung disease (especially COPD). The fingertips are also likely to enlarge. (See Fig. 3.5)
Furrowing (Beau's lines)	This can be the result of systemic problems or traumatic injury. A ridge will appear across the nail that extends to the nail bed.
Thickening	This can be the result of chronic fungal infections in the nail beds. *Candida albicans* is one of the most difficult to treat. Removal of the nail is often necessary.
Paronychea	This is the result of an infection around the nail, thus causing erythema and tenderness.
Linear markings	Some people have hairline type markings under the nail. They are usually white. Their etiology is unknown and they are generally not problematic.

Hair. The hair on the scalp is inspected routinely in a complete physical and in an acute situation if it pertains to the problem. The hair is observed for color, amount, quality, and distribution.

The hair on a newborn is called *lanugo.* Lanugo is the fine hair of fetal life and it is found primarily on the shoulders, back, and extremities. During the first few months of life the baby loses this hair as well as the hair on his head that he is born with. The hair on his head is then replaced by his permanent hair. While it is coming in, the quality is usually fine and thin.

Permanent hair may normally be black, brown, red, yellow, or various shades of these colors. Hair fibers are formed into straight, wavy, helical, or spiral filaments, depending on the structure of the protein molecules that make up the hair. This variation in hair fibers makes hair texture range from straight to kinky or wooly.

There are few notable changes in a child's hair once his permanent hair has come in. The hair color may change in children as they get older, but the texture and curl will not change much.

Prior to puberty, body hair will become more pronounced in several areas. (Note, however, that absence of body hair is not uncommon among people of Asian descent.) In both sexes hair will appear in the axilla and genitalia. Hair present on the legs will darken and thicken. For cosmetic reasons many American women shave the axillary and leg hair.

In the middle years, graying of the hair on the head may begin in both sexes. This usually starts with a gradual "salt and pepper" pattern at the hairline. Balding is more apparent in men and is most common among people of European and Near Eastern ancestry. Some men may note a receding hairline as early as in their twenties; however, patterns will vary. Because balding is a genetic trait, the amount of hair loss as well as the time it begins may reflect family patterns.

As women age, they too may note a thinning of the hair on the head. This is often aggravated by years of stretching it on rollers, teasing, or blow-drying. After menopause, pubic, axillary, and leg hair may lessen, too. Some adult women may also be aware of the appearance of facial hair. This occurs most commonly over the upper lip and under the chin.

Men may note loss of hair on the extremities as the years go by. This varies among individuals. Generally speaking, the amount of body hair, including growth and loss, can often be attributed to genetic predisposition.[8,9]

REFERENCES

1. Quevedo, W., Fitzpatrick, T., Pathak, M., & Jimbow, K. Role of light in human skin color variation. *American Journal of Physical Anthropology*, 1975, *43*, 393–408.
2. Cage, G. Eccrine and apocrine secretory glands. In T. Fitzpatrick, et al. (Eds.), *Dermatology in general medicine*. New York: McGraw–Hill, 1971.
3. Roach, L. Color changes in dark skins. *Nursing*, 1972, *2*, 19–22.
4. Williams, R. The clinical and physiological assessment of black patients. In D. Luckraft (Ed.), *Black awareness: Implications for black patient care*. New York: American Journal of Nursing Co., 1976, 16–26.
5. Rubin, B. Black skin. *RN*, 1979, 31–35.
6. Branch, M., & Paxton, P. *Providing safe nursing care for ethnic people of color*. New York: Appleton–Century–Crofts, 1976.
7. Wasserman, H. *Ethnic pigmentation: Historical, physiological and clinical aspects*. Amsterdam: Excerpta Medica, 1974.
8. McDonald, C., & Kelly, P. Dermatology and venereology. In R. Williams (Ed.), *Textbook of black-related diseases*. New York: McGraw–Hill, 1975, 513–592.
9. Ewing, J., & Rouse B. Hirsutism, race and testosterone levels: Comparison of East Asians and Euroamericans. *Human Biology*, 1978, *50*, 209–215.

BIBLIOGRAPHY

Behrman, H., Labow, T., & Rozen, J. *Common skin diseases: Diagnosis and treatment* (2nd ed.). New York: Grune & Stratton, 1971.

Fitzpatrick, T. B., Arndt, K. A., Clark, W. H., Jr., Eisen, A. Z., Van Scott, E. J., & Vaughn, J. H. (Eds.). *Dermatology in general medicine*. New York: McGraw–Hill, 1971.

Pillsbury, D. *A manual of dermatology*. Philadelphia: Saunders, 1971.

Sauer, G. *Manual of skin diseases* (3rd ed.). Philadelphia: Lippincott, 1973.

EXAMPLE OF A RECORDED HISTORY AND PHYSICAL

SUBJECTIVE:

Chief Complaint: "My skin has been itchy for 3 days."

HPI: This 16-year-old female considers herself to be in "good health." Three days ago noticed she was scratching a lot around the elastic waist of her panty hose. She did not pay attention to it. However, as she was about to bathe that evening, she noticed "tiny, flesh-colored bumps" where she had been scratching. The itch increased that night. She applied some calamine lotion but got no relief. The following day, the itching and same bumps appeared on her wrists, between the fingers of her left hand, in the axillary folds, and in the left groin. Last night the itching was so bad "I almost went crazy. I tried dry skin lotions and hot baths. Nothing helped."

Patient has never had this problem before. She has used no new soaps, perfumes, or detergents. No new clothes, night clothes, bed linens. She is taking no medications presently and has taken none in the last 6 weeks. She has eaten no unusual foods or in unusual restaurants. No pets. She did visit some friends last weekend who "found a little puppy and decided to give it a home." No known allergies to foods, medications, or environmental irritants.

OBJECTIVE: T. 98.6°F orally; P. 80 radial; R. 16; B.P. 124/72 sitting.

Skin: Multiple papules and pustules; white-gray in color in a linear configuration along left flank area at waist, right and left anterior axillary folds, left groin folds, flexor surface of right and left wrist, and between the digits of the left hand. Some crusting and redness along the waist. No edema or discharge in these areas.

Microscopic: Skin scraping of axilla; mite present.

4

The Head, Face, and Neck

Much of the examination of the head, face, and neck is general inspection and palpation. A good deal of observing can be done while eliciting the history. However, if this is the only time that inspection is implemented, it is likely to be superficial and abnormalities may be missed. To complete the evaluation of the head, face, and neck, one must include the examination of the eyes, ears, mouth, nose, and sinuses. These areas are covered in other chapters.

HISTORY

There are several questions to ask in reviewing the head, face, and neck. One can usually combine the questions regarding the head and face and then follow with the review of the neck.

A general inquiry about the patient's hair is a good place to begin. How does he describe his hair? Thick? Thin? Plentiful? Lacking in spots? Coarse? Fine? Has he noticed any changes recently? Unusual loss? Is the loss in one spot or all over? Is there a difference in consistency or texture? Is there a change in color or shine. (i.e., either natural or unnatural)? Does the patient chemically treat his hair (i.e., permanents, straighteners)? And last, how often does the patient have to wash his hair? This may produce information about the oiliness or dryness of the hair.

Questions regarding the scalp range from problems with lumps or bumps to itching, scaling, or dandruff. A lump on the head may have been due to traumatic injury. If so, how it was incurred needs to be investigated. A mass on the head may also be some form of a cyst. In either case it is important to get a description of how long it has been there as well as the location, size, associated pain, discharge (describe), and previous history of the problem. Itching, scaling, or dandruff may have various etiologies. Information should be elicited on the area involved, the length of time the problem has existed, and any known cause of the problem (allergy to hair products, incomplete rinsing of shampoos, stress, chronic skin conditions, etc.). If any other abnormalities have occurred in the past, a brief discussion of what the problems were, known causes, symptoms, treatment, and any recurrences should be recorded.

Relevant to the review of this system is any history of loss of consciousness, seizures, dizziness, headache, trauma, or facial pain. A loss of consciousness may have occurred for several reasons. A traumatic injury may have caused the patient to become unconscious. If this has happened, the patient should be questioned about the existing circumstances: when and where the incident happened, what activity the patient was involved in at the time, what was done for the patient, how long he thinks he was "out," and any residual effects of the injury.

Seizures may or may not cause a loss of consciousness. If a seizure occurred one time as a result of a high fever when the patient was a child, that is different from a history of seizures through the years. It is important to have the patient describe what he means by the word and what exactly happened to him. People may refer to this as a "spell," so a mutual understanding of what is being described is necessary. Any treatments as a result of the episode(s) should be recorded.

Dizziness can be a symptom and a complicated problem, too. A very helpful question to ask regarding dizziness is: "Do you feel like the room is spinning around you (vertigo) or do you feel lightheaded?" Rotational dizziness is due most often to vestibular dysfunction and in this instance the patient will describe the sensation of the room spinning around him. The patient may also describe the sensation that he is spinning, rather than the room.

People who have headaches are often very frustrated. Finding a cause and a successful treatment often follows years of pain and various opinions and treatments. If headaches are a problem, a thorough pain history should be obtained, including location, radiation, duration, intensity, associated activity, aggravating and alleviating factors, accompanying symptoms, and past diagnosis and treatments. Allergies, past history of traumas, stress, and the menstrual cycle may also be related. In any case, if the eight areas of investigation are applied, much valuable information can be collected.

With the exception of the question about parents noticing a child's head growing in infancy and toddlerhood, questions concerning the head are basically the same for all ages.

A more specific investigation of the face and its problems includes not only what it is, but also where on the face the problem is located. Common complaints that are likely to be mentioned are edema; pain; discoloration; unusual movements, such as tics or twitching; and lesions, such as moles and pimples. Remember that positive responses require a more detailed inquiry.

The history regarding the neck follows easily in this systematic approach. The patient should be asked if he has any pain or stiffness or has noticed any lumps in his neck. If he has pain or stiffness, he is then asked where exactly and with what movements the discomfort is associated. If he notices a lump, the nurse should inquire as to the location, size, and amount of tenderness and ask if there has been a recent diagnosis of a systemic infection. This information plus additional questions from the eight areas of investigation will give a more complete picture.

The patient should be asked if he has ever been told he has a thyroid problem. If he has, he may have been told whether his thyroid was overfunctioning or underfunctioning. That knowledge will be very helpful. There may have been blood tests or other diagnostic studies done to confirm the diagnosis. The nurse should find out what the patient specifically recalls about when they were done, what was suspected, and what the results were. Were medications ordered following the tests? If so, what kind and how much did the patient take? Are they still being taken? If not, why not? Were any other treatments implemented, such as surgery or radiation? What was its course and outcome? All these data add to the very important data base that the patient provides.

ANATOMY

The skull is a relatively round, boney structure. It is made up of both the facial and the cranial bones (Fig. 4.1). All the cranial bones of the skull are joined by suture lines. The *frontal bone* is the bone called the forehead. It attaches to the *parietal bone* on the anterior aspect of the skull at the *coronal suture line*. The *sagittal suture line* falls in the middle of the parietal bone. Posteriorly, the *lambdoidal suture line* lies horizontally and serves as the connection between the parietal and the occipital bone. The *squamosal suture line* joins the temporal and parietal bones on the lateral aspects of the head. An

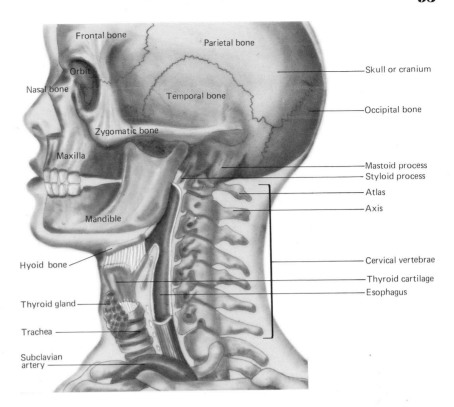

FIGURE 4.1. Major structures of the head and neck. (From Heagarty, M., Glass, G., King, H., & Manly, M. *Child health: Basics for primary care.* New York: Appleton–Century–Crofts, 1980, p. 118)

additional suture line may occur across the occipital bone in American Indian children and between the frontal bones in children of West European descent.[1] Suture lines, especially the coronal, sagittal, and the lambdoidal, have a ridge-like feeling when palpated at birth, but should be smooth and no longer palpable by 5 to 6 months.

The other portions of the skull that are not completely ossified at birth are called *fontanelles.* These areas are present at birth and are often referred to as "soft spots." There are two important fontanelles: the *anterior* and the *posterior* (Fig. 4.2). The diamond-shaped anterior fontanelle is located at the union of the frontal and parietal bones. The exact size is not as important as its presence so that the brain can grow as it should during the first year of life. The fontanelle is about 3 cm long by 4 cm wide and closes gradually anywhere between 8 months and 2 years of age. The joining of the parietal and occipital bones is the posterior fontanelle. This triangular soft spot closes by 3 months of age and may even be closed at birth.

The size of the head is a crucial statistic at birth and during infancy and early toddlerhood. An average-size baby should have a head measurement of 13 to 14 inches (35 cm). During the first year of life the head grows about 4 inches. At birth the head is about 2 cm larger than the chest. As the child grows, this proportion reverses, but not during the first year of life. Abnormal growth rates can be indicative of serious problems. Some terms commonly used to describe head size are as follows.

Normocephalic: A head size within normal limits.
Macrocephalic: An inappropriately large head for age and body size.
Microcephalic: An inappropriately small head for age and body size.

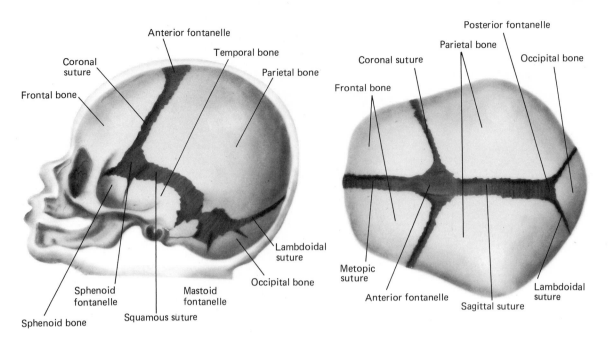

FIGURE 4.2. Fontanelles at birth. (From Heagarty, M., Glass, G., King, H., & Manly, M. *Child health: Basics for primary care.* New York: Appleton–Century–Crofts, 1980, p. 119)

The facial bones are also connected by suture lines, although these are normally not palpable at any time. The facial bones are not moveable, with the exception of the *mandible.* The mandible is the lower jaw. It is the longest bone of the face and contains the sockets for the lower teeth. The upper teeth come out of the *maxillary bone,* which surrounds the nose. Attached to the maxillary bone is the *zygomatic bone;* the two jointly form the lower rim of the orbit of the eye. The maxilla and frontal bone meet as well. Together they surround the *nasal bone,* which is the boney portion of the nose. These are the skull bones accessible to external inspection and palpation.

The neck has a variety of structures that are readily accessible to physical examination. They are the *sternocleidomastoid* and *trapezius muscles,* the *trachea,* the *carotid arteries* and *jugular veins,* the *thyroid gland,* the *thyroid cartilage* and the *cricoid cartilage,* and the *lymph nodes of the neck.*

There are two major neck muscles: the sternocleidomastoid and the trapezius. The sternocleidomastoid longitudinally extends from the mastoid process to the clavicle. The trapezius begins at the occipital area and reaches to the shoulder region (Fig. 4.3). The positions of these two muscles are such that they form invisible triangles. The anterior portion of the neck represents the anterior triangle and the posterior triangle involves the posterior region. This description is helpful when trying to learn proper techniques of palpation of the lymph nodes and the thyroid gland.

There are several structures in the anterior portion of the neck with which the examiner must be familiar. The *hyoid bone* is the most superior boney structure in the neck that can be palpated in the midline area. It is the support for the tongue and its muscles. Moving down, the next firm structure that can be felt is the *thyroid*

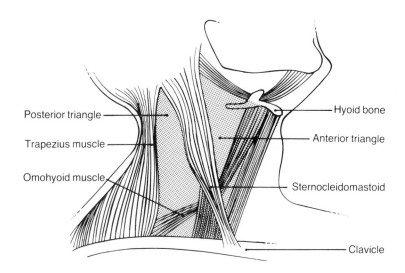

FIGURE 4.3. Anterior and posterior triangle of the neck.

cartilage. It is the largest cartilage of the larynx. Below the thyroid cartilage is the *cricoid cartilage,* often referred to as the "Adam's apple." This cartilaginous landmark is narrower than the thyroid cartilage. Both ascend when a person swallows. The *trachea* lies under these cartilages and is the pipe of respiration. It is about 5 inches in length. The *thyroid gland,* the only endocrine gland accessible to physical examination, is in this same general vicinity. It lies adjacent to the tracheal rings 2–3–4. The lateral lobes of the thyroid gland are connected by a spongy tissue called the *isthmus.* It, too, ascends with swallowing (Fig. 4.4).

Most of the palpable lymph nodes in the body are located in the neck. The lymph nodes palpable in this region are (Fig. 4.5):

1. Occipital: In the occipital region of the head where the trapezius and the occiput meet.
2. Postauricular: In front of the mastoid process but behind the auricle.
3. Preauricular: In front of the tragus.

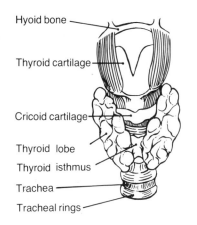

FIGURE 4.4. Major structures of the neck, anterior view.

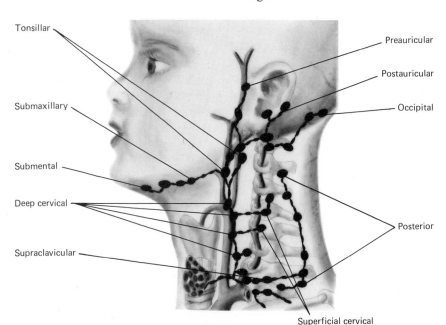

FIGURE 4.5. Lymphatics of the neck. (From Heagarty, M., Glass, G., King, H., & Manly, M. *Child health: Basics for primary care.* New York: Appleton–Century–Crofts, 1980, p. 118)

4. Tonsillar: 2 cm below and inferior to the angle of the mandible in the hollow of loose skin.
5. Submaxillary: Along the mandible halfway from the angle to the chin.
6. Submental: Underneath the chin.
7. Deep cervical: Under the sternocleidomastoid.
8. Superficial cervical: Also under the sternocleidomastoid, but slightly more posterior.
9. Posterior: Below the superficial cervical and along the anterior aspect of the trapezius.
10. Supraclavicular: Above the clavicle, along the base of the sternocleidomastoid.

Circulation of blood to the head and neck is supplied primarily by the *external* and *internal carotid arteries.* The *internal* and *external jugular veins* are also located in the neck. The twelve cranial nerves are responsible for innervating the head and neck. Both the circulatory and the neurologic aspects will be discussed in detail in later chapters.

PHYSICAL ASSESSMENT

For the head, face, and neck, the following techniques of examination are used: inspection, palpation, percussion, and auscultation. Both inspection and palpation are used throughout the exam, while auscultation is only used to check over the major arteries and thyroid for bruits (see Chap. 9). Percussion and/or palpation are used to assess tenderness of the paranasal sinuses (see Chap. 7). The equipment needed by the examiner is her eyes and hands, good lighting, a stethoscope, a glass of water, and a tape measure.

Because of the nature of the examination of the head, face, and neck, inspection and palpation are discussed together. As always, it is best to begin with a general inspection.

The Head

The hair on the head is inspected for quality, amount, and distribution. "Coarseness" and "fineness" are terms used to describe the quality of the hair. The amount and distribution of the hair may vary with age. The hair of a newborn is likely to fall out during the first few months of life and be replaced with the fine, soft hair of infancy and toddlerhood. Hair grows at different rates and differs in quality among individual children. The hair of childhood, adolescence, and young adulthood grows at a relatively consistent rate. As middle age and old age approach, many people will notice a loss and a thinning out of the hair. Men especially have a problem with alopecia (loss of hair). Balding has a genetic predisposition and not much can be done about it. Women notice a change in the amount and thickness of their hair during and after menopause.

The scalp is inspected by separating the hair at various spots and taking a thorough look at the skin under the hair. Look for scaliness, lesions, or irregularities. Scaliness on the scalp may be indicative of a common condition such as *dandruff.* This often occurs in the winter months, when skin tends to be dryer. *Seborrhea* is another condition commonly found on the head and is a result of an overproduction of sebum (from the sebaceous glands). Seborrhea presents as greasy, scaly, patches and is found in places on the body where hair follicles are located. It can be caused by stress and

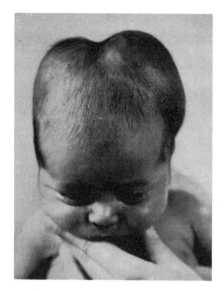

FIGURE 4.6. Cephalohematoma involving both parietal bones in an infant 13 days old. (From Rudolph, A., Barnett, H., & Einhorn, A. (Eds.). *Pediatrics* (16th ed.). New York: Appleton–Century–Crofts, 1977, p. 1827)

tension in addition to genetic predisposition. This problem can usually be controlled by topical medication and/or shampoos and by trying to decrease the psychosocial stresses that may be associated with it.

Next the scalp should be observed for lumps, bumps, and lesions. Moles are often found on the head. If they are elevated above the skin surface, combing and shampooing the hair may cause them to bleed. This information may be elicited in the history, but if not, these matters should be investigated when a lesion is found.

A lump on the head may be a sebaceous cyst (see Chap. 3). It will feel like a firm, well-defined mass under the skin surface. These cysts are usually not painful and, if small enough, are not bothersome. Size should be noted for comparative purposes. Traumatic injury may also cause a bump on the head. These bumps will vary in size, depending on the type of injury incurred. Tenderness over the involved area is likely to be elicited in a recent injury.

In newborn infants, asymmetry of the head may be present. There are two conditions which can cause this. *Caput succedaneum* is a soft tissue injury which happens during birth, causing edema and ecchymosis of the presenting position of the baby's head during a vertex delivery. This usually resolves gradually during the first few days of life. *Molding*, which is an overriding of the parietal bones, may accompany caput succedaneum. This too, will resolve without treatment during the first weeks of life.[2]

The other asymmetrical abnormality on the head of a newborn is a *cephalhematoma* (Fig. 4.6). This is a subperiosteal hemmorhage which limits itself to one cranial bone (and is thus unilateral[2]). It does not appear until several hours after birth and gradually increases in size. There is no discoloration with a cephalhematoma. It looks bizarre and is very frightening to parents. They need a lot of reassurance and support. Fortunately, this, too, resolves without treatment during the first few weeks of life.

The skull is inspected and palpated for size, shape, and tenderness. Abnormal skull size is most likely to occur in infancy, unless there is a congenital anomaly (Fig. 4.7).

In order to ascertain the proper size of the baby's skull, the head circumference is measured in all children under 2 years of age. A paper tape or cloth tape with both centimeter and inch calibrations will do fine. It is important that the child is still while taking this measurement. It may be helpful to have the parent hold the child's head. The tape is placed around the child's head. The occipital bone and frontal bone are used for landmarks in placing the tape. The widest span is the correct measurement (Fig. 4.8) The number is then plotted on a standardized growth chart (Fig. 4.7). As long as the measurement falls within the established norms for the appropriate age, then the head size is considered within normal limits. Because all standardized growth charts currently available in the United States are based on statistical averages for Caucasian children, growth assessment of racially distinct children requires particular attention. For example, the head circumference of newborn children of Asian descent is normally nearly 1 cm narrower than that of black or Caucasian children (see Chap. 2 for additional information on growth differences).

Next the anterior and posterior fontanelles are inspected and palpated. If they are still open, the nurse should approximate the size. Any bulging or depression of these areas should be noted. A

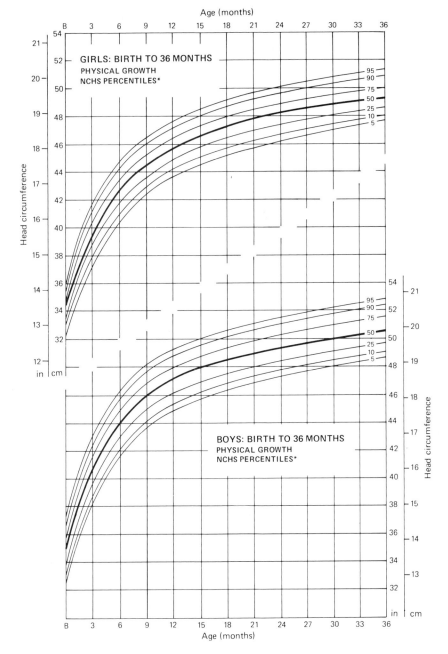

FIGURE 4.7. Head circumference in boys and girls (standardized chart)—birth to 36 months. (Reprinted with permission from Ross Laboratories, Columbus, Ohio, C. 1976 Adapted from National Center for Health Statistics: NCHS Growth Charts, 1976. Monthly Vital Statistics Report. Vol. 25, No. 3 Supp. (HRA) 76-1120. Health Resources Administration, Rockville, Md., June, 1976. Data from The Fels Research Institute.)

bulging fontanelle may indicate intracranial pressure. In a dehydrated child the fontanelles will appear depressed or sunken. While still palpating the head, the suture lines should be checked. If they are still palpable, a ridge-like sensation will be felt, and nothing more.

Face

In both adults and children the face should be inspected for color, facial hair, symmetry, expression, tics, swelling, and any unusual conditions of the skin. Palpation of any lumps, lesions, or other raised abnormalities is necessary. Some facial abnormalities may be due to systemic conditions. The skin may have the classic pallor of fatigue or anemia, or it may have the yellow tones of jaundice. The shape of the face may be "puffy" in advanced hypothyroidism or

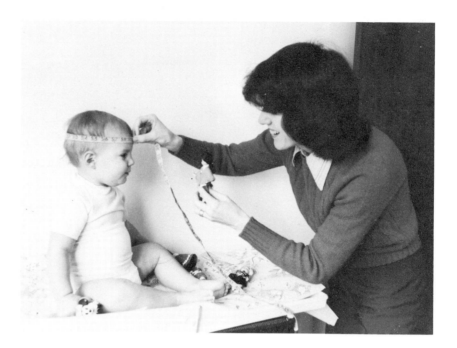

FIGURE 4.8. Measuring circumference of infant's head.

Cushing's disease. Branch and Paxton point out that in examining black patients this characteristic broadening of facial characteristics with hypothyroidism may be obscured by the health professional's notions about racial characteristics of the face.[4] Periorbital edema may be a clue to kidney malfunction. There are also certain signs that accompany cranial nerve damage. For instance, one side of the face may droop. The condition is known as Bell's palsy and involves the seventh cranial nerve. Ptosis of the eyelid is another manifestation of cranial nerve damage (see Chap. 3). If any acne, moles, and/or unusual facial hair exists, a thorough description is necessary. When acne is a problem, it is important to keep track of where the lesions are located. In addition lesions should be described by color, size, and type (see Fig. 3.4). The nurse should also note whether or not they are blackheads, white heads, or cysts and whether there is permanent scarring. The details are noteworthy if week-to-week or month-to-month change is being assessed. Accurate, detailed descriptions are the only way improvement or deterioration of a condition can be documented.

Acne does not usually begin until adolescence and in most cases will resolve during young adulthood. It has several degrees of severity. The more serious types can be treated systemically. The milder forms are approached with topical treatments. In either case the crisis of altered body image is prevalent in the teenagers with the problem.

Any facial lesion, especially if it is isolated and elevated, should be described in detail. It should be described in terms of color, location, size, tenderness, discharge, crustation, and type of surface (e.g., pitting in the center).

Neck

Inspection of the neck begins this portion of the exam. The structures and any abnormalities will be easier to see if the patient raises his chin and tilts his head backward. Good lighting is also necessary. The nurse should look for any asymmetry, swelling, obvious

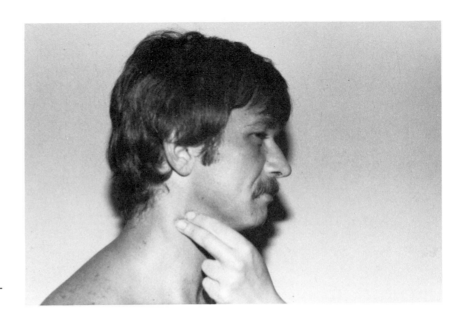

FIGURE 4.9. Palpating the anterior cervical lymph nodes.

lymph nodes, masses, or lesions and palpate any of these enlargements. She should also note size, tenderness, color, shape, and mobility of any palpable masses.

Palpation of the lymph nodes and thyroid gland follows. A systematic approach for palpation of the lymph nodes is a must! If a meticulous method is not implemented, it is likely that portions of a lymph node chain will be missed. To feel the nodes, the pads of the first three fingers of both hands are used. The skin is rolled, not pushed, over the underlying tissue (Fig. 4.9). If the nurse pushes too hard, any palpable nodes will be obliterated. If a gentle but firm technique is used the enlarged nodes will be felt easily. Flexing the neck slightly midline will facilitate the exam. The patient should be asked if there is any tenderness.

The examiner should proceed in the following manner. She should start with the occipital nodes and move to the postauricular and preauricular nodes. She should follow with palpation of the tonsil-

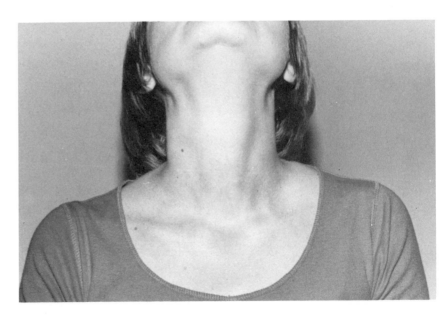

FIGURE 4.10. Major structures of the neck—anterior view.

lar, submaxillary, and submental. In the neck she should feel for the superficial cervical, deep cervical, and posterior cervical nodes. She should complete the exam by palpating the supraclavicular region.

In a well developed adult, lymph nodes are generally not palpable. In a child, a thin adult, or someone who has had mononucleosis they may be easier to feel. However, if while palpating these lymph nodes a lump or lumps are discovered, then the following information must be noted: location, mobility, size, shape (edges well defined), consistency, or tenderness. Tenderness, however, often indicates an acute inflammatory response to a viral, fungal, or bacterial infection. Hard, immobile, irregularly shaped, nontender nodes often involve a malignancy.

The Thyroid

The thyroid gland is extremely difficult to inspect and palpate. Most health care providers agree that the normal thyroid gland is not always palpable. However, people with thin necks are likely to have a normally functioning thyroid gland which can be felt. Authorities also feel that a slightly enlarged thyroid gland is not necessarily pathologic.

The thyroid is inspected for enlargement and nodules; palpated for size, tenderness, and masses or nodules; and auscultated for bruits. Palpation of the thyroid gland involves both an anterior and a posterior approach. Both methods should be used to assure accuracy.

In order to inspect and palpate the thyroid and its lateral lobes, one must be able to locate specific landmarks (Fig. 4.10: see also Fig. 4.4). The hyoid bone is the first landmark. It is slightly inferior and under the mandible. This bone is attached to the tongue's posterior surface. The hyoid has a firm, boney sensation when felt (Fig. 4.4). The firm and immobile thyroid cartilage is then found. It sits below the hyoid bone and above the cricoid. The cricoid (Adam's apple) is a mobile cartilaginous ring that ascends when one swallows. The thyroid isthmus is a soft, spongy band that lies across the trachea below the cricoid (Fig. 4.4).[2]

Once the landmarks have been located, inspection of the thyroid can proceed. Good lighting must be available for this portion of the exam. The examiner stands in front of the patient. She asks him to hyperextend his chin slightly and then to swallow. Any obvious enlargement, masses, or asymmetry should be noted. While looking at the trachea, the nurse should note if there is deviation from the midline. Checking for tracheal deviation includes palpation as well.

The patient will need a glass of water. This will make swallowing easier while the examiner is displacing the thyroid during palpation.

Posterior Examination of the Thyroid. The nurse stands directly behind the patient and has him relax his neck by bending it slightly towards his chest (Fig. 4.11). The patient is asked to take a sip of water and hold it in his mouth. The nurse locates the cricoid and, directly below it, the isthmus. The patient is told to swallow the water and the examiner feels the isthmus ascend. The thyroid lobes are on either side of the isthmus about 1 cm away. The nurse palpates and follows the lobes as they curve behind the trachea to check for nodules. The patient is asked to take another swallow of water. The examiner then rests her thumbs at the nape of the patient's neck.

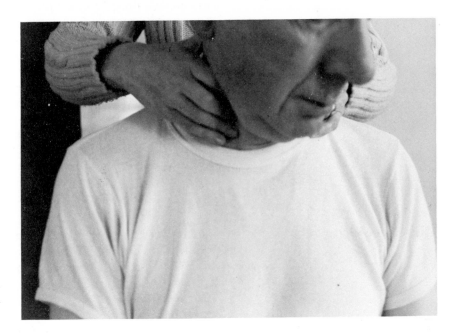

FIGURE 4.11. Proper placement of hands for posterior examination of the thyroid.

To examine the left thyroid lobe the patient is told to flex his head slightly to the left. With the first two fingers of her right hand, the examiner gently pushes the thyroid cartilage to the left (Fig. 4.11). The examiner's left hand is on the left side of the patient's neck. Her left thumb is placed deep behind the sternocleidomastoid muscle. The first and second finger of this hand should be placed along the anterior edge of the sternocleidomastoid directly across from the isthmus (Fig. 4.11). The muscle is retracted slightly with the fingers. The patient is asked to swallow the sip of water. The thyroid lobe will ascend under the examiner's fingers at this time. If an enlargement or irregularity exists, it will be felt during this ascension. The procedure is repeated for the right thyroid lobe.

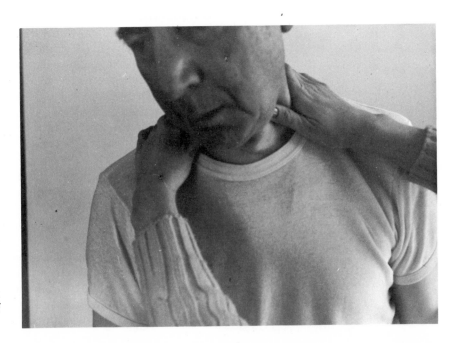

FIGURE 4.12. Proper placement of hands for anterior examination of the thyroid.

Anterior Approach. The sternocleidomastoid and other landmarks are located once more. The examiner should be standing in front of the patient. To palpate the right lobe she should have the patient flex his head to the right. This time the thyroid cartilage is displaced to the right with the examiner's right thumb (Fig. 4.12). She then places the first two fingers of her left hand deep behind the sternocleidomastoid. The patient is asked to swallow another sip of water. As he swallows, the thyroid lobe will ascend under the examiner's left thumb. The procedure is reversed to examine the left lobe.

In addition to any enlargement, the nurse should note any tenderness or specific nodules. If the gland is enlarged she should be sure to listen over each lobe with the stethoscope for bruits (see Chap. 9). This accentuated flow sound may be heard over an abnormal thyroid gland.

Examination of the carotid arteries and jugular veins will be discussed in the chapter on cardiovascular assessment.

REFERENCES

1. Barnicot, N. Biological variation in modern populations. In G. Harrison, et al. (Eds.), *Human biology.* 1977, pp. 181–300.
2. Vaughn, V., & McKay, J. *Nelson textbook of pediatrics* (10th ed.). Philadelphia: Saunders, 1975, p. 352.
3. Alvear, J., & Brooke, O. Fetal growth in different racial groups. *Archives of Disease in Children,* 1978 53, 27–32.
4. Branch, M., & Paxton, P. *Providing safe nursing care for ethnic people of color.* New York: Appleton–Century–Crofts, 1976.

EXAMPLE OF A RECORDED HISTORY AND PHYSICAL

SUBJECTIVE:

Chief Complaint: "I have had pain behind my left eye for 2 hours."

HPI: This 20-year-old female considers herself to be in "perfect" health. Suddenly, 2 hours ago, while sitting and watching T.V., a "sharp, stabbing, shooting" pain began behind her left eye. She never has had anything like this before. The pain goes from behind her eye straight through to the back of her head. She noticed earlier in the evening that when she was doing dishes she saw "some green rings" in front of her eyes and that the light above the sink seemed unusually "bright."

She took three aspirin when the pain began, "because it was so bad," and vomited them 10 minutes later. She then tried to lie down but was unable to lie still. When she got up to vomit again she felt "very weak and clammy."

She has no dizziness, blurry vision, neck stiffness, ear, or tooth pain. There has been no recent trauma, emotional upset, or history of ↑ B.P. She takes no medications (including birth control pills). She has never had a seizure or loss of consciousness. She has no allergies, sinus problems, or recent upper respiratory illness. Her last menstrual period was 1 week ago and unremarkable.

Her mother and brother have severe headaches. "Now I know what they go through." In the past she has had occasional headaches three to four times/year that are relieved by aspirin. The pain now is "crippling and I couldn't do anything if I had to."

OBJECTIVE: T. 99°F axillary; P. 72 radial; R. 24; B.P. (R) 140/80 lying, (L) 138/82 lying.

Head: No tenderness over skull. No lesions or masses.

Face: Wrinkling of forehead and squinting eyes. No asymmetry, tics. No tenderness over tempomandibular joint.

Neck: Supple, full range of motion, no palpable lymphnodes.

Ears: Bilaterally—no tenderness with palpation; canal clear; TM—no redness, bulging, retraction, or distortion of landmarks.

Eyes: Left eye—ptosis of lid, some tearing, no redness of sclera, PERRLA;* fundus—no hemorrhages, exudate, A-V nicking, dilated vessels; disc visualized, borders well defined; macula visualized. Right eye—unremarkable (external features → fundus exam)

Nose: Nasal mucosa pink → red. No drainage or polyps. Paranasal sinuses—frontal and maxillary nontender.

Mouth: Dentition—no obvious caries or misplaced teeth; gums—no lesions, bleeding, tenderness, or retraction.

Neurological: MENTAL STATUS—oriented to time, person, place; CRANIAL NERVES—II (vision not tested), III (motor-somatic), V, VI, VII (motor), all intact; MOTOR—walks without difficulty, gait normal; SENSORY—see Cranial nerves above; DEEP TENDON REFLEXES. (See stick figure illustration below.)

*Pupils equal, round, and reactive to light and accommodation.

5

The Eye

Of all the senses, vision is perhaps the most important. The eyes allow us to move freely in our environment without incurring harm. They also allow us to perceive the emotions of those people around us so that we can react accordingly. To maintain their integrity, the eyes, should be carefully assessed throughout the life cycle. A vision examination is an integral part of every physical examination.

Most ophthalmologists recommend a complete eye examination every 3 to 5 years for all patients under 40. More frequent examinations are necessary if the family history is positive for diabetes, hypertension, blood dyscrasia, glaucoma, or other eye diseases. Also, the patient who has a known or suspected systemic disease (e.g., leukemia, sickle cell anemia, hypertension, diabetes) or is on medication known to affect vision (e.g., Myambutol) should be referred for more frequent eye examinations. Once the patient is over 40 he should have a complete eye examination every 2 years to screen for the presence of glaucoma, which exists in 2 percent of patients over this age.[1]

HISTORY

A sound subjective data base is obtained on any patient who presents for a general assessment of his eyes or has a related complaint. An overview of the system includes questions regarding changes in visual acuity; blurring of vision; spots; lacrimation; photophobia; itching; pain; inflammation; date of last examination; the use of glasses; and family history of glaucoma, cataracts, diabetes, hypertension, or blood dyscrasias. The nurse investigates further to detect common eye problems that may vary according to the patient's age. Frequent concerns include visual disturbances, congenital defects, and infectious or inflammatory problems. Two serious problems that require screening are cataracts and glaucoma.

To adequately assess visual impairment, the nurse should be aware of developmental patterns. The parent of a 6-week-old infant should be able to report that the child can fixate on an object. By 8 to 10 weeks the child should be able to follow and bat at objects. If the child is unable to perform these tasks, a vision problem is suspected. The parent of a toddler should be asked if the child is continually bumping into objects. The nurse should also inquire if the parent has noticed crossing of the eyes, squinting, or holding objects very close. The school-age child may complain of headache, painful eyes, blurred words when reading, inability to see the blackboard, squinting, frequent blinking, and double vision. All of these are symptoms of poor visual acuity and warrant further investigation.

Common Eye Abnormalities

Strabismus is one of the most common congenital conditions that interferes with vision (see the section on ocular motility). The primary complaint of strabismus will be that the child's eyes appear crossed. Additional complaints include squinting, blinking, tilting of the head in order to focus, and difficulty with coordination. It is wise to elicit any family history of strabismus because it is often seen in siblings.

Presbyopia is a condition in which there is a loss of elasticity of the crystalline lens. This results in a loss of the lens's ability to accommodate to nearby objects. Presbyopia begins around 45 years of age. To check for the presence of this symptom, the nurse asks the patient if he has noticed any difficulty reading newsprint, thus needing to hold the paper at arm's length. If he gives a positive response, presbyopia should be suspected.

Some of the more common infectious and inflammatory processes include *conjunctivitis*, *dacryocystitis*, *hordeolum*, and *iritis*.

Conjunctivitis is inflammation of the conjunctiva and may be due to mechanical, chemical, allergic, bacterial, or viral factors. Symptoms include tearing, redness, itching, and mucopurulent discharge. In addition, the parent or patient may report that the eyelids are matted together and appear crusty after sleeping.

Dacryocystitis is obstruction of the nasolacrimal duct. The patient will complain of tearing and discharge from the lacrimal duct at the inner canthus.

Hordeolum (sty) is an infection of the hair follicles and glands of the anterior lid margin, usually due to staphylococcus. Redness, swelling, and tenderness are the typical symptoms.

Iritis is inflammation of the iris caused by local or systemic infections. Characteristic symptoms are lacrimation, pain, and photophobia.

Cataracts and *glaucoma* are typically considered eye problems of the aged, but may occasionally be found in young persons. The transparency of the lens is lost with cataracts so that light rays are blocked. Congenital cataracts are due to malformation of the lens. This may be seen in an infant whose mother had rubella in the first trimester of pregnancy. Senile cataracts are the result of the aging process. Cataract patients may give a history of decreased visual acuity, diplopia, spots, and blurred vision.

Glaucoma is an increase in intraocular pressure due to a disturbance in the circulation of the aqueous fluid. It is the greatest cause of blindness in people over 40 and can be controlled if detected early. The National Society for the Prevention of Blindness gives the following as danger signals of glaucoma:

1. Frequent changes in glasses, none of which are satisfactory.
2. Blurred or foggy vision that clears up for a short period of time.
3. Loss of peripheral vision.
4. Appearance of rainbow-colored rings around lights.
5. Difficulty in adjusting to dark rooms.
6. Difficulty in focusing on close work.

ANATOMY

The *orbit* of the eye is a cavity formed by the frontal, maxillary, zygomatic, lacrimal, sphenoid, ethmoid, and palatine bones. The eye occupies the anterior portion of the orbit, the posterior portion being composed of nerves, blood vessels, and adipose tissue, which serve as a cushion to the eye. There are six muscles for each eye which begin at the bones of the orbit and insert in the outercoat of the eye. The four *rectus muscles* are the *superior, inferior, medial,* and *lateral.* These muscles direct the eyeball in the direction which their names indicate. The two oblique muscles are the *superior oblique and inferior oblique.* These two muscles rotate the eyeball on its axis. The muscles of the eyes work together to hold the eyes parallel, making binocular vision possible. Cranial nerves III, IV, and VI innervate these muscles.

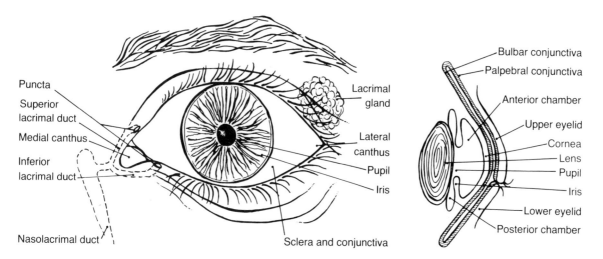

FIGURE 5.1. External structures of the eye.

The anatomy of the eye can be divided into the external structures and the fundus. Included in the external structures are the *eyelashes* and *lids*, the *lacrimal apparatus, conjunctiva, sclera, cornea, anterior chamber, iris,* and *pupils* (Fig. 5.1). The *fundus* includes the *retina, choroid, fovea centralis, macula, optic disc,* and *retinal vessels* (Fig. 5.2).

The eyelids serve to protect the eye. The space between the lids is called the *palpebral fissure*. When the eyelids are open, the upper lid covers a small part of the cornea. The *inner* and *outer canthi* are the points where the upper and lower lids meet. A tarsus plate of dense connective tissue gives shape to the lid. Within the tarsus plate are *Meibomian glands*. Sebaceous glands are located along the lid margins. *Epicanthic folds* are vertical folds of skin covering the inner canthus. These folds are found in infants all over the world. They are present in up to 20 percent of children of European descent, but generally disappear within the first year of life. They are most common in Oriental individuals, usually persisting for life. Figure 5.3 depicts the anatomical differences between eyes with and without epicanthic folds.[2]

The lacrimal apparatus consists of the *lacrimal gland, lacrimal ducts,* and *lacrimal sac*. The lacrimal gland is an almond-size structure located temporally and slightly above the eye. Its function is to secrete tears which flow over the surface of the eyeball and drain through the puncta at the lid margins into the lacrimal ducts and sac.

The *conjunctiva* is a thin transparent membrane which lines each eyelid and the anterior surface of the eye. It is divided into the *bulbar* and the *palpebral* conjunctiva. Where the eyelids meet the eyeball, the conjunctiva bends around to line the inside surface of the eyelids and becomes the palpebral conjunctiva (Fig. 5.1).

The *sclera* and *cornea* compose the fibrous coating of the eyeball. The sclera is the outer protective, supporting layer of the eye. It is the "white" of the eye viewed through the conjunctiva. In front of the eyeball the sclera bulges and changes from a white, opaque membrane to the transparent cornea. Light enters the eye through the cornea.

The area between the cornea and iris is the *anterior chamber*. It

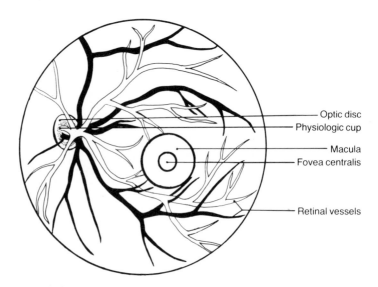

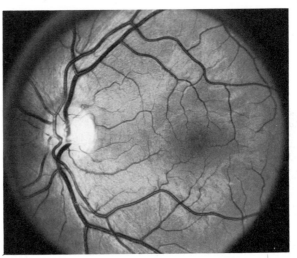

FIGURE 5.2. Fundus of the eye. (Photograph courtesy of Alan Campbell)

is filled with fluid called the *aqueous humor.* This fluid is drained off into the circulatory system through the *canal of Schlemm.*

The *iris* is a circular muscle that regulates the amount of light entering the eye. The color of the iris varies from person to person, but is usually the same in both eyes. The round hole in the center of the iris is the *pupil,* which allows the entrance of light.

Behind the iris and pupil is the crystalline *lens.* This is a transparent structure which bends the rays of light in order to focus an image on the *retina.*

The retina is the internal layer of the eye. It is the nervous coat and is only observable with the use of the ophthalmoscope. At the posterior retina the surface shows a slight depression called the *fovea centralis,* which is the region of most acute vision. The area immediately surrounding the fovea centralis is the *macula* (Fig. 5.2). The *optic disc* lies to the nasal side of the macula. The disc is the point of exit for the optic nerve of the eye. The small depression just temporal to the center of the disc is the *physiologic cup* (Fig. 5.2). The disc has no visual receptors and thus creates a blind spot. The retinal arteries and veins come from the depths of the disc and become smaller as they branch into the periphery of the fundus. The retina lies on the *choroid,* which is the middle layer of the eye. It is a thin, highly vascular membrane.

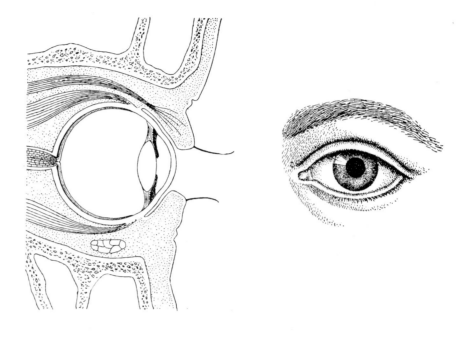

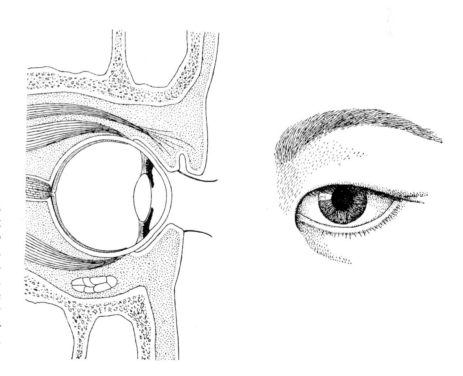

FIGURE 5.3. "ALMOND" EYE OF MONGOLOID RACES is among latest major human adaptations to environment. The Mongoloid fold, shown in lower drawings, protects the eye against the severe Asian winter. Drawings at top show the Caucasian eye with its single, fatty lid. (From Howells WW. The Distribution of Man, *Scientific American*, September, 1960, p. 124)

Visual Pathways

To focus a clear image on the retina, light must first pass through the cornea, anterior chamber, pupil, and lens. Images formed on the retina are upside down and reversed left to right. For example, an object seen in the lower nasal field of vision will form an image on the upper temporal portion of the retina (Fig. 5.4).

The nerve fibers in the retina are preserved in the optic nerves. On entering the cranial cavity the optic nerves unite to form the *optic chiasma*, which are then continued as the *optic tract*. Visual impules are thus transmitted to the occipital lobe of the cerebral cortex.

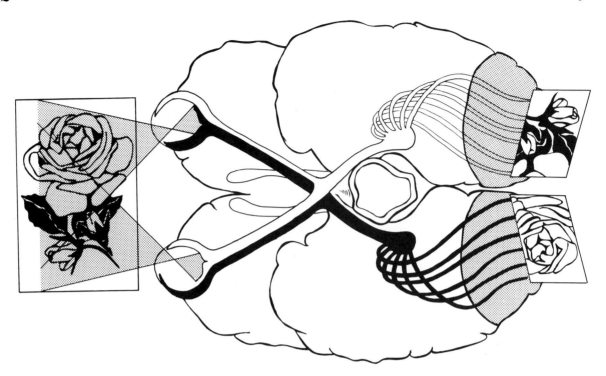

FIGURE 5.4. Left and right visual pathways.

The optic nerve fibers from the medial (nasal) halves of the retina cross in the optic chiasma to the opposite side of the brain. The optic nerve fibers from the lateral (temporal) halves remain uncrossed. Therefore, the right optic tract contains fibers only from the left half of each retina. Ultimately, the right occipital lobe receives impulses from the right half of each eye and the left occipital lobe receives impulses from the left half of each eye.

EXAMINATION OF THE EYE

A systematic approach to the examination of the eye includes measuring visual acuity, testing ocular motility, examining visual fields, inspecting external structures, and visualizing the fundus. The equipment needed for this assessment is a Snellen eye chart, a penlight, an index card (for an eye cover), a wisp of cotton, and an ophthalmoscope.

Visual Acuity

A good place to begin assessing the eye is by screening for refractive errors. Vision is not very acute at birth, but by 6 weeks of age visual acuity can be estimated by observing the way a child follows a light. To examine a child 6 months to 3 years, the nurse observes how the child fixates to light and maintains that stare when the opposite eye is covered and uncovered.[3] At about the age of 3 years a child is old enough to cooperate with instructions necessary to identify pictures on a chart or to use the Snellen illiterate E chart. During the early school years refractive errors can be identified by use of the Snellen alphabet chart.

When using the Snellen eye chart, the patient is tested with his corrective lenses, if he wears them. One eye is tested at a time; the eye not being tested is covered. Afterwards both eyes are uncovered, so that three readings are recorded. The chart is placed 20 feet from the patient and he is asked to identify the letters from the first line down. Recorded on the chart is the last line at which he identifies 4 out of 6 symbols or letters correctly. The score is read as a fraction. The numerator is the distance the patient is from the chart and the denominator is the distance the normal eye can read the chart. For example, if the patient's vision is 20/100 he can see at 20 feet away from the chart what a normally sighted person can see at 100 feet from the chart. Visual acuity gradually increases during childhood until 6 years of age, when normal vision of 20/20 is obtained. The higher the denominator, the greater the vision problem. Generally, if the patient screens 20/40 or worse, a referral is made for follow-up care.

If the patient is unable to read the largest letter on the chart, he should be checked to see if he can perceive finger movement. The fingers should be visible about 12 inches in front of his eyes. One can also try to direct a penlight into his eyes. The eye that cannot distinguish the light is considered totally blind.

Near vision is usually not tested unless the patient has a complaint or is over 40 years old, when presbyopia commonly occurs. Using a newspaper to test near vision is adequate. If the patient has reading glasses, he should be tested with them, holding the printed page about 14 inches away. Again, three readings are recorded.

The visual acuity test is simple to perform and can detect a variety of problems. In addition to detecting errors of refraction, it tests the function of the second cranial nerve.

Ocular Motility

Ocular motility refers to the alignment and coordination of the eyes. Strabismus is faulty alignment of the eyes, most commonly due to impairment of the function of the rectus muscles. More than 1 percent of children are born with this problem or will develop it.[4] Caucasian patients tend to have higher rates of convergent strabismus (esotropia), while divergent strabismus (exotropia) is more common in Oriental patients.[5] In the first few months of life there may be an occasional "wandering" of the eyes. However, by 3 months of age the child should have developed a normal binocular pattern. Any child with deviation of the eyes after the age of 3 months should be referred to an ophthalmologist.

Normally, images viewed fall on opposite parts of the retina in each eye (Fig. 5.4). Images are then passed on to the brain as two sets of nervous impulses that are fused into one. Double vision *(diplopia)* occurs in strabismus because this fusion is faulty. To overcome this problem, the child learns to avoid using the eye that deviates. It must be pointed out that the vision is being suppressed during the time eyesight is developing. If it is left untreated, the eye becomes *amblyopic.* Amblyopia is permanent impairment of vision due to disuse. Therefore, early diagnosis of strabismus is essential.

Some children, particularly those of Asian ancestry, may have *pseudostrabismus.* This results when an epicanthic fold hides a portion of the medial aspect of the eyes, causing the illusion of crossed eyes. This can be differentiated from true strabismus by the corneal light reflex test (Hirschberg's test).

There are three tests that can be done on all patients over 6

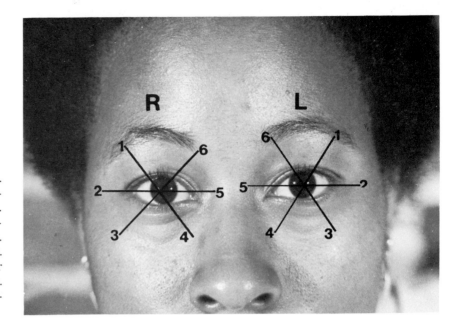

FIGURE 5.5A. Right eye (R). 1. Superior rectus (3rd). 2. Lateral rectus (6th). 3. Inferior rectus (3rd). 4. Superior oblique (3rd). 5. Medial rectus (3rd). 6. Inferior oblique (4th). Left eye (L). 1. Superior rectus (3rd). 2. Lateral rectus (6th). 3. Inferior rectus (3rd). 4. Superior oblique (4th). 5. Medial rectus (3rd). 6. Inferior oblique (3rd).

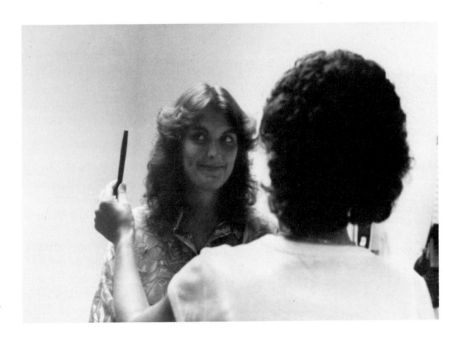

FIGURE 5.5B. Testing the cardinal fields of gaze.

months of age to test ocular motility: the *corneal light reflex test* (Hirschberg's test), the *six cardinal positions of gaze,* and the *cover–uncover patch test.*

Corneal Light Reflex Test. The alignment of the eyes is easily assessed by observing the reflection of light upon the cornea. The examiner darkens the room and has the patient look straight ahead as the light from a penlight is directed to the bridge of his nose. Normally, the light reflection is symmetrically situated in the same place on both eyes. Deviation of the light indicates faulty alignment.

Six Cardinal Positions of Gaze. Weakness of the extraocular muscles is best detected by moving the eyes through the six cardinal positions of gaze. These positions are used because they specifically identify the debilitated muscle if the eye does not return to position. In addition, the six cardinal fields of gaze test the function of the III (oculomotor), IV (trochlear), and VI (abducens) cranial nerves (Fig. 5.5A).

The patient is positioned directly in front of the examiner, holding his head in a fixed position. He then follows the tip of the examiner's penlight with his eyes only. The penlight is held a comfortable distance in front of the patient and the eyes are taken through the six cardinal fields of gaze in a slow, orderly manner, pausing periodically to note *nystagmus* (Fig. 5.5B). This is an uncontrolled and rhythmic movement of the eyes. A few beats of nystagmus on extreme lateral gaze, called *end-positional nystagmus*, is a normal finding demonstrated in many patients. Infants up to 3 months of age may have intermittent periods of nystagmus. If any other nystagmus is observed, there is need for further investigation and referral. It can result from vestibular, neurologic, or ocular dysfunction.

The Cover–Uncover Patch Test. This is a more sensitive method of determining poor alignment of the eyes. The patient fixes his vision on the tip of a penlight held approximately 5 to 6 inches in front of him. The examiner then covers one of the patient's eyes while observing the uncovered eye. Normally, the uncovered eye remains stable. If it moves to fix upon the penlight, it was not straight before the other eye was covered. As the examiner removes the cover patch, the previously covered eye is observed for movement. The well aligned eye will be focused on the penlight. If there is weakness of the muscle, the eye will turn out while covered. When the eye is uncovered there will be a quick inward movement to bring it back to alignment. Each eye is tested several times to confirm findings. (Fig. 5.6).

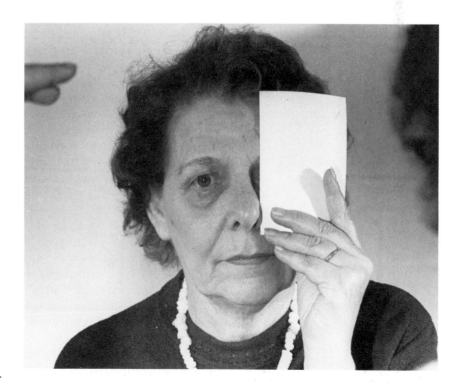

FIGURE 5.6. Cover–uncover test.

Visual Fields

Examination of the visual fields, which is a test of the second cranial nerve, measures the function of the visual pathways. A rough estimate of the visual fields is obtained by *confrontation testing*.

The examiner is the control in confrontation testing; thus it is assumed that she has good visual fields. The patient and the examiner face one another approximately 2 feet apart, situated at the same level. The patient is asked to cover one eye with a card and to look directly at the bridge of the examiner's nose. The examiner covers her own eye as the control—she covers her right eye, for example, when the patient covers his left. The examiner tests the nasal, temporal, upward, and downward fields by bringing into vision from various points in the periphery a small object or constantly moving finger (Fig. 5.7). When examining the patient's left eye the examiner extends her right arm to test the temporal fields and her left arm to test the nasal fields. This pattern is reversed for the right eye. The patient tells the examiner when the moving object comes into his peripheral vision. The object should be equidistant from the examiner and the patient, so that both see it at the same time. An exception is encountered when examining the temporal field, in which case it is difficult to bring the object far enough peripherally so that it is out of the patient's field of vision. In this case, the examiner should start with the object behind the patient, at a point where the examiner is able to see the object. Normally, the visual fields have a full range of vision, without any obvious blind spots.

Confrontation testing does not detect small lesions or early changes in the visual pathway. If the patient complains of decreased peripheral vision, he must be referred for more sophisticated screening. More accurate measurements can be made with the use of the tangent screen or perimeter.

External Examination

A systematic approach to examining the external eye is essential or findings will be missed. A sound knowledge base of anatomy is necessary as the examiner moves from the outer structures of the eye to the inner portions. The external structures are assessed in the following order: eyebrows, eyelids, eyelashes, lacrimal apparatus, conjunctiva, cornea, anterior chamber, iris, and pupil. The examination begins with inspection and proceeds to palpation.

The examiner should still be standing directly in front of the patient. She should carefully inspect the eyelashes, eyelids, and the lacrimal apparatus. She begins by inspecting the eyelashes for presence, color, condition, and position. Normally, the eyelashes are evenly distributed and curve outward.

The eyelids are examined for position, color, edema, signs of infections, and ability to close. When the eyes are open, the lids are positioned so no sclera is visible above the corneas. The following are abnormalities related to the lid. Drooping of the eyelid, *ptosis*, can result from a variety of causes, including congenital underdevelopment of the lid muscle, inflammatory edema, or early impairment of the third cranial nerve. *Ectropion* is an outturning of the lid. If the lower lid is involved it will droop due to loss of firmness and elasticity of the lid connective tissue. This leads to excessive tearing. Inversion of the lid so that the eyelashes are in contact with the conjunctiva is called *entropion*. This may result from progressive relaxation of the lid muscles due to aging. This condition is common

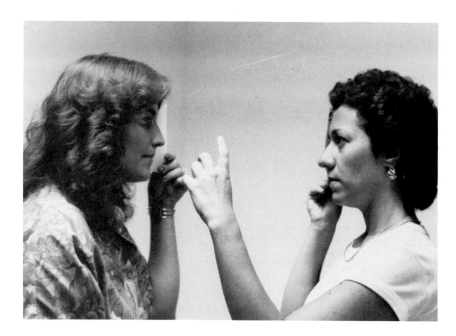

FIGURE 5.7. Testing the visual fields.

among Oriental patients and is harmless unless causing a corneal abrasion.[6] Faulty positioning of the eyelids is more common in the elderly. An *epiblepharon* or Mongolian fold is a horizontal skin fold in the upper eye and may indicate Down's syndrome or other pathology. This is not to be confused with the vertical epicanthal folds normally occurring in Asian individuals.[6]

The eyelids are inspected closely for any color changes. Slightly raised, yellowish plaques observed along the nasal portions of one or both eyelids may indicate a lipid disorder, but they can also occur in healthy individuals. This condition is called *xanthelasma.* Edema of the eyelids may point to either systemic or local disease. Some of the causes for edema are nephrosis, heart failure, thyroid deficiency, allergy, or an infectious process of the area.

The eyelids can be the site of infection. A sty or *hordeolum* results from infection of the sebaceous glands of the upper or lower lids. A *chalazion* is an infection or retention cyst of the Meibomian glands within the tarsal plates of the eyelid. A chalazion is not always obvious on inspection, so palpation of the eyelids is necessary.

Before beginning palpation of the eye, the examiner should be sure that her fingernails are short and that the patient has removed his contact lens to prevent injury to the eye. The examiner first places her index finger at the inner canthus of the eye. Using gentle palpation she then slides the examining finger across the closed lid, noting any raised areas. The eyes are then palpated to determine *intraocular pressure* (Fig. 5.8). The patient is asked to look down as the examiner places the tips of both index fingers on the upper lid over the sclera (not over the cornea). Pressure is applied with one finger, pushing the eyeball into the intraorbital region. The finger is quickly removed as the opposite finger palpates the rebound of the depressed eyeball. A spongy, soft consistency indicates decreased tension, as in dehydration. A hard consistency of the eyeball is indicative of increased intraocular tension, as in glaucoma.

The *lacrimal apparatus* is examined. The lacrimal gland is inspected for edema, then palpated gently (Fig. 5.9A). Normally, this

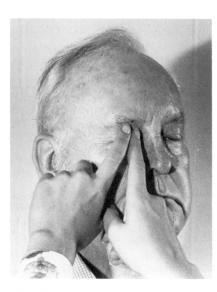

FIGURE 5.8. Palpating for intraocular pressure.

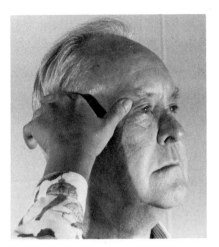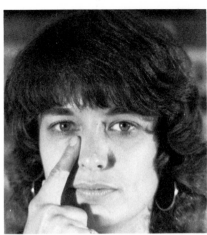

FIGURE 5.9 Left. Palpating the lacrimal gland. **Right.** Palpating the lacrimal duct.

gland is not felt. Next, the lacrimal apparatus is inspected for edema between the lower eyelid and nose, and for evidence of increased tearing. These findings indicate blockage of the nasolacrimal duct. Should the passage of tears from the nasolacrimal duct to the nose be obstructed, finger pressure on the lacrimal sac will cause regurgitation of fluid. The fingertip is placed inside the lower inner orbital rim, not on the side of the nose (Fig. 5.9B). Pressure is applied and the finger is moved inferiorly to observe for fluid. *Dacryocystitis* is the term used for infection and blockage of the lacrimal duct.

Next the orbit of the eye is inspected. A sunken appearance to the eye is called *endothalmos* and is seen in the person who is malnourished or dehydrated. *Exophthalmos*, the outward bulging of the eyeball is frequently associated with thyroid disease.

The conjunctiva consists of two components, the bulbar conjunctiva and the palpebral conjunctiva. To separate the lids so that the *bulbar conjunctiva* can be inspected, the examiner places her index finger on the patient's upper orbital rim and her thumb on the patient's lower rim. The eye should never be pressed when separating the lids. The patient is then instructed to look up, down, and to both sides. Except for a few capillaries, one should see the white of the sclera coming through the transparent conjunctiva. The sclera may be jaundiced, indicating a liver problem, or excessively pale, as in anemia. The sclera also offers an excellent site for detecting petechiae. Inflammation of the conjunctiva is called conjunctivitis and may be due to mechanical, chemical, allergic, bacterial, or viral factors.

In the complexion of blacks, changes that are hard to detect may be initially observed in the eye. However, the nurse should be aware that many blacks normally have a yellowish discoloration in the subconjunctival fat and sclera which could mislead the nurse into thinking they are jaundiced. In this case the hard palate should also be assessed for color changes.

Examination of the *palpebral conjunctiva* is a difficult skill and is done only if a problem is indicated. This exam involves eversion of the upper lid. The patient is instructed to look down as the examiner grasps the eyelashes between her thumb and index finger and pulls downward and forward. The upper border of the lid is pushed down with a small cotton swab which everts the eyelid (Fig. 5.10). When the lid is everted, the lashes are held to the brow by the

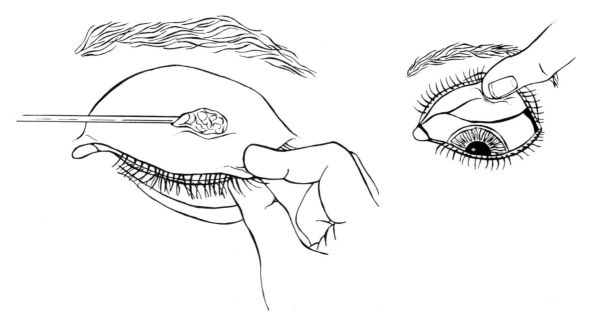

FIGURE 5.10. Examination of the palpebral conjunctiva.

examiner's finger so that the palpebral conjunctiva is visualized. To return the lid to place, the upper eyelashes are grasped and pulled gently forward.

The *cornea* is carefully inspected for abrasions and opacities. Using a penlight, an oblique light is directed onto the surface of the cornea. Normally the cornea is smooth and transparent; irregularities are detected by noting defects appearing in the light reflections of the normal surface. A thin, grayish white ring at the margin of the cornea may be observed. This is called *arcus senilis* and is normal in elderly patients, but should not be seen in young adults.

Corneal sensitivity (cranial nerve V) is tested by touching a wisp of cotton to the cornea and observing the quick closure of the lid. This test is performed by instructing the client to look straight ahead and bringing the cotton in from behind him when he is unaware. If the patient blinks after the cornea is touched, one can assume the fifth cranial nerve is intact.

The anterior chamber is the area immediately behind the cornea and in front of the iris. This chamber is inspected for its depth. At the same time that the cornea is observed with the oblique light, the underlying anterior chamber is examined (Fig. 5.11). Normally no shadows of light will be observed on the iris. Illumination will cast a crescent-shaped shadow on the far side of the iris if it *is* anteriorly displaced. This indicates a shallow anterior chamber and a predisposition to glaucoma.

The *pupils* and the *iris* are assessed together. The pupils are examined for shape, equality, color, accommodation, and reaction to light. The pupils are normally round, equal, and black in color. The health of the iris is determined by noting the regularity of the pupil. *Miosis* is constriction of the pupil which can result from drugs such as morphine or pilocarpine (used in patients with glaucoma) or from inflammation of the iris. Miosis also occurs normally during sleep. *Mydriasis* is enlargement of the pupils, which can be caused

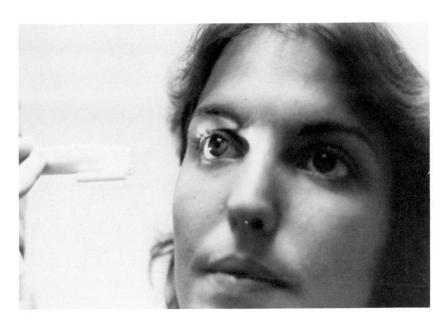

FIGURE 5.11. Examination of the anterior chamber of the eye.

by injury, glaucoma, systemic poison, or dilating drops. Miosis and mydriasis occur normally in accommodation to light changes.

Approximately 5 percent of the population have nonpathologic unequal pupils, or *anisocoria*. The examiner should, however, be aware that this can be a result of various central nervous system disorders. If the pupil appears cloudy or discolored, the probable cause is a cataract.

The *pupilary reflexes* include the *direct reaction to light*, the *consensual reaction to light*, and the *reaction to accommodation*. These reflexes are a test of the function of the third cranial nerve. To test the direct and consensual pupilary reactions, the patient is asked to focus his gaze on the bridge of the examiner's nose. The examiner brings a light in from the side, directing it on the pupil. The pupil receiving increased illumination constricts directly. The opposite eye constricts consensually. In monocular blindness, the blind eye will not react directly to illumination and the opposite eye will not react consensually. If the good eye is illuminated, it will react directly and the blind eye consensually.

To test for accommodation, the examiner holds a penlight about 4 inches from the bridge of the patient's nose. The patient is asked to look alternately at the top of the penlight and at the far wall directly behind the penlight. Then, the examiner brings the penlight in toward the patient's nose. The pupils constrict when looking at the top of the penlight, dilate when looking at the wall, and converge as the penlight is brought towards the nose.

Ophthalmoscopic Examination

That portion of the eye posterior to the lens which is observed through the pupil is called the *fundus* of the eye. The fundus includes the *retina, choroid, fovea, macula, disc,* and *retinal vessels* (Fig. 5.12). These structures are inspected with the use of an ophthalmoscope.

It takes much time and practice to become proficient in observing the fundus. The purpose here is to explain the technique of using the ophthalmoscope and to describe the normal fundus. The

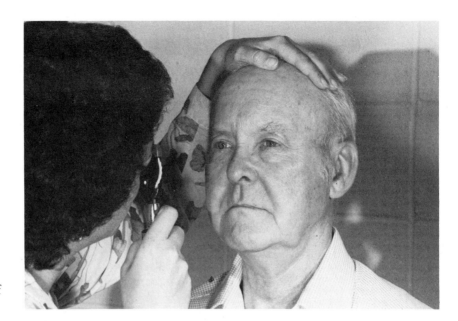

FIGURE 5.12. Examination of the eye with the ophthalmoscope.

*Refer to the directions supplied with the ophthalmoscope for a detailed explanation of the proper use of the dial.

nurse is not expected to identify the specific findings seen in the abnormal eye, but simply to become familiar with normal findings and describe abnormal findings adequately.

To adequately inspect the fundus, the room should be darkened so that the pupils dilate. If the patient is wearing contact lenses, they may be left in. However, it is easier to examine the eye if the patient takes off his glasses. The examiner usually keeps her contacts in and may or may not choose to wear glasses. To prevent the eye from moving around during the examination, the patient is instructed to focus in on a specific point on the wall. The examiner selects the largest round light on the ophthalmoscope. The dial of the ophthalmoscope is set, at +8 to +10 diopters indicated by black numbers.* This will allow visualization of the structures in front of the fundus as the examiner moves in toward the fundus. For clear visualization of the fundus of a farsighted person, the examiner uses the black diopters. However, for the nearsighted person the ophthalmoscope will need to be moved into the minus diopters signified by red numbers.* To examine the patient's left eye, the examiner takes the ophthalmoscope in her left hand and puts it comfortably to her left eye keeping both eyes open while examining the fundus. The examiner should become proficient with both her right and left eye and her right and left hand when examining the eye. The examiner stands approximately 15 inches from the patient and about 15 degrees lateral and shines the light on the patient's pupil. An orange glow is observed in the pupil called the *red reflex*. The color of the normal fundus ranges from orange to vermilion. With darker skin colors, the fundus may be brown or purplish.[8] Any opacities suggest cataracts. As the examiner moves closer to the patient, the dial is moved to successively lower numbers and possibly into the red numbers to focus on the retina. The order of observation in the examination is as follows: the optic disc and cup, the retinal blood vessels, the periphery, and the macula (Fig. 5.2).

The *optic disc* is evaluated for color, shape, size, margins, and its physiologic cup. The disc is a yellowish pink, round structure. Everything within the fundus is measured in terms of disc diameters

(DD). For example, a finding seen in the fundus could be described as 2 DD in size, 2 DD away from the disc at 6 o'clock. The margins of the disc are more or less regular, frequently with scattered pigment overlying the margins (*pigment crescents*). The margins may be surrounded by a white ring called the *scleral crescent.* Occurring more often in blacks than caucasians, both of these are normal findings. Just temporal of the center of the disc, the physiologic depression (or cup) is noted. It may be quite large, but normally it never extends completely to the disc margin.

Three serious problems to look for when examining the disc are *papilledema, optic atrophy,* and *glaucoma. Papilledema* is edema of the optic disc and thickening of the retinal vessels due to increased intracranial pressure. Blurring of the disc margin, observable depression, and a reddened disc are signs of this condition.

Optic atrophy results from death of the optic nerve. With the death of the nerve fibers the tiny disc vessels disappear. This results in paleness of the disc. When there is a question of the presence of optic atrophy, the eyes should be compared. Normally the two discs appear similar. This problem can destroy sight.

Glaucoma results from increased intraocular pressure which almost pushes the optic disc out of the eye. The nurse will observe a retinal vessel which may disappear at the disc edge and then reappear in the depths of the cup. The disc appears pale due to optic atrophy.

In the depths of the disc the central artery and vein will appear. Assessment of the *retinal vessels* is useful with patients who have hypertension, arteriosclerosis, and diabetes. The retinal vessels are examined for size, color, and arteriovenous crossings. Arteries have two-thirds to four-fifths the diameter of veins. A narrow band of light, the arteriolar light reflex, is reflected from the center of the arteries. Normally this light reflex is about one quarter the diameter of the blood column. With hypertension there is a narrowing of the arteriolar blood column and the light reflex. Eventually with hypertension there is a thickening of the vessel wall so that the wall is less transparent. This causes changes of the blood in the vessel, giving it a copper color. Normal veins are darker in color than arteries and do not have a prominent light reflex. Arteries and veins may cross and entwine each other, but normal arteries do not indent or displace veins.

The blood vessels are followed peripherally in each of four directions. The periphery is an orange color, but is lighter in fair people and darker in black people. It is explored for hemorrhages and exudates. Hemorrhages are typically red or dark in color. They are obvious signs of disease. Hemorrhages are described in terms of location, size, shape, relationship to retinal vessels, and color (Fig. 5.13). Exudates are residues of edema and blood substances which are incompletely absorbed due to poor retinal circulation.[9] Cotton wool patches are exudates with a fuzzy outline (Fig. 5.14). Like hemorrhages, exudates are signs of disease. They are described in terms of size, shape, color, and location.

Last of all, the *macular area* is examined. This is the sensitive area of vision, and examination requires focusing the light directly on it. This is uncomfortable for the patient, which discomfort allows only a few seconds of observation. The macula is located approximately 2 DD away from the disc temporally. It is a small circular

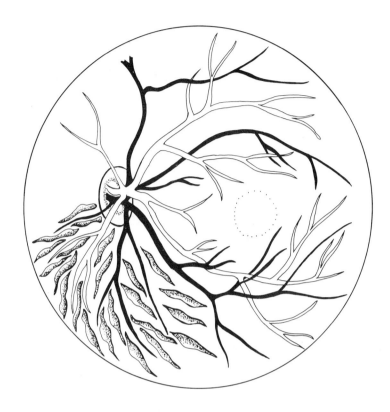

FIGURE 5.13. Linear hemorrhage.

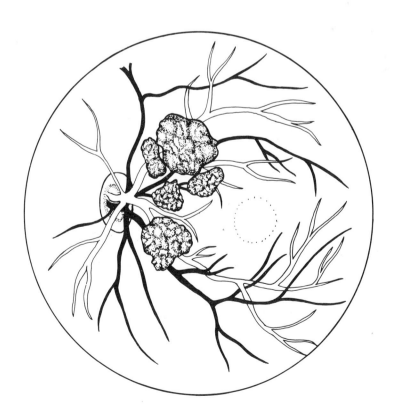

FIGURE 5.14. Cotton wool patch.

structure, 1 DD in size. The minute glistening spot of reflected light seen in the center of the macula is the *fovea centralis*. Macular lesions, including edema, hemorrhages, and exudates, appear much the same as they do throughout the fundus. However, a comparatively small lesion on the macula can seriously interfere with vision. A large peripheral lesion may cause no disturbance to the patient.

REFERENCES

1. Office Ophthalmology. *Patient care*, June 15, 1979, p. 53.
2. Alexander, M., & Brown, M., *Pediatric history taking and physical diagnosis for nurses.* New York: McGraw-Hill, 1979.
3. Hughes, J.G. *Synopsis of pediatrics.* St. Louis: Mosby, 1975, p. 965.
4. Hughes, J.G. *Synopsis of pediatrics.* St. Louis: Mosby, 1975, p. 973.
5. Ing, M. & Pang, S. *The racial distribution of strabismus.* Hawaii Medical Journal, 1973, pp. 22–3.
6. Alexander, M. & Brown, M. *Pediatric history taking and physical diagnosis for nurses.* New York: McGraw-Hill, 1979.
7. Roach, L. Color changes in dark skins. *Nursing, 2,* 1972, 19–22.
8. Wasserman, H. *Ethnic pigmentation: Historical, physiological, and clinical aspects.* Amsterdam: Excerpta Medica, 1974.

EXAMPLE OF A RECORDED HISTORY AND PHYSICAL

SUBJECTIVE:
   Chief Complaint (Reason for Visit): "Tearing from the right eye began yesterday."

   HPI: This 9-month-old white female has been seen regularly for well baby examinations and has been without problems. Yesterday the child's mother noticed that she was rubbing her right eye. Her mother attributed this to the fact that the child had just awakened from a short nap. This morning, when the child awoke, the eye was matted together with a "green, crusty" substance. Her mother cleaned it with clear water and then noticed that the eye was reddened and tearing. The left eye has been clear. The child has had no fever, lethargy, apparent light sensitivity, irritability, runny nose, cough, or exposure to irritants. No one else in the family is experiencing these symptoms. Her father has a history of allergy to ragweed and cats. She has no known allergies.

OBJECTIVE: T. 99.2°F rectally.
   Eyes
   Lids: Right—clear, tearing, green crusting on lower lid; no edema; left—no tearing, crustation, or edema.
   Conjunctiva: Right—erythematous; left—no erythema.
   Cornea: No clouding, enlargement, or irritation, bilaterally.
   Sclera: White, bilaterally.
   Pupil: Pupils equally round and react to light (PERRLA), bilaterally.

Alignment: Light reflex equal, bilaterally.

Iris: Brown, round, bilaterally.

Lens: No clouding, bilaterally.

Lacrimal apparatus: No discharge from the inner canthus, no swelling of the lacrimal glands, bilaterally.

Funduscopic examination: Red light reflex present, bilaterally.

Ears: Canals clear; tympanic membranes pearly gray, landmarks present, bilaterally.

Oral Cavity: Tonsils not enlarged, pharynx without redness or exudate.

Chest: No adventitious breath sounds.

6

The Ear

The ear is one of the few organs of the body that can be evaluated rather simply. An accurate assessment of the ear is crucial at any age because an oversight of any abnormality may cause lifelong damage. In general, ear dysfunction has one of four origins: an acute illness, a mechanical problem, a neurologic disorder, or a traumatic injury.

Acute ear problems occur most commonly in children. Although adults can acquire the same types of infections or viruses, youths are much more frequently bothered. The most typical acute ear problems are blockage of the eustachian tubes (serous otitis), middle ear infections (otitis media), and inflammation of the external canal (otitis externa). Further descriptions of these problems can be found at the end of the chapter.

Mechanical dysfunctions have relatively simple explanations. A build-up of cerumen (ear wax) is the most common mechanical problem. This causes an obstruction in the external canal which results in a hearing loss. Such extra growths as tumors, chondromas, and exostoses (the latter two are boney nodules in the canal) can occur, but are less likely and not generally obstructive.

Neurologic disorders will cause some degree of hearing loss. They may be congenital, acquired, or inherited. Congenital hearing losses are often found in children who were exposed to rubella in utero, especially in the earlier months of pregnancy. Babies who are small, premature, and have congenital kidney disease or liver dysfunction run a greater chance of having hearing problems. Acquired hearing losses can come from such diseases as mumps and meningitis and from severe adverse reactions to the administration of drugs—i.e., streptomycin, kanamycin, and gentamycin. Although most inherited hearing problems do not manifest themselves until adulthood, it is important to elicit a good family history as early as possible. If accurate information is given to the provider, earlier intervention can take place and may ultimately prevent severe damage. It should be remembered that some hearing loss may be part of the normal aging process and cannot be prevented.

Traumatic injury to the ear is most likely to occur in children and adolescents. Children are notorious for inserting unusual objects in their ears. Some foreign bodies can be very destructive, so prompt removal is necessary. Teenagers who are active in contact sports need to be especially protective of their ears. The components of the external ear are relatively close to the surface and can be permanently damaged by a traumatic blow. Another source of traumatic stress to the eardrum involves occupational hazards, such as exposure to loud noises. Men and women exposed to constant loud machine noises have a high potential for hearing loss. Similar damage can be done by frequent, close exposure to loud music.

THE HISTORY

There are two perspectives to explore in the review of this system: present complaints and past problems. In terms of present concerns, the patient should be asked if he has any ear pain, itching, discharge, tinnitus (ringing in the ears), or change in hearing ability. Investigation of past problems includes a history of ear infections, excess cerumen, or a hearing loss at any time. It is also important to ask about any family history of hearing losses.

If the patient states he has ear pain, the examiner should try to determine its location and quality. Does the pain feel close to the surface or is it deeper in the head? Can the patient elicit the pain by pushing on his ear? Is the pain sharp and stabbing or nagging and aching? Does it stay in one place? Does it come and go, or is the pain always present? Does changing the position of the head make it worse or better? What has been done so far? Has the pain ever occurred before? What was done for it then? Was the problem resolved with the treatment (medication) administered? Were there any symptoms, such as a cold or sore throat, preceding the ear pain? Did any trauma occur?

If itching is a complaint, the patient should be asked where he feels the sensation. It is also helpful to find out about the patient's showering practices and frequency of swimming. Some people who get water in their ears when showering or who swim on a regular basis may acquire local irritation in the ear canal. For the same reason, the method of maintaining ear hygiene may irritate the canal. Excessive or inappropriate use of "Q-Tips" may cause skin breakdown, which can cause itching. The nurse should inquire as to whether this has been a problem in the past, what was done for it, and whether the problem was resolved. The etiology of this symptom can also be infectious, so asking the patient if he knows anyone with similar symptoms may provide useful information.

When discharge is the complaint, it is necessary to find out what the substance is. Blood will be a pink or red color. Pus is usually white, yellow, or green. The amount of discharge and the existence of any odor is important to note. Pain and discharge will often accompany one another. In the case of discharge leaking from behind the tympanic membrane, the classic story includes a description of severe pain which stopped suddenly after a popping sensation. This was followed by awareness of discharge on the pillow. (In such a case, the tympanic membrane has ruptured.)

If a patient has ringing in the ears, a key area to investigate is aspirin ingestion. Many times a sign of high serum salicylate levels will be tinnitus. A careful investigation of onset, frequency, associated phenomena, medication history (and amount), recent activities (sports, air travel, etc.), and allergy history may shed some light on the cause.

A decrease in hearing can be very disconcerting. The problem usually has an insidious onset. The etiology is probably mechanical or neurologic. Mechanical problems are usually attributed to an ear-wax build-up and can be resolved easily. The neurologic loss is much more complicated and is often not correctable; thus any information elicited can be helpful. The nurse should inquire about the type of hearing loss (low-pitched or high-pitched sounds), how long it has been going on, the history of noise exposure (certain occupations are especially hazardous in this way—musicians, construction workers, and policemen are at increased risk), and a family history of the same.

As concerns past problems, if frequent ear infections are mentioned, further investigation is needed. How often does the patient consider "frequent" to be? Who diagnosed the problem? How was the patient treated? Some people have had their tonsils removed or have had ear tubes inserted to help combat ear infections. If either of these procedures were implemented, the nurse should find out if that ended the problem. Sometimes these turn out to be temporary solutions. The nurse should also inquire as to whether or not there was any permanent hearing loss due to the repeated infections.

If excess earwax has been a long-term concern, the patient should be questioned about what he has done about the problem and how often the treatment is necessary. Some people put mineral oil in their ears (or a similar oil-based solution) and then have them irrigated periodically. Others just wait until they notice a hearing loss and then seek treatment. Many patients have a sensation of decreased hearing when they have an upper respiratory infection. Therefore, differentiating between the causes is a necessary part of the history.

When a patient states that there is a family history of hearing dysfunction, exact information regarding who it was that had the problem and when in his or her life the problem occurred is helpful. If there is any known reason for the problem, such as repeated ear infections or trauma, then that should be investigated as well. The patient may know of the treatment that was used (e.g., a hearing aid) and the success or failure of the treatment. Such data are worthy of recording in the permanent record.

Finally, the patient should be asked if he has ever had a hearing test, when the last one was, and what the results were. All of this information can help the nurse anticipate what she might find objectively as she continues the assessment of the ear.

ANATOMY

The ear is a sensory organ which is divided up into three parts: the *external ear*, the *middle ear*, and the *inner ear*.

The external ear includes the *auricle* (pinna) and the external canal (Fig. 6.1). The auricle is a cartilaginous material. The combination of the elastic cartilage and the skin covering the auricle gives it a firm but pliable consistency. There are landmarks to note on the pinna (Fig. 6.2). The *helix* and *antihelix* make up the most obvious curves on the superior aspect. The *tragus* is the protruding feature at the entrance of the external canal. This curved canal, which ends abruptly at the *tympanic membrane*, is about 2.5 cm (1 inch) long (Fig. 6.1). In an adult the outer portion of the canal is cartilaginous and the more inferior section is boney. In young children the canal

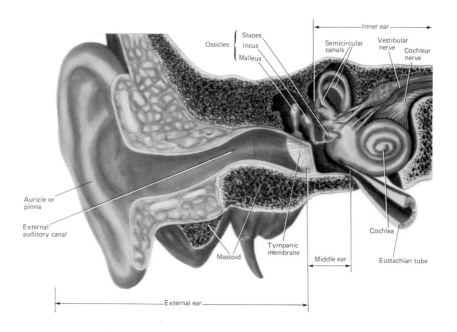

FIGURE 6.1. Structures of the ear. (From Heagarty, M., Glass, G., King, H., & Manly, M. *Child health: Basics for primary care.* New York: Appleton–Century–Crofts, 1980, p. 128)

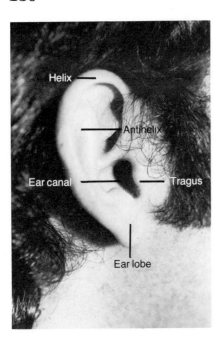

FIGURE 6.2. Landmarks of the external ear.

is totally cartilaginous, as bone formation of the nature found in adults has not taken place yet. The skin covering the length of the canal has fine hairs and many glands and nerve endings. The fine hairs are more visible on some people than on others. In fact, in many they cannot be seen at all. These hairs may provide some degree of protection and keep out some foreign substances, but their physiologic function is minimal. The glands are wax producing and secrete cerumen (earwax). This wax is a lubricative and protective substance produced in varying amounts, depending on the individual. Cerumen is classified as wet (sticky) or dry (flaky). Wet earwax, generally found in Caucasian and black clients, is tan or brown. Dry earwax, common among clients of Asian or American Indian descent, is colored a light to brown gray.[1]

The confirmation of the existence of several nerve endings is most easily made during the otoscopic exam. When the nerve endings are stimulated, they cause a painful sensation. This is especially apparent in children. Therefore, extreme caution must be taken while examining the ear (see discussion in Physical Assessment section). The *mastoid process* is not exactly part of the external ear, but it is an important landmark. It is the boney prominence behind the ear (Fig. 6.2).

The middle ear is an air-filled cavity which begins at the *tympanic membrane.* This membrane is a circular, pearly gray, opaque membrane which lies at an angle (Fig. 6.3). The superior aspect is more anterior than the lower rim of the drum. There are several visible landmarks to note on the eardrum. The *cone of light* is a triangularly shaped reflection that lies diagonally at about 5 o'clock in the right ear and 7 o'clock in the left. At the inferior end of the cone of light lies the *malleus.* This is one of the bones of the *ossicles* (see discussion of the ossicles below) and is embedded in the tympanic membrane. There are three portions of this bone that can be seen: the *umbo,* which appears attached to the cone of light; the *handle of the malleus,* which extends to the superior aspect of the tympanic membrane; and the *short process,* which looks like a small circle at the end of the handle. The taut folds which surround the malleus and the cone of light are the *pars tensa* (Fig. 6.3). Along the attic of the eardrum lies another section of taut membrane called the *pars flaccida* (Fig. 6.3).

There are three ossicles in the middle ear: the *malleus,* the *incus,* and the *stapes* (Fig. 6.3). These are the bones of sound transmission. The malleus is the most easily seen of the three. Less frequently, the others can also be viewed; however, the incus is more accessible to inspection than the stapes.

The *eustachian tube* is another portion of the middle ear (Fig. 6.1). It connects the middle ear cavity to the nasopharynx. The tube functions as an air pressure stabilizer between the external atmosphere and the internal air pressure. The eustachian tube does not function as well in children as in adults. As the child gets older, the tube assumes a more mature form and function. It is believed that, for this reason, ear infections decrease as the child matures.

The inner ear houses the end organ receptors of hearing and balance. The *cochlea* is a structure shaped like a seashell that is essential to the transmission of sound (Fig. 6.1). The *vestibule* and *semicircular canals* are the receptors for equilibrium. The inner ear is inaccessible to examination by inspection. One can evaluate the function of the inner ear with specific hearing and balance testing.

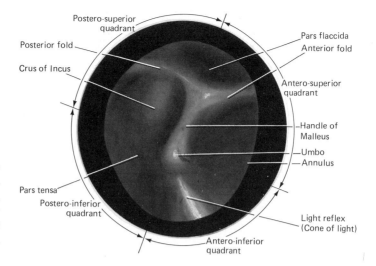

FIGURE 6.3. Tympanic membrane as seen with the otoscope. (From Heagarty, M., Glass, G., King, H., & Manly, M. *Child health: Basics for primary care.* New York: Appleton-Century-Crofts, 1980, p. 129)

Physiology of Hearing

A detailed discussion of the physiology of hearing goes beyond the scope of this book. However, a brief review is necessary to understand the physical assessment of the ear.

There are two basic methods of sound transmission: air conduction and bone conduction. In air conduction a sound is heard when:

1. A stimulus is sent to the external canal.
2. That stimulus reaches the tympanic membrane.
3. Most of the sound waves then cross the tympanic membrane to the ossicles.
4. The sound travels from the ossicles to the oval window (the opening to the inner ear).
5. The cochlea, which contain the organ of Corti (the organ of hearing), pick up the vibrations.
6. The stimulus then travels to the auditory nerve in the auditory cortex (the eighth cranial nerve).

In bone conduction, the vibrations are transferred to the auditory cortex via bone. In this method, the skull bones carry the sound directly to the eighth cranial nerve.

PHYSICAL ASSESSMENT

Inspection and palpatation are the techniques of examination used for the ear. Auditory acuity is also evaluated during this portion of the exam.

The examination begins with inspection of the auricles for placement and symmetry, lesions, skin abnormalities, and discharge. The auricles should be level with one another. Where the superior aspect of the pinna attaches to the head, there should be a straight line from the lateral canthus of the eye. Low-set ears may indicate chromosomal abnormalities (mongolism) or renal disease. Typical lesions that appear on the pinna are sebaceous cysts, moles, and tophi (subcutaneous deposits of uric acid on the ear). The cysts may enlarge periodically and will disappear without treatment. Moles may occur around the ear rather than on it, but in any case are observed for change in color, size, or shape. The most likely skin abnormality to occur on or behind the external ear is seborrhea. The skin appears to be flaky and scaling. This is usually seen behind the ear or in the area of the *concha* (Fig. 6.2).

Palpation of the external ear precedes inspection with the otoscope. Any tenderness and inflammation can be detected by pulling slightly on the auricle in an up, down, and backward motion; by pushing on the tragus; and by applying slight pressure to the mastoid process.

Inspection of the remaining parts of the ear requires the use of the otoscope. However, because of the sensitivity of the external canal, young children find this exam unpleasant. For this reason, it is recommended to postpone the otoscopic exam until the end of the child's physical.

In beginning the otoscopic exam there are a few helpful points to keep in mind. First, the head of the patient is always tipped slightly away from the examiner. Second, the auricle is pulled in a specific direction, depending on the age of the patient, so that the auditory canal straightens out. In a young child the shape of the canal is such that it is straightened by pulling the auricle down. In an adult, the pinna is pulled up and back (Fig. 6.4). Both these

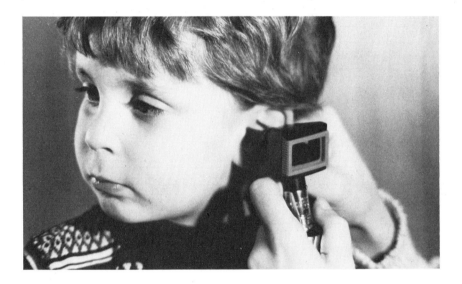

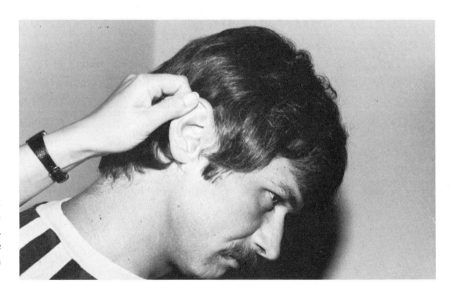

FIGURE 6.4 Top. Pulling down on the auricle to straighten the external canal in the child. **Bottom.** Pulling up and back on the auricle to straighten the external canal in the adult.

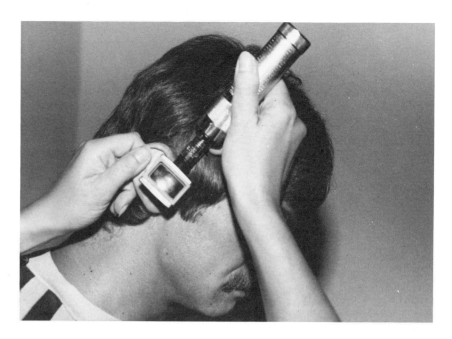

FIGURE 6.5. Alternate method of holding the otoscope.

techniques facilitate the visualization of the tympanic membrane. The third point relates to the size of the speculum tip. The largest tip that will fit in the ear without causing discomfort should be used. This helps to assure the examiner maximum visualization of the tympanic membrane.

Now that the patient's head is tipped away from the examiner and the auricle is pulled in the appropriate direction, the otoscope is gently inserted into the ear canal. There are two methods for holding the otoscope. Figure 6.5 shows the instrument held upside down with the examiner's finger between the patient's head and the instrument. This is helpful with squirmy children, as they are not bumped with the otoscope. (Figures 6.6 and 6.7 show suggestions for gaining children's trust for using the otoscope)

The canal is inspected for cerumen, foreign bodies, inflammation, redness, scaling, exostoses, and other lesions. At the end of the canal the eardrum is spotted and its landmarks are identified. The most obvious feature is the cone of light. The umbo, the handle of the malleus, and the short process can be viewed as an extension of the cone of light. The pars tensa and pars flaccida are checked for position, lesions, bulging, and retraction. All 360° of the anulus are inspected carefully. The otoscope and the examiner's body will have to be moved slightly to see all these features. The position, color, and gloss of the eardrum are noted in addition to any lesions or unusual markings. The otoscopic exam is not complete until all the landmarks are seen. If cerumen is in the way and there is no way to see around it, then it must be removed before any final assessment can be made. Generally, wet (sticky) earwax is best removed with a curette; dry (flaky) earwax is best removed by irrigation with lukewarm water.

Auditory Acuity

This portion of the physical examination begins when the patient and the interviewer begin talking. If the patient has difficulty hearing the examiner's voice, then an obvious hearing loss exists. However, there are more specific hearing tests available to confirm

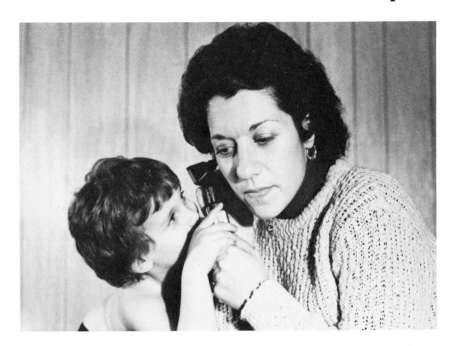

FIGURE 6.6. Helping the child become familiar with the otoscope.

any suspicion of a hearing loss or to establish normal hearing patterns.

Gross hearing is tested first. This is done by simply whispering numbers to the patient while standing at his side. One ear is tested at a time. The patient is instructed to place a finger in one ear. While standing 1 or 2 feet away, the examiner whispers three numbers. Nonconsecutive numbers should be whispered so that the patient will not anticipate which number will follow. It is also important to be certain that the examiner's lips cannot be read while reciting the numbers. Another method of testing gross hearing is to ask the patient to listen to a ticking watch. The watch is held about 3 inches away from the patient's ear. The patient then says whether or not he can hear it. The sound is higher pitched than that of the human voice.

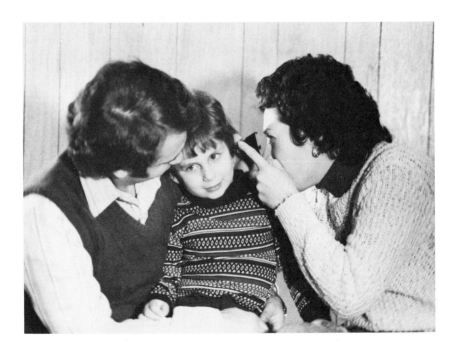

FIGURE 6.7. Gaining trust by examining the child on the parent's lap.

Assessing the conduction of sound through air and bone comprise the next set of hearing tests. Air conduction is the process by which sound reaches the acoustic nerve as it travels through the canal and the middle ear to the inner ear. In bone conduction, the vibrations are carried via the skull or mastoid process to the eighth cranial nerve. Air conduction is more sensitive than bone conduction. A tuning fork (either 256 cycles, 512 cycles, or 1024 cycles per second) is needed to evaluate air and bone conduction.

The Weber Test

The Weber test assesses bone conduction by testing the lateralization of sounds. The tuning fork will vibrate when the examiner taps it against his hand while holding onto it at the base. The vibrating fork is then placed on the top of the patient's head (Fig. 6.8). The patient is then asked where he hears the noise. With normal hearing the sound will be heard in both ears or localized in the center of the head. If there is a conductive hearing loss, the sound will be heard better in the poor or damaged ear. A conductive loss represents an inability of the vibration to reach the inner ear. This can be due to an obstruction of the ossicles. This type of loss can be imitated by putting a finger in one ear and then speaking. The voice will be louder in the ear with the finger inserted in it. The finger represents a conductive disturbance. Obstruction in the ear canal will obliterate room noise, thus increasing bone sensitivity. When a sensorineural hearing loss exists, there is damage either to the eighth cranial nerve or to the inner ear. In a sensorineural disturbance the Weber will lateralize to the ear without a problem. The ear without any nerve or inner ear damage will always hear better.

The Rinné Test

The Rinné test compares air conduction to bone conduction. It should be remembered that air conduction is more sensitive. In other words, sound vibrations will last longer via air conduction, if there is no disturbance. To perform this test, the vibrating tuning

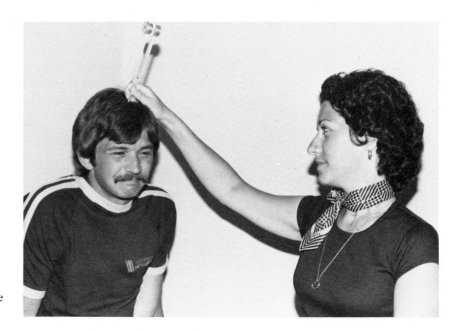

FIGURE 6.8. Performing the Weber test.

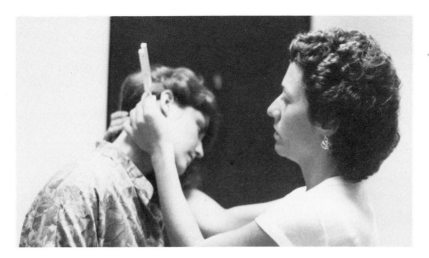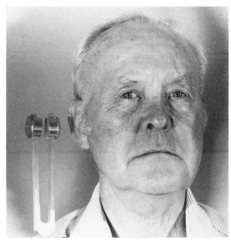

FIGURE 6.9. Performing the Rinné test.

fork is placed on the mastoid process of one ear (Fig. 6.9). The patient is asked to say when he can no longer hear the vibrations. The fork, which is still vibrating, is then placed in front of the ear canal. If necessary, the nurse should push the patient's hair away. The patient is asked once again to say when he can no longer hear the sound. The sound will disappear eventually, although it will take about twice as long to go away as when the fork was on the mastoid process. The same procedure is repeated with the other ear. If air conduction time is longer than bone conduction time (AC > BC), which is normal, the test is considered positive. This is one of the few tests in our classification of terms for which "positive" is the desired result (Chart 6.1).

In the Rinné test a conductive loss will reveal a bone conduction time equal to or longer than air conduction time. In the case of sensorineural disturbance, air conduction time will be greater than bone conduction time because in the damaged ear the nerve will pick up air vibrations more readily than bone vibrations.

Of course, the most precise test is that which measures hearing at various decibels. This testing is called audiometry and can be done without much difficulty with the appropriate equipment. Many ambulatory care facilities and primary care offices have the necessary machine available. The testing should be done annually. If children have it performed in school, there is no need to repeat it. For adults, annual testing can detect early signs of a hearing loss. If treatment can be initiated to prevent further loss, then the sooner intervention takes place, the better. For the geriatric population

CHART 6.1

Tuning Fork Tests for Normal Hearing, Conductive Hearing Loss, and Sensorineural Hearing Loss

	Weber (Bone Only)	Rinné (Air-Bone)
Normal	Not lateralized	Positive AC > BC
Conductive loss	Lateralized to poorer ear	Negative BC ≥ AC
Sensorineural loss	Lateralized to better ear	Positive AC > BC

From DeWeese, D. D., and Saunders, W. H. *Textbook of otolaryngology* (4th ed.). St. Louis: Mosby, 1973, p. 305.

audiometry is essential. Most hearing losses in the elderly are due to sensorineural deterioration. The ability to hear high frequencies is the first to diminish. Lower frequency hearing remains intact longer. The only test refined enough to detect these changes is audiometry.

Abnormal Findings in the Ear

The external ear canal is a place in which localized infections or traumatic injury may occur. Disorders in this region are referred to as *external otitis*. Symptoms of infectious process in this region usually indicate a viral or occasionally a bacterial etiology. The chief complaint is often itching or pain. The objective findings may include pain while pushing on the tragus or palpating the auricle. The external canal may be erythematous and inflamed. There may also be flaking of the skin.

In traumatic injuries, which usually occur from overzealous hygiene practices or a foreign body lodged in the canal, the chief symptom is likely to be sudden pain in this area. The otoscopic exam will reveal redness, edema, bleeding, or the foreign body itself.

Any infectious process of the middle ear is called *otitis media*. The two most common forms of otitis media are *acute* and *serous*.

Acute otitis media usually begins with redness on the ear drum or hyperemia of the blood vessels. The next phase may be retraction of the landmarks. Retraction is the result of absorption of air in the Eustachian tubes, changing the appearance of the tympanic membrane. This shortens the malleus and the short process and accentuates the pars tensa and pars flaccida. The cone of light will bend. In the most infectious stages of this condition, the tympanic membrane will bulge forward and be vividly reddened. The landmarks will be obliterated. This occurs commonly in children and is extremely painful. If the pressure behind the eardrum is too great, a perforation can occur. Perforations usually happen along the peripheral margins. The pain disappears immediately. The appearance of a minuscule hairline will be evident at the site of perforation. Pus or blood may be seen in the canal. Because of the advances of antibiotic therapy, perforations occur much less frequently today. Appropriate intervention usually takes place prior to this occurrence. It is therefore obvious that any reddened ear warrants immediate attention.

If a clear, sterile substance builds up behind the tympanic membrane as a result of a blockage in the Eustachian tube, a condition called *serous otitis* exists. The fluid appears amber in color and one can sometimes see a fluid line or bubbles behind the transparent ear drum. This condition usually occurs along with an otitis media or an upper respiratory condition. Patients commonly complain of "voices sounding like my head is in a bucket" or "ear-popping." There is much debate over the method to be used for treatment.

REFERENCE

1. Matsunaga, E. The dimorphism in human normal cerumen. *Annals of Human Genetics*, 1962, *25*, 273–286.

BIBLIOGRAPHY

DeWeese, D., & Saunders, W. *Textbook of otolaryngology* (4th ed.). St. Louis: Mosby, 1973.

EXAMPLE OF A RECORDED HISTORY AND PHYSICAL

SUBJECTIVE:

Chief Complaint: "I've had ringing in my ears for 1 month."

HPI: This 35-year-old male considers himself in "fair health," but has never had any problems with his ears prior to 1 month ago, when the "ringing in both ears" began. The high-pitched noise is constant "from morning until night," but seems more intense after riding the subway to and from work.

There is no discharge, dizziness, blurry vision, headache, pain, known hearing loss, history of excess earwax, or recent cold, fever, allergies or other acute illness. There is no prior history of this or of any family members with the same problem. Patient has taken no medications or applied any home remedies to relieve the problem.

Patient works in factory, where he has worked for 7 years. The noise level is considered safe by OSHA, although he states some people wear ear plugs anyhow. Patient takes aspirin (10 gr) about three times a week for "my joint stiffness." He does not consider this problem disabling, just a "nuisance."

OBJECTIVE: T. 98.8°F orally; P. 86 radial; R. 20; B.P. (sitting) (R) 116/72, (L) 120/78.

Left Ear: No lesions, discharge, scaling, or tenderness of external ear. No cerumen or other substances in canal. Tympanic membrane: Light reflex bright and not diffuse. No redness, bulging, or retraction. A white rim appears around anulus. Landmarks visible.

Right Ear: 0.5 cm flesh-colored, nontender nodule on helix. No discharge. No other lesions, scaling, discharge, or tenderness of external ear. Moderate amount of brown cerumen in canal. Tympanic membrane: Light reflex bright and not diffuse. No redness, bulging, retraction, or scarring. Landmarks are visible.

Rinné: BC > AC bilaterally.

Weber: Lateralization of vibrations to (R) ear.

Gross Hearing: Unremarkable. Can repeat whispered numbers and hear watch tick from 4″ away.

7

The Nasopharynx

The nasopharyngeal region includes the oral cavity, the nose, and sinuses. For the purpose of simplifying the assessment of these regions, they are divided into two sections: (1) the mouth and throat and (2) the nose and sinuses.

THE MOUTH AND THROAT

The oral cavity has many functions. It has a sensory division, which is responsible for gustatory and pain responses, and a motor component, which provides the ability to talk, chew, swallow, and gag. From a review of these features it is easy to see that the mouth can harbor various problems. Some are simple, acute, and easy to provide care for, such as a sore throat or a broken tooth. Other problems, such as a lesion discovered under the tongue or on the gum, may be life-threatening.

A good percentage of the less severe problems can be controlled if preventive care is obtained and practiced. The semiannual or annual visit to the dentist may serve as one of the best available modes of prevention. Practicing thorough oral hygiene will help to keep dental expenses at a minimum. The teaching of oral hygiene methods is an excellent area for nursing intervention. Although detailed checking for caries (cavities) is beyond the scope of nursing expertise, observing for more evident deformities or lesions and evaluating the hygiene practices of our patients are both certainly appropriate.

Sharp observation skills, a bright light, and a tongue depressor comprise the basic equipment necessary for this exam. On occasion a glove or finger cot will be needed to palpate a lump or abnormality.

After a thorough review of this system and a look at the anatomic structures of the oral cavity, the physical examination can begin.

History

The subjective review of this system includes questions on anything from the ability to taste, talk, and swallow to the existence of pain.

Just asking a patient if he has pain in his mouth is too general. Taking a more specific direction will provide more information. The patient should be asked whether he has pain in his teeth, gums, throat, or tongue. As always, if any of these answers are positive, a thorough history using the eight areas of investigation is necessary.

Specific health-oriented questions that involve the oral cavity should be asked, including questions on the date of the last dental exam, the general condition of the teeth, the presence of caries, and the types and frequency of hygiene measures used (i.e., brushing, flossing, use of a water pick). In addition, certain problems are common to the oral cavity and their existence or nonexistence should be reviewed. These include soreness, bleeding, or ulcerations of the lips, tongue, or gums; halitosis or fruity-smelling breath; hoarseness; a change in the ability to taste; and any recent extractions and the reasons for them.

If ulcerations or a history of them exists, then further data are needed:

1. Where are the ulcers (usually) located?
2. How often do they appear?

3. When they occur, is there any association to colds, viruses, stress, or time of the year?
4. What treatment is used and how successful is it?

A complaint of *frequent* sore throats may arise during the interview. A precise history of what the patient means by this will give the nurse a better picture. The patient needs to be definite in terms of the number of sore throats that occur in a year's time. The definition of frequency will vary among individuals. Once a common understanding of this word is established, several other questions should follow:

1. Describe the throat pain. Where is the pain? What does it feel like? Is there difficulty with swallowing?
2. Is care usually sought for the problem? Is a throat culture usually obtained? What is the usual diagnosis (i.e., strep vs. viral)?
3. What is the treatment prescribed? Are antibiotics given? If so, what kind? How long are they taken? Do they help?
4. Does the "sore throat" happen in one season more than another? Does it seem worse upon arising? What is the humidity in the room where the patient sleeps? Is there an allergy history? Does the patient smoke? Is occupation or the working environment related?

Anatomy

The *lips* begin the region known as the oral cavity (Fig. 7.1). The portion called the *posterior pharynx* terminates the area. The *buccal mucosa* lines the inside of the mouth along the lateral walls. This mucosa extends from the floor to the roof of the mouth. The roof of the mouth consists of the *hard and soft palate*. The hard palate is the bony structure directly above the tongue. The soft palate begins slightly anterior to the *uvula*. This is the short, elongated, pink, finger-like projection attached to the soft palate medially on the *anterior pharynx*.

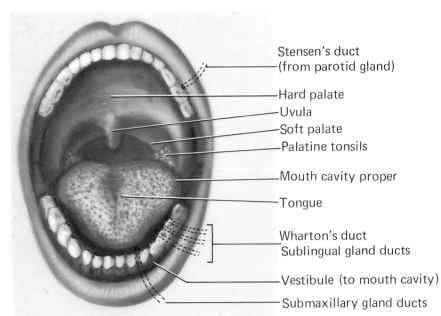

FIGURE 7.1. The oral cavity. (From Heagarty, M., Glass, G., King, H., and Manly, M. *Child health: Basics for primary care.* New York: Appleton–Century–Crofts, 1980, p. 129)

Stensen's duct (from parotid gland)
Hard palate
Uvula
Soft palate
Palatine tonsils
Mouth cavity proper
Tongue
Wharton's duct
Sublingual gland ducts
Vestibule (to mouth cavity)
Submaxillary gland ducts

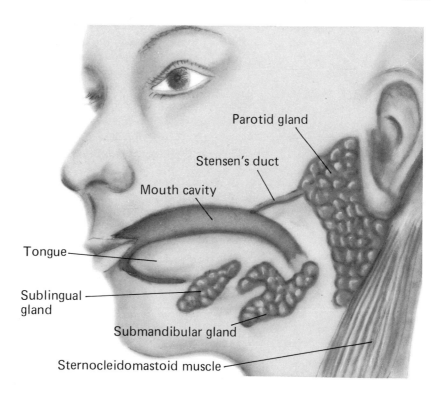

Parotid gland

Stensen's duct

Mouth cavity

Tongue

Sublingual gland

Submandibular gland

Sternocleidomastoid muscle

FIGURE 7.2. Position of the salivary glands. (From Heagarty, M., Glass, G., King, H., and Manly, M. *Child health: Basics for primary care.* New York: Appleton–Century–Crofts, 1980, p. 129)

The *tongue* is a mass of muscles. *Papillae* (tastebuds) located on the tongue's surface are divided into salt, sweet, bitter, and sour. The tongue is attached to the floor of the mouth by the *frenulum.* Under the tongue lies one of two pairs of salivary ducts that are visible in the mouth. These are called the *submaxillary ducts* (Wharton's ducts). The other salivary ducts that open into the mouth are opposite the second molar along each maxilla (Fig. 7.2). These are the *parotid ducts* (Stenson's ducts). These ducts are the endpoints of the salivary glands: the parotid and the submaxillary glands. Altogether there are three pairs of salivary glands in the oral cavity. The last one is called the *sublingual,* and its ducts are inaccessible to examination.

The amount and classification of teeth varies among different age groups. All teeth erupt from the *gingiva.* Although the first teeth, the *deciduous teeth,* do not erupt until 5 to 6 months of age, they form during the sixth week of fetal life. There are 20 deciduous teeth; the first to appear are usually the lower incisors. The last to erupt are the deciduous molars, and these should be in by 2½ years of age.

The *permanent teeth* form during the sixth month of fetal life and do not appear until 6 or 7 years of age. The third molars, or *wisdom teeth,* are the last of the permanent teeth to emerge, making their appearance in most at the age of 17 or 18 years. These teeth are notorious for becoming impacted or coming in crooked, and eventually may require extraction.

Many population differences in dentition have been documented. Gross tooth size of incisors, canines, premolars, and molars varies widely from group to group. Some groups have larger anterior teeth, others have larger posterior teeth. Tooth morphology also differs. For example, the rear surfaces of the incisors of many American Indian and Asian populations are "shovel-shaped." Finally, the number of teeth occurring in any individual is also a population variable. Some people from the Pacific have an entire extra set of molars; American Indians and Asians often have a congenital absence of the third molars.

The posterior section of the mouth begins at the soft palate and uvula. Together these form the anterior pharynx (Fig. 7.1). The arch-like sides that extend to the tongue from the soft palate are called the *anterior pillars*. The *tonsils* and *posterior pillars* comprise the *posterior pharynx*. The portion of the pharynx described above is known as the *oropharynx*.

Physical Assessment

Inspection is the primary method of examination used for the oral cavity. Any abnormal findings in the anterior portion of the mouth can be palpated, too. The patient who wears dentures is asked to remove them so that the gums can be inspected thoroughly. This is also true for people who wear partial plates.

The correct approach in examining the oral cavity is to start with the outer features and move to the inner aspects: the *lips* to the *posterior pharynx*. The following structures are examined in the oral cavity:

1. Lips.
2. Teeth.
3. Gingivae.
4. Tongue.
5. Buccal mucosa.
6. Hard palate.
7. Anterior pillars.
8. Uvula.
9. Tonsils.
10. Posterior pillars.

The lips are inspected for position, color, symmetry, moisture, and lesions (ulcerations or fissures). The most common abnormal findings involve color, texture, and lesions. The normal red color of the lips is likely to change if the patient is anemic, short of breath, or very chilled. Decreased hemoglobin concentration in the blood may cause pallor of the lips. The bluish lip color that is seen on someone who is cold or dyspneic is referred to as *cyanotic*. Because the lips of some black individuals normally have a bluish hue, it is important to know the patient's baseline lip color if this site is to be used in detecting cyanosis.

In the winter months lips may get chapped due to the cold air or wind. This is aggravated by frequent licking of the lips. The lips become dry and rough and the skin thus appears to be peeling or cracking.

Ulcerations on the lips are often due to a herpes virus (see Chart 3.3). This relatively painful and annoying lesion will appear as a small vesicle on the edge of the lip. It will ooze and eventually form a crust. Another typical lesion of the lips occurs at the junction of the upper and lower lips. Drying and chapping of this area causes this and a small fissure results. Such painful lesions are more common in the winter months. Malignant lesions of the oral cavity may also occur on the lips. In malignancy, the history often reveals years of smoking a pipe or cigars. Those who do not smoke are not necessarily immune to this type of cancer, although its incidence is proportionately higher among such smokers.

The teeth are checked for their state of repair, obvious caries, displacement, color, position, and extraction sites. In children it is important to check the deciduous teeth as they are erupting and to note the order in which they are coming in. It is also important to note when these teeth begin to fall out and to make sure that the permanent teeth appear shortly thereafter.

The importance of good oral hygiene cannot be overemphasized. The earlier a child learns to care for his teeth, the better. Toddlers love to imitate adults and setting a good example is certainly a good way to get them started. If a child sees his parent or sibling practicing good hygiene techniques, then he is likely to do the same. At any age, it is important to reinforce and teach patients about oral hygiene.

The gingivae are examined for color, edema, retraction, bleeding, and lesions. Healthy gums have a pink, moist, and smooth appearance. There is no edema or pulling away of the gums from the teeth (retraction). When the gingivae become red and edematous and the patient states that they bleed easily and feel irritated, *gingivitis* may exist. This is a relatively benign problem if taken care of promptly. If neglected, it can turn into *pyorrhea*. This condition is advanced gingivitis. If untreated, the retraction eventually becomes so marked that the roots of the teeth may be exposed.

Patients taking Dilantin should have regular examinations of the oral cavity, with special attention to the gums. Long-term use of this drug may cause problems, the most common being *gingival hyperplasia*. The gums enlarge and extend to the point of covering portions of the teeth.

With a bright light the nurse should inspect the tongue for color, size, position, lesions, coating, and surface texture. There are some variations in tongue surfaces that should be described:

1. *Hairy tongue:* In this condition, hairs seem to be growing out of the surface of the tongue. Actually, the hair-like protrusions are brown or black filliform papillae. Hairy tongue is a chronic condition and cannot be cured in most people.
2. *Geographic tongue:* The tongue in this condition resembles a one-dimensional topographic map. Smooth, reddened areas are located sporadically on the dorsum. These areas have no papillae, thus giving the tongue an irregular texture. Geographic tongue is harmless and does not warrant treatment.
3. *Fissured tongue (scrotal tongue):* This is a familial condition which is generally not a problem, occurring in up to 40 percent of some populations. The tongue looks exactly as the name implies, with fissures of various depths on the dorsum of the tongue. Occasionally food will get caught in the fissures and may cause some mild irritation. There is no treatment for this; most problems can be avoided with good oral hygiene.

The tongue and oral mucosa may exhibit hyperpigmentation. Darkly pigmented tongues occur in 10 to 50 percent of Caucasians and in up to 90 percent of black populations.

The amount and regeneration of papillae are of interest because they vary throughout the life span. Although the number of taste buds varies among different populations, they are generally most abundant in infants and children.[1] The papillae are also most sensitive to stimuli at these ages. As children become adults the number of papillae decrease. By the time a person is beyond middle age, the tastebuds have deteriorated even farther. The most important reason to note this is in an attempt to understand a person's sense of taste. Because of the large number of papillae, children have an acute sense of taste, and to them rich foods (i.e., SPINACH!!) probably taste entirely different than they do to adults. Elderly people suffer from just the opposite problem. Their food does not taste terribly interesting unless it is rich or highly seasoned because of the decreased number of papillae. Thus it is common to see older people highly salt and season their foods.

To further inspect the tongue and its undersurface, the nurse asks the patient to lift his tongue. She then observes for symmetry with movement. The area under the tongue is examined for lesions, distribution of superficial veins, attachment of the frenulum, and the presence and patency of Wharton's ducts.

Oral cancer is a potentially fatal disease if not discovered early. In its early stages a cancerous lesion may look like a minute ulceration. Therefore, meticulous inspection of the area under the tongue is essential. Many dentists and hygienists consider this inspection part of routine health maintenance. This is certainly a good practice, but the inspection should be done as thoroughly during a physical exam. Much of the oral cancer of the mouth is found in this region.

Varicosities are another abnormality that can occur under the tongue. These are most likely to be seen in the elderly. They are of virtually no significance and do not require treatment. Some authorities feel they may be related to a deficiency of the cardiovascular system.

The buccal mucosa is evaluated for moisture, color, lesions (canker sores), and pigmentation. Because the buccal mucosa and the tongue may exhibit less pigmentation than any other body areas in dark-skinned individuals, this may be an excellent site for detection of cyanosis, jaundice, or ecchymosis. However, there are two frequently occuring nonpathologic conditions in the oral mucosa which also lead to color changes. The first is hyperpigmentation of the oral mucous membranes. In Caucasians, the incidence of hyperpigmentation may reach 10 percent by age 50; in Blacks, 50 to 90 percent will show mucous membrane hyperpigmentation by the fourth decade. In both groups, there is a higher incidence in darker-hued individuals. A second frequently occurring variation in oral pigmentation results from a condition termed leukoedema. This presents on the buccal mucosa as a benign grayish white lesion. This condition is present in nearly 50 percent of Caucasians and 90 percent of Blacks. Figure 7.3 shows leukoedema in a Black patient.[2,3]

The presence of the parotid ducts should also be noted and can be found opposite the area of the second molar at the level of the maxilla. They look like the top of a straight pin and are the same color as the mucosa.

Canker sores commonly occur on the buccal mucosa. These small white ulcerations are viral in origin and can be very painful. Many people notice that the lesions appear when fatigue, stress, or a systemic infection exist.

If a child presents with a brief history of a cold, cough, and fever, the examiner should check the buccal mucosa for white,

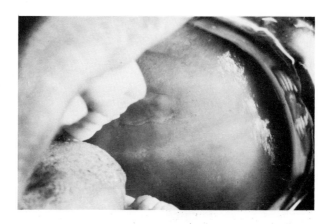

FIGURE 7.3. Moderate leukoedema observed in a 20-year-old Negro female. Notice the diffuse grayish-white opacity of the buccal mucosa which radiates along the occlusal line (From Martin, J. M. Epidemilogy of leukoedema in the negro. *Journal of Oral Medicine, 28* No. 2:41, 1973)

patchy, spotty areas. These are called *Koplick's spots* and appear 48 hours before the arrival of the measles (rubeola). The nurse should inquire about the child's immunization status and about how old the child was when he received the MMR (measles, mumps, and rubella) vaccine.

The dome-shaped hard palate is observed for its shape and the presence of any extra bony prominences. In black individuals the color changes of jaundice are especially prominent at the junction of the hard and soft palates. However, instead of the classical yellow hue, the palates of jaundiced blacks are often a muddy yellow or greenish-brown in color.[2] Occasionally there may be a bony growth on the roof of the mouth. This is known as *torus palatinus* and is found along the midline of the hard palate. Palatine tori are common in Asian people (up to 77 percent) and less common in Blacks and Caucasians.[2,4] The extent of the extra growth determines whether treatment is required. Rarely is it necessary to do anything about torus palatinus.

In newborns and infants small retention cysts can occur on the hard palate. These are small, yellow-white, pearl-like nodules that are most frequently found on the posterior aspect. These are called *Epstein's pearls* and will resolve without treatment within the first few weeks of life. Similar cysts occur on the gums of infants and can be mistaken for teeth. Patient education is important so the parents understand what they are and that they are harmless.

Examination of the pharynx begins with inspection of the anterior pillars and uvula. The entire pharynx should be observed for color, edema, petechiae, ulcerations, and exudate. After the anterior pillars are examined, the uvula is visualized for length, deviation from the midline, movement, and symmetry. The patient is asked to say "ah" and the uvula and soft palate should rise (see the section on Cranial Nerve X in Chapter 15). Not infrequently, the uvula has an unusual shape. The most common deviation is called a *bifid uvula* and it looks like it has been partially severed in the midline. This may have clinical significance and should be reported, especially when it occurs in children. A bifid uvula may indicate a submucous cleft palate, which implies that there is a deficient muscle of the palate.[5] Incidence of cleft uvula varies dramatically among populations. In American Indians it is seen in 1 of every 9 to 14 individuals; among Blacks it is extremely rare (1 in 300); and in Caucasians the frequency lies in between that of the other groups.[4]

Observation of the pharynx continues to the tonsils and posterior pillars. To visualize these areas, the examiner should have the

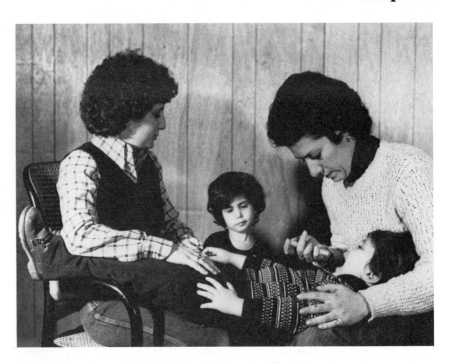

FIGURE 7.4. Gaining trust by examining the child on the mother's and the examiner's laps while looking at the child's pharynx.

patient say "ah" or "eh." Although the "eh" sound is harder to make with the mouth open, it gives the examiner a better look at the posterior pharynx (Fig. 7.4).

The tonsils may appear enlarged on examination. This does not necessarily indicate pathology. If a benign state of tonsilar enlargement exists, the tissue will be the same pink color as the rest of the oral mucosa. Enlarged tonsils of this nature are called *hypertrophied.*

Pharyngitis. The term pharyngitis has many implications. Obviously, when the word is defined for its actual meaning, it is simply "inflammation of the pharynx." Unfortunately, pharyngitis is not that simple.

A viral pharyngitis may be very minor or it may cause as many unpleasant symptoms as a bacterial infection. Symptoms of a less intense sore throat may cause mild discomfort with swallowing, a low grade fever, rhinorrhea, lethargy, etc. A more severe sore throat may cause marked throat pain and difficulty in swallowing, an erythematous and exudative pharynx, swollen glands, overall weakness, etc. Both can be the description of a viral infection.

The etiology of pharyngitis can be documented by obtaining a throat culture (a strep screen). If this is positive—in other words, if growth on the culture plate occurs—then a diagnosis of a streptococcal infection can be made.

Most bacterial throat infections are caused by strep and may cause absolute misery. On the other hand, it is easy to be fooled by the lack of intense symptoms. However, in general, a strep throat will manifest with a cherry red exudative pharynx. One can also expect to elicit in the history the following: acute onset, abdominal symptoms (nausea, vomiting, diarrhea), an elevated temperature, and swollen glands (especially in the anterior cervical chain).

The treatment differs for a viral pharyngitis and a strep throat. Antibiotics are warranted for a strep infection. In some instances, antibiotics are given for prophylactic purposes, whether strep exists or not. This is not usually done for a healthy adult, and a great deal of patient education is necessary to help the patient understand the reason for just treating with the supportive measures. It is easy to be deceived by a pharyngitis. Therefore, the patient with more than a minor sore throat irritation should be referred for a throat culture and proper treatment.

THE NOSE AND PARANASAL SINUSES

Various problems can occur with the first portion of the respiratory system—the nose. Chronic nasal stuffiness, postnasal drip, allergies, traumatic injury, and bleeding are some of the complaints often elicited. When questioning a patient about his nose and related symptoms, the nurse must remember that there are few patients who, when asked about some of these annoyances, will have a totally negative history. Therefore, precise questions must be asked to eliminate unnecessary information.

History

An overall review for this area includes inquiry about: problems with sinus pain; postnasal drip, nasal obstruction, discharge, or stuffiness; frequent colds; allergies; and epistaxis (nosebleeds). When the history for any of these problems is positive, further data are required. For instance, if the patient states he has a history of "nosebleeds," certain information should be elicited:

1. What exactly does the patient mean by a "nosebleed?"
2. How much blood is there? Less than a teaspoon? More than a tablespoon? Does the blood seem to "run" out? For how long? What color is the blood: red, brown? Are there clots? Is only one nostril involved?
3. How frequently do they occur?
4. When was the last episode? What was the patient doing when it occurred? What is he usually doing when they start?
5. What measures are taken to stop the bleeding? Has treatment been sought in the past? Describe what was done and the outcome.
6. What medicine is the patient taking? How much? How often?
7. Does the patient have any illnesses (i.e., hypertension)?
8. Is there anyone in the family with the same problem?

If allergies exist, then an allergy history should be elicited. The nurse should find out what the patient is allergic to, how that was determined (i.e., scratch tests), how the allergy manifests, what treatment is implemented, what time of year seems to be the worst, and what (if any) environment aggravates or alleviates the problem.

To complete the review of the nose and sinuses, the patient should be asked if there is any history of trauma (including an explanation about the course of events) and whether he has noticed change in his ability to smell.

Anatomy

The nose has two main functions. It is the air conditioner of the respiratory system and it enables us to use our sense of smell. The nose, in conjunction with the paranasal sinuses, filters, warms, and moistens the air. The sinuses also act as voice resonators and help to reduce the weight of the skull.

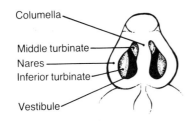

FIGURE 7.5. External structures of the nose.

To describe the nose anatomically, it is most logical to start with the external structures. The *vestibule* is the first identifiable feature and it is an opening which surrounds the *nares* (Fig. 7.5). The vestibule is separated medially by a skin-covered cartilaginous structure called the *columnella*. This is the bottom of the bony structure which separates the nares, called the *septum*. Both cartilage and bone comprise the septum. The bottom of the septum is cartilaginous. As it progresses up towards the orbital area, it becomes more bony. The lining of the nares is mucosa covered with cilia. The nasal mucosa appears red and more vivid in color than the oral mucosa due to the rich blood supply feeding the area. If this lining lacks the characteristic red color or appears gray-blue and boggy, then there is probably a strong allergy history.

The *turbinates* branch off the septum. These are bony, vascular structures with a meatus in between each turbinate. Each meatus is named for the turbinate below it; thus we have the superior turbinate, the middle meatus, the middle turbinate, the inferior meatus, and the inferior turbinate (Fig. 7.6A). In fact, the reason one gets a "stuffy" nose with sinus problems or excessive tearing is because the middle meatus drains the sinuses and the inferior meatus drains the nasolacrimal duct.

Paranasal Sinuses. The eight paranasal sinuses are air-filled cavities with ciliated mucous membrane linings (Fig. 7.6B). Only the *frontal* and *maxillary* sinuses are accessible to examination. The *ethmoid* and *sphenoid* sinuses are visible only with skull films. The frontal sinuses are located above the eyebrow in each eye. They are separated by the septum. These sinuses are absent at birth and do not develop until 7 or 8 years of age. The maxillary sinuses are the largest of all the sinuses. They can hold up to 20 cc of fluid. These sinuses lie along each maxilla and are present at birth.

Physical Assessment

The nose is inspected and palpated. The paranasal sinuses are palpated, percussed, and transilluminated. Equipment used for examination of the nose and paranasal sinuses includes a nasal speculum and a head lamp, or else an otoscope with the wide, short speculum tip and a bright penlight.

Nose. The outside of the nose is inspected and palpated. Any unusual skin markings, obvious deviation of the septum (asymmetry), discharge, or flaring of the nares should be noted. If recent trauma has occurred, there may be edema or discoloration as well. The area should be palpated for tenderness, swelling, and structural deviations.

Next the nasal mucosa, septum, and turbinates are examined. For this portion of the exam, the otoscope with the nasal speculum tip is needed. The examiner places her hand on the patient's head and gently guides it backward. With her hand firmly placed on the patient's head, she can control the degree of movement and stabilize herself as well as the patient. After the patient's head is at the angle desired, the instrument is inserted about 1 cm (Fig. 7.7). The septum should not be touched. Like the ear canal, the septum has many nerve endings and is very sensitive when touched.

The anterior aspect of the nose is examined first. The mucosa is inspected for color, lesions, discharge, swelling, and evidence of

POSITION OF SINUSES

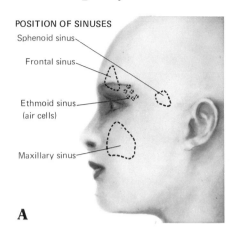

A

FIGURE 7.6. (A) The position of the sinuses. (B) The structure of the nose and pharynx. (From Heagarty, M., Glass, G., King, H., and Manly, M. *Child health: Basics for primary care.* New York: Appleton–Century–Crofts, 1980, pp. 128, 129)

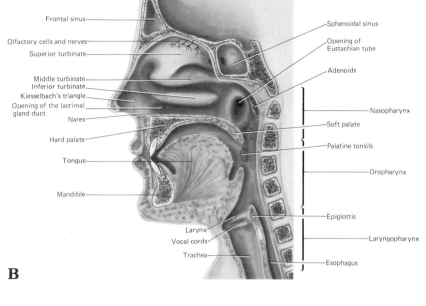

B

bleeding. The nasal septum is checked for deviation, lesions, and superficial blood vessels. To visualize the turbinates, the examiner tips the patient's head back a little more. This should reveal the turbinates without having to insert the speculum any farther. The examiner should see the inferior and middle turbinates, which are separated by the middle meatus. This area is inspected for edema, polyps, and change in color.

Paranasal Sinuses. The frontal and maxillary sinuses are palpated and percussed for tenderness. There are two accepted methods. The first method involves the application of gentle pressure over the frontal sinuses and then the maxillary sinuses (Fig. 7.8). Pain elicited on palpation of any area indicates some degree of irritation. Immediate percussion (see respiratory system technique of exam Chapter 8, p. 167) is the other method used to detect tenderness.* The examiner simply taps the palmar aspect of the index or second finger lightly over each sinus. Once again, tender areas may be indicative of a blocked sinus.

Transillumination is a technique used to detect abnormalities in the shape and size of the sinuses, but its success and reliability are questionable. Without an extremely dark room and a very bright penlight, the exam is not worth the time it takes to perform.

*In this method of percussion no pleximeter is used.

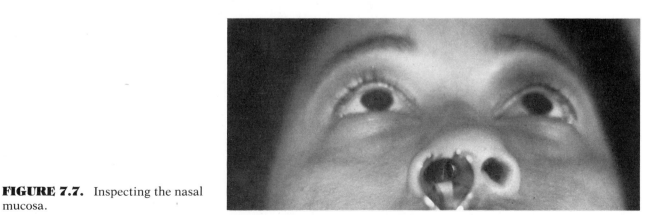

FIGURE 7.7. Inspecting the nasal mucosa.

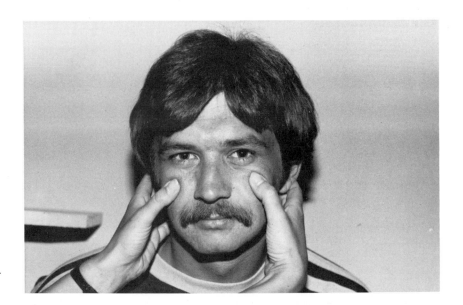

FIGURE 7.8. Palpating the maxillary sinuses.

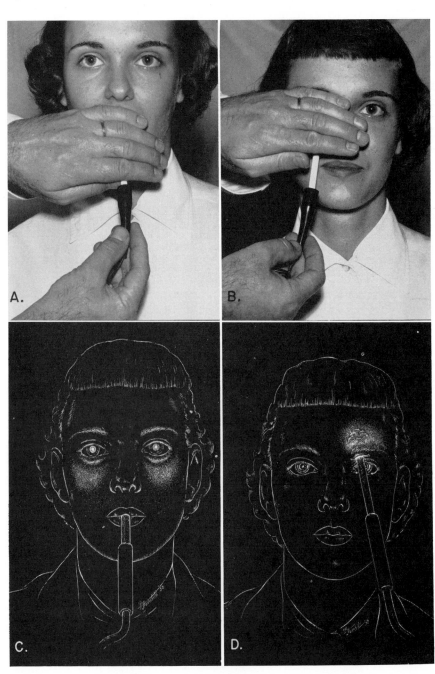

FIGURE 7.9. Technique of transillumination of the paranasal sinuses: (A) the maxillary sinuses, (B) the frontal sinuses, (C) illumination of the maxillary sinuses, (D) illumination of the frontal sinuses. (From Saunders, W. E. Ears, nose, and throat. In Prior, J. and Silberstein, J. *Physical diagnosis: The history and examination of the patient* (5th ed.). St. Louis: Mosby, 1973, p. 167)

Normally the sinuses are asymmetrical in shape and size, so unless there is a question of significant obstruction or inflammation, there will be no findings. However, to check for blockage of the maxillary sinuses, the examiner simply places the lit penlight in the patient's mouth. The patient is then instructed to place his lips tightly around the penlight (Fig. 7.9). Both maxillary sinuses will illuminate with a pink cast. A red reflex will appear in the pupil as well. If either sinus is blocked, the light will not be seen through the cheek.

To check the frontal sinuses, the lit penlight is placed under the eyebrow in the periorbital arch. The examiner must be careful not to burn the patient. These sinuses are tested one at a time. If they are not infected or blocked, their illumination will also give off a pink cast (Fig. 7.9).

REFERENCES

1. Spuhler, J. Genetics of three normal morphological variations: Patterns of superficial veins of the anterior thorax, peroneus tertius muscle, and number of villate papillae. *Cold Spring Harbour Symposia on Quantitative Biology*, 1950, *15*, 175–189.
2. McDonald, C., and Kelly, P. Dermatology and venereology. In R. Williams (Ed.), *Textbook of black-related diseases*. New York: McGraw–Hill, 1975, pp. 513–592.
3. Martin, J., and Crump, E. Leukoedema of the buccal mucosa in negro children and youth. *Oral Surgery*, 1972, *34*, 49–58.
4. Jarvis, A., and Gorlin, R., Minor orofacial abnormalities in an Eskimo population. *Oral Surgery*, 1972, *33*, 417–426.
5. DeWeese, D., and Saunders, W. *Textbook of otolaryngology* (4th ed.). St. Louis: Mosby, 1973, p. 36.

EXAMPLE OF A RECORDED HISTORY AND PHYSICAL

SUBJECTIVE:

Chief Complaint: "Sore throat for 2 days."

HPI: (History given by mother and son.) This 11-year-old male considers himself "basically healthy." Woke up yesterday and noticed that he had "difficulty swallowing" and a "burning" pain in the back of his throat. The pain worsened as the day went on. He did nothing for it and went to school. This morning he awoke and the pain was more intense and his right ear hurt "inside" his head. No discharge. Took temperature and it was 100.6°F orally. He also complains of nasal stuffiness and clear drainage of 1 week duration. Today he feels tired, slept most of the day, and has no appetite. He has no dizziness, headache, cough, nausea, vomiting, or diarrhea. Mother gave him two adult aspirin this AM. He has also been taking throat lozenges every 3 hours or so. He gets about two sore throats every winter. Last winter, he had four sore throats and two were cultured and diagnosed as "strep." He is allergic to penicillin, gets a "rash all over his body." His sister had a strep throat, diagnosed 1 week ago. He feels he cannot go to school as long as he feels this badly.

OBJECTIVE: T.101°F orally; P. radial 76; R. 18; B.P. (sitting) 110/70.

Ears: Left and right: No discharges and no tenderness with palpation of external ear. Canals clear. Right tympanic membrane: Redness throughout drum; landmarks not visible—retraction. Left tympanic membrane: Unremarkable.

Nose: Clear drainage in each nares. Mucosa red. No inflammation or polyps. Paranasal sinuses (frontal and maxillary) nontender.

Throat: Anterior and posterior pillars red. No tonsils. Exudative patch on left posterior pillar.

Neck: Supple. Enlarged palpable, tender lymph nodes along right anterior cervical chain. Kernig's sign and Brudzinski's sign negative.

Chest: Regular respirations. No retraction. No tenderness on palpation or dullness to percussion. No adventitious breath sounds.

Abdomen: Bowel sounds audible in all four quadrants. Soft. No tenderness or masses on palpation. Liver span 6 cm, nontender. Spleen not palpable or tender.

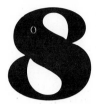

8

The Respiratory System

Every system in the body interfaces with the respiratory system in one fashion or another. For instance, the color and quality of the nailbeds and the generalized color of the integumentary system are affected by the O_2–CO_2 balance in the body. The amount of oxygenated blood circulating throughout the body depends not only on the quality of the lung tissue, but also on the "health" of the veins and arteries of the cardiovascular system. Thus the nurse, to make an accurate evaluation of the respiratory system, must understand all its interfacings.

Any degree of change within this system can cause significant problems for the patient. The nurse must be able to quickly assess alteration of respiratory status. In addition to doing a thorough history and physical, she must be able to distinguish between acute and chronic signs. The patient with a chronic obstructive pulmonary disease often depends on the nurse to make decisions and act quickly in order to prevent an acute attack or severe distress.

As with all the other systems, the evaluation of the respiratory system begins with a complete history.

HISTORY

A general overview of this system includes questions about chest pain with breathing; coughs; shortness of breath; night sweats; frequent upper respiratory infections; any history of emphysema, pneumonia, bronchitis, asthma, hemoptysis, or tuberculosis; when the last chest x-ray was taken and the results, if known; and smoking habits. The review of this system is not lengthy if there are no present concerns.

A frequent complaint involving the respiratory system is a cough. There are several questions to ask regarding this problem:

Onset: When did it begin? Did it start suddenly or gradually?

Sequence and chronology: Has it been consistently present? Did it stop for a period of time and restart? Is it worse at night? Does the cough awaken the patient or keep him from going to sleep?

Quality: Is it high-pitched or low-pitched? Barky? Is it non-productive or productive? If productive: How much sputum (more or less than a tablespoon)? What color (green, yellow, white, clear)? Blood-tinged (tan or pink—lightly stained; red, brown, copper—more heavily stained; fresh blood will be bright red, occult blood will be more brown)? Consistency (thick or thin)? Odor (describe)?

Setting: Work? Home? What is the ventilation system like? (This may overlap with *aggravating factors*.)

Aggravating factors: Pollen? Animal dander? Cigarette smoke? Occupation—both environment and type of work? Temperature change? Stress?

Alleviating factors: Rest? Medications? Position? Alteration of the environment? Relief of stress?

Associated phenomena: Chest pain? Fever? Allergies (including dairy products)? A recent cold or postnasal drip? Ear pain or stuffiness? Cyanosis? Nausea, vomiting, diarrhea? Changes in the volume or rate of breathing? Fatigue or weakness?

As concerns the past history of the respiratory system, the patient should be asked if he ever had pneumonia, bronchitis, asthma, tuberculosis, or hemoptysis. If any positive responses are given, the following course of inquiry should be pursued:

1. Who treated the problem?
2. With what was it treated?
3. Was a hospitalization necessary?
4. Did the problem resolve quickly or did it linger?
5. Were there any complications?
6. Give a short description about the course of the disease.

The patient should be asked if any other family members have a similar problem or other problems pertaining to the respiratory system. This is also a good time to inquire about smoking habits. If the patient does smoke, he should be asked what, how much, and for how long. Does he have a smoker's cough? If so, he should be asked to describe it. Finally, the patient should be questioned about his last chest x-ray, when it was, the reason for it, and what the results were.

In children the most frequent complaints involve recurrent colds, chronic cough, and allergies. The evaluation of these types of problems follows the same principle of inquiry, using the eight areas of investigation to decipher between relevant and irrelevant data.

In the adolescent, young adult, and middle-aged person, most of the problems concerning the respiratory system include acute infections, a continuing problem with allergies, or, less commonly, a chronic disease.

In the geriatric patient the most common problems are chronic obstructive pulmonary disease and a general decrease in the efficiency of the respiratory system. The gradual decline in efficiency occurs in the vital capacity and the air exchange of the lung tissue. The amount of oxygen circulating in the bloodstream of the young adult can be as much as 60 percent greater than the amount in the bloodstream of an elderly person. Thus "shortness of breath and fatigue," which are frequent complaints of the older patient, may be due to nothing more than a less efficient respiratory system.

ANATOMY

The respiratory system begins at the nares and ends at the diaphragm, where the lower lobes of the lungs lie. However, for the purpose of this chapter only the thoracic cavity will be discussed, including the area extending from the trachea through both lung fields.

Pathology in the respiratory system is often localized. In order to be able to describe the boundaries of an involved area, certain imaginary and anatomic landmarks must be used.

Landmarks

The chest is assessed laterally, anteriorly, and posteriorly. Imaginary vertical lines are drawn on both aspects from the shoulder to the pelvis. These divide the thorax lengthwise (Fig. 8-1). Actual lines called pigmentary demarcation lines may appear on the anterior chest and arms. These lines are considered normal pigmentary variants and are common in Oriental and American Black patients. Figure 8.2 illustrates patterning of pigmentary demarcation lines.[1,2]

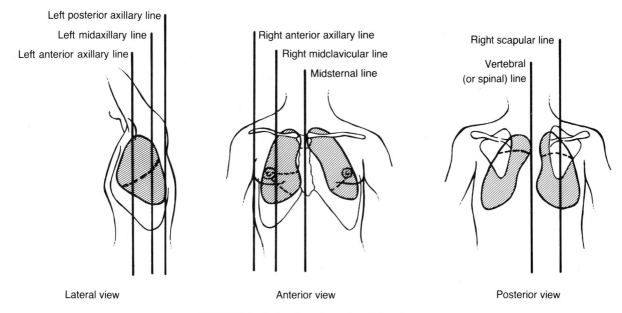

FIGURE 8.1. Landmarks of the thorax.

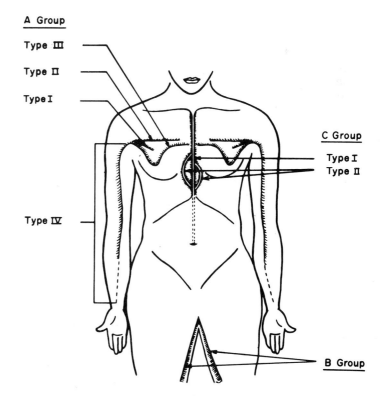

FIGURE 8.2. Demarcation lines of pigmentation (feathered and hyphenated) found in Japanese, after Miura. (Ventral axial lines of inner thigh, to which Group B may correspond, are usually shown in posterior view.) (From Sebmanowitz, V. J. & Krivo, J. M., Comparison of Negroes with Japanese. *British Journal of Dermatology*, 1975).

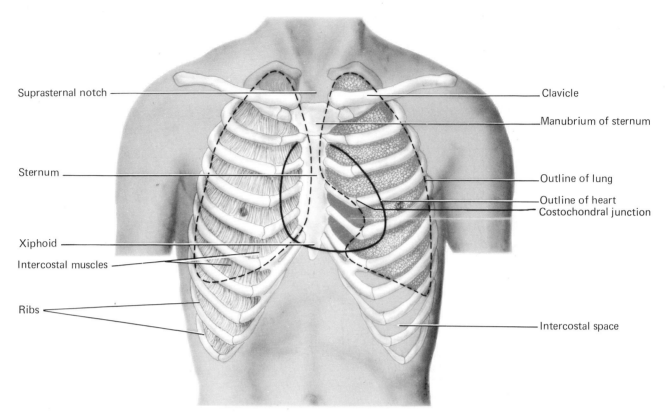

FIGURE 8.3. The thorax: thoracic cage and position of organs within it. (From Heagarty, M., Glass, G., King, H. & Manley, M., *Child health: Basics for primary care.* New York: Appleton–Century–Crofts, 1980, p. 138).

The other set of landmarks used to describe the chest are not imaginary lines, but bony prominences which help the examiner count ribs and rib spaces. Counting the ribs aids in mapping out the location of specific organs, consolidations, tumors, etc. This landmark system is also helpful when learning to examine the heart.

Anterior Thorax. The easiest bony landmark to find is the *suprasternal notch* (Fig. 8.3). This U-shaped curve is at the top of the *manubrium.* The ridge-like feature below the manubrium is the *sternal angle* (or *angle of Louis*). This ridge adjoins the second rib. The intercostal space immediately below the second rib is the second intercostal space (also known as ICS). All intercostal spaces are named for the ribs above them.

The body of the sternum is attached to the first seven ribs which is shown in Fig. 8.3. By using the 2ICS as the starting point, it is not difficult to then locate the next four ribs and their respective intercostal spaces.

The *xiphoid process* is the bony prominence at the bottom of the sternum. The eighth, ninth, and tenth ribs terminate medially at the costal margin. An imaginary angle called the *costal angle* describes the area between the costal margins. The eleventh and twelveth ribs are free-floating and do not articulate with anything anteriorly. The other anatomic features of the rib cage that deserve mention here are the *costochondral junctions.* These are located in the middle of each rib (Fig. 8.3). This junction is formed during fetal

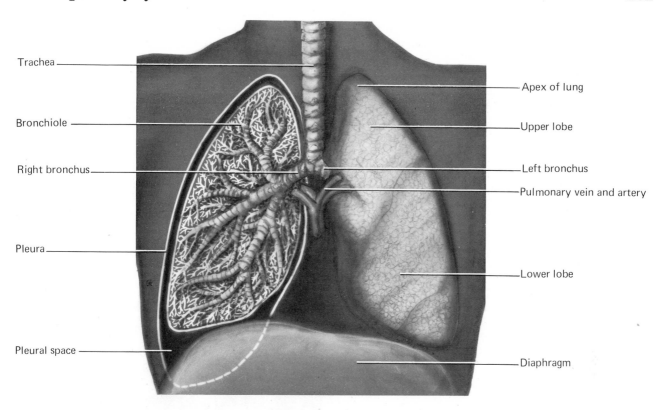

Trachea

Bronchiole

Right bronchus

Pleura

Pleural space

Apex of lung

Upper lobe

Left bronchus

Pulmonary vein and artery

Lower lobe

Diaphragm

FIGURE 8.4. Structure of the lungs. (From Heagarty, M., Glass, G., King, H., & Manly, M. *Child health: Basics for primary care.* New York: Appleton–Century–Crofts, 1980, p. 138).

development and is often a site for an inflammatory response or traumatic injury in the thoracic area.

Posterior Thorax. Of the bony landmarks used to classify boundaries on the posterior aspect of the chest, the spinal column is the most obvious feature. When the patient flexes his head forward, a bony prominence can be palpated at the base of the neck called the *vertebrae prominens.* This is the spinous process of C_7. The easily palpable but not quite as prominent protuberance below C_7 is T_1. It is also reasonable to estimate that the second to eighth ribs lie directly under the scapular area.

Lungs. After locating all these landmarks, the examiner should be able to picture where the lungs lie. They extend from just above the clavicles (3 cm above) to about the level of the diaphragm shown in Figure 8.4. Anteriorly the lower lobes end at the sixth rib at the midclavicular line (also known as MCL) and at the eighth rib at the midaxillary line. Posteriorly, T_{10}, T_{11}, and T_{12} mark the lower base of the lungs. The precise range is affected by the depth of inspiration.

There are three lobes of the right lung and two lobes of the left. Fissures divide each lung into specific regions. The *oblique fissure* bisects the lung posteriorly at T_3 and extends to the fifth rib anteriorly at the midclavicular line. Since the right lung has upper, middle, and lower lobes, it has an additional fissure. The *right horizontal fissure* separates the right-upper lobe (RUL) and the right-middle lobe (RML). It extends anteriorly from the fifth rib at the midaxillary line to the fourth rib at the midsternal level.

PHYSICAL ASSESSMENT

All four techniques of examination are used to assess the respiratory system. Both the anterior and the posterior aspects of the thorax are evaluated. For two reasons, the posterior aspect is usually examined first. First, the examiner will have just completed the head and neck exam, which may have included the posterior approach to the thyroid. Second, the patient is still sitting up and this is the proper position for examining the posterior chest. Assessment of the anterior thorax follows when the examiner is standing in front of the

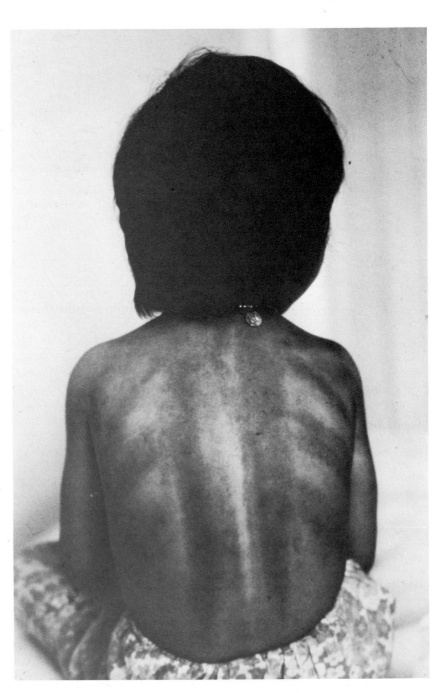

FIGURE 8.5. Symmetrical purpura caused by coin-rubbing. (From: Yeatman, G.W., et al. Pediatrics 58 (4):617, October, 1976. Copyright American Academy of Pediatrics, 1976.)

patient again and the patient assumes the supine position. The patient then remains in this position for the cardiovascular exam.

It is important that the total thorax is exposed and that the room is well lit. The only equipment needed is a stethoscope with a diaphragm, a ruler, and a marking pen. Whether examining the anterior or the posterior chest, the order is as follows: inspection, palpation, percussion, and auscultation.

Examination of the Posterior Thorax

Inspection. The skin should be examined for lesions, rashes, moles, discoloration, and edematous areas. While marked bruising may indicate pathology or child abuse, bruising of a Vietnamese child's posterior thorax is a common result of the folk treatment *Cao Gio* (Fig. 8.5) This practice is commonly used for treating colds and consists of stroking a child's oiled back with the edge of a coin.[3]

The thoracic contour should be assessed next. The examiner should note any irregularities in shape, whether congenital or from newly developing problems.

The *anterior–posterior* diameter (A–P diameter) should be visually estimated. This is done by comparing the shoulder-to-shoulder breadth to the lateral span. In caucasian adults, the average A–P ratio is approximately 1:2. In infants this ratio is equal. By 5 or 6 years of age this ratio is the same as that of an adult. The chest of a child is measured through the first year of life. Precise measurements can be taken with a tape measure. The tape measure is placed around the thorax, using the nipples as landmarks (Fig. 8.6). As a person ages, major changes in the A–P diameter will most likely be signs of pulmonary disease. There are special terms used to describe abnormalities of the chest contour (Fig. 8.7 and Chart 8.1).

The rate, rhythm, regularity, and quality of respiration are observed next. The rate is also counted at this time (Chart 8.2). If any irregularities are noted, they are described (Chart 8.3).

Palpation. The thoracic cavity is palpated for tenderness, masses, lesions, extent of thoracic expanse, and vocal fremitus. Any specific

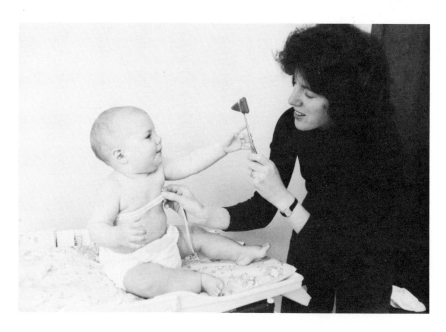

FIGURE 8.6. Measuring chest circumference on an infant.

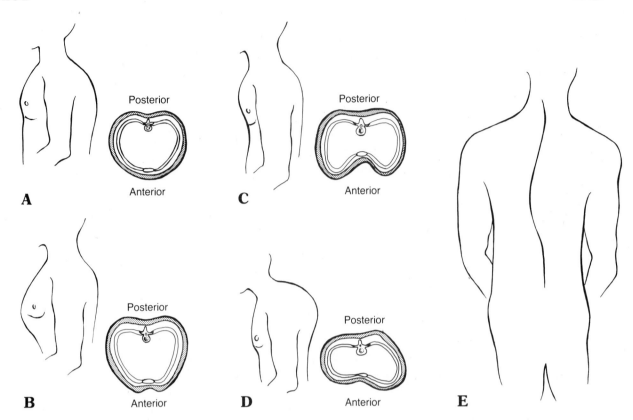

FIGURE 8.7. Abnormalities of the chest contour: (A) barrel chest, (B) pigeon chest, (C) funnel chest, (D) kyphosis, (E) scoliosis.

CHART 8.1

Abnormalities of Chest Contour

Abnormality	Description
Barrel chest	The A–P diameter is about equal; typically seen in emphysema
Pigeon chest (pectus carinatum)	The sternum juts anteriorly and the chest looks like that of a chicken
Funnel chest (pectus excavatum)	The sternum points posteriorly; this may cause abnormal pressure on the heart, which could affect function
Lumbosacral deformities (kyphosis and scoliosis)	May cause other defects, depending on the degree (see Chap. 14)

CHART 8.2

Normal Respiratory Rates

Adult	12–20/min or 16–20/min
Older child	12–20/min
6 months–2 years	Up to 30/min
Infants	Up to 45/min

CHART 8.3

Description of Abnormal Respiratory Patterns

Irregularities	*Description*
Tachypnea	Rapid superficial breathing ↑ 20
Bradypnea	Slow deep breathing ↓ 12
Apnea	Cessation of breathing
Hyperventilation	Fast, deep, and constant breathing: offsets O_2–CO_2 imbalance, causing dizziness, etc.; often a stress-related reaction
Kussmaul's	Deeper than normal respiration; often seen in acidosis
Cheyne–Stokes	Often in a critically ill patient; regular episodes of apnea occur within a regular breathing pattern
Stertorous breathing	Rattly snoring type of respiration; often heard in the terminal states
Dyspnea	A subjective complaint of difficulty in breathing
Orthopnea	A subjective complaint; air gets "stuffy" when patient is sleeping and he feels a need to sit up or sleep on extra pillows

areas of chest pain should always be palpated to see if pain can be elicited or if there is a mass. Any unusual lesions or rashes should be felt for consistency and elevation. The exact location, size, color, shape, and mobility should be described thoroughly.

Assessing the *thoracic expanse* is neither difficult nor time-consuming and reveals significant information about the symmetry of breathing. To palpate thoracic expanse, the examiner places her thumbs around the posterior costal margins at the level of the tenth rib. Thumbs should be placed equidistant from the spinal column to measure symmetry (Fig. 8.8). The patient is then asked to take a deep breath. The examiner observes the movement of her thumbs while the patient inspires. The thumbs should separate symmetrically. The regularity of breathing can also be watched while doing this test.

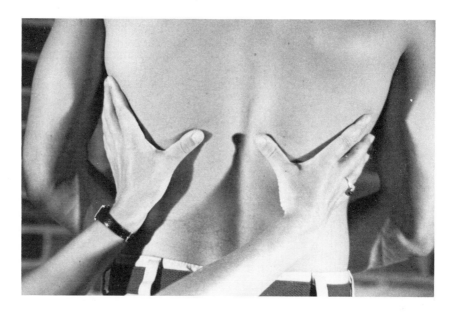

FIGURE 8.8. Palpating the thoracic expanse.

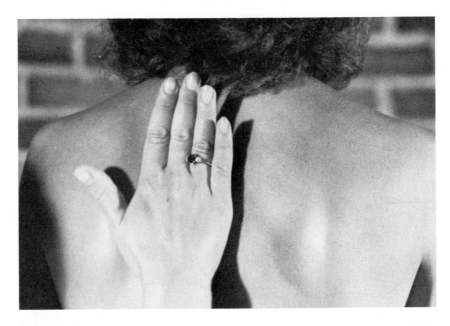

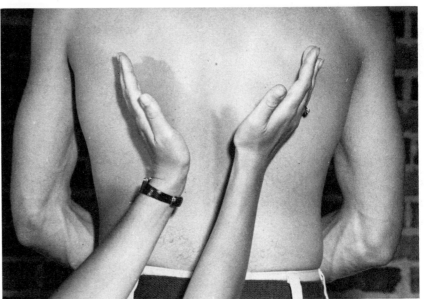

FIGURE 8.9. Palpating for vocal fremitus.

Vocal fremitus is defined as palpable vibrations through the lung fields. These vibrations are most easily felt when the patient says a word like "99" and the palmar aspects of the examiner's hands are placed on either side of the spinal column (Fig. 8.9). The ulnar side of the hand may also be used. One or both hands may be used, but one hand is preferable. (This omits any discrepancies in the findings if there is a difference in the sensitivities of the examiner's hands.) The examiner moves back and forth from one side to another, covering first upper lobes, then the lower lobes. The vibrations will be strongest around the tracheal bifurcation and the major bronchus. Although this is a gross test, symmetry of fremitus is expected in the normal, healthy lung.

In an infant, palpation for vocal fremitus is not carried out routinely. However, if it is necessary and an abnormality is suspected, it can be done when the baby cries.

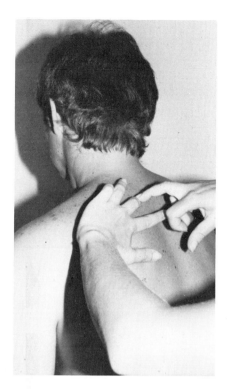

FIGURE 8.10. Indirect percussion method.

Fremitus is altered under the following conditions:

1. Decreased fremitus: A low voice, an obstructed bronchus COPD, pleural effusion.
2. Increased fremitus: A mass, a consolidated area (as in pneumonia or other inflammatory processes).

The level of the diaphragm can be estimated to be around T_{10}, where vocal fremitus stops. Determining this level is the first step in measuring *diaphragmatic excursion*.

Percussion. Percussion is used to determine whether an area is filled with air, fluid, or a solid material. This method of examination involves a "tapping" gesture on the skin (usually the abdomen and thorax) which sets the underlying organs into motion. The result of this tapping creates a sound and a vibratory sensation known as a *percussion note*. These notes can be elicited from areas up to 7 cm deep. However, an abnormality should be about 2 to 3 cm for it to give a positive percussion note.

The most commonly used technique of percussion is called the *indirect* or *mediate* method. This term indicates that an object lies between the examiner's percussing finger and the skin surface (usually the second finger of the examiner's other hand).

There is a cardinal rule to remember about percussion. Effective technique depends on loose wrist motion. The procedure is as follows:

1. The examiner lays the second finger of her left hand over the area being percussed. The first and third fingers are elevated so they are not touching the skin (Fig. 8.10) The second finger of the left hand is known as the pleximeter (the hands are reversed if the examiner is left-handed).
2. With the other hand, the examiner extends and flexes her wrist rhythmically, using the middle finger as the "hammer" or plexor.
3. This motion (proceeding at 3 to 5 cm intervals down the thorax) is repeated two or three times over each area (Fig. 8.11).
4. The percussion sounds are compared—those of one side of the chest to those of the other.

Since this is a gross assessment, any asymmetry of percussion notes warrants further investigation. Two points to remember are: short nails are a must and percussion over bone will cause a great inaccuracy.

There are five notes that can be elicited. Each sound has its own intensity, pitch, and duration (Chart 8.4). Percussion notes are relatively consistent throughout the age groups. However, in infants one finds the lung fields more hyperresonant than resonant. This is due to the close proximity of the lungs to the chest wall, as well as to the large amount of the surface area of the baby's body that the thorax occupies.

In addition to this general orientation, the posterior thorax is percussed for *diaphragmatic excursion*. This span estimates the ele-

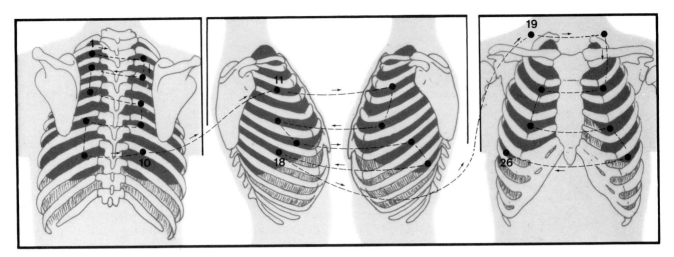

FIGURE 8.11. Sequence of percussion and auscultation. (From Heagarty, M., Glass, G., King, H., & Manly, M. *Child health: Basics for primary care.* New York: Appleton–Century–Crofts, 1980, p. 139).

CHART 8.4

The Five Percussion Notes

	Relative Intensity	Relative Pitch	Relative Duration	Example of Location
Flatness	Soft	High	Short	Thigh
Dullness	Medium	Medium	Medium	Liver
Resonance	Loud	Low	Long	Normal lung
Hyper-resonance	Very loud	Lower	Longer	Emphysematous lung
Tympany	Loud	*	*	Gastric air bubble or puffed-out cheek

*Distinguished mainly by its musical timbre.

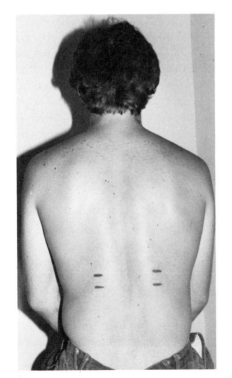

FIGURE 8.12. Markings showing percussed levels of diaphragmatic expanse.

vation and lowering of the diaphragm during breathing. (The examiner should keep in mind that the diaphragm descends with inspiration and ascends with expiration.) The procedure is as follows:

1. The patient takes a deep breath and holds it.
2. The examiner begins percussing downward along the midscapular line from the bottom of the scapula at about 3 cm intervals.
3. The point where the percussion note changes from resonance to dullness is noted and marked with a pen.
4. The patient is then asked to expire forcefully and hold his breath.
5. The nurse percusses upward from dullness to resonance, and the point of change is marked with a pen (Fig. 8.12).

The distance between these points is measured and the procedure is repeated on the opposite side. The average span of the diaphragm is 3 to 5 cm. It is normally slightly higher on the right side.

Auscultation. Auscultation is used to determine the existence of air, fluid, or solid mass in the lung. Any presence of the latter two will obstruct air flow to some degree, thus creating various auscultatory sounds. An overall decrease in air exchange will cause a lessening in the volume of the breath sounds. This can be the result of a disease process or the aging process in general.

To determine the status of the lungs, the examiner listens for normal breath sounds, adventitious (abnormal) breath sounds, and voice sounds. To auscultate the posterior thorax, the examiner simply places the diaphragm of the stethoscope on the chest at the points in Figure 8.10. The patient is asked to breathe in and out through his mouth slowly and deeply (more deeply than normal). Many consecutive deep breaths can cause light-headedness. The patient should be given a chance to rest between breaths, if necessary.

An array of breath sounds can be heard throughout the lungs. They will seem louder and more "raspy" in infants and young children. The sounds are named for their location over a specific region of the lung. They are evaluated in terms of their intensity, quality, pitch, duration, location, rate, and rhythm.

The three normal breath sounds are: *vesicular, bronchovesicular,* and *bronchial* (or tubular). Vesicular sounds are heard over most of the lung as a soft, low-pitched sound in which inspiration is longer than expiration. Bronchovesicular breath sounds are heard most clearly where the bronchi and trachea are close to the chest wall and along the scapular area. They are heard as a medium-pitched sound in which inspiration and expiration are about equal. Bronchial breathing produces a loud, high-pitched, blowing sound in which expiration is longer than inspiration. This is heard over the trachea; if it occurs anywhere else in the lung fields, it is always indicative of disease.

Adventitious breath sounds are often heard along with normal breath sounds. The most common abnormal sounds are: *rales, rhonchi,* and *friction rubs.*

Rales are noises that are created when air is traveling through vessels that have abnormal moisture in them (Fig. 8.13). These are noncontinuous noises that do not usually disappear with coughing. They are most frequently heard during inspiration. Rales are divided into three categories: *fine, medium,* and *coarse.* The gradation depends on the amount of moisture and the airway involved. The larger the airway, the louder the rale will be.

Fine rales sound like two hairs rubbing together next to the ear. They usually represent moisture in the alveoli. Fine rales can be heard in disease processes involving the alveoli, such as pneumonia or congestive heart failure.

Medium rales are about one degree louder than fine rales. The sound is that of opening a can of soda. These can be heard over the bronchioles, which are larger airways.

Coarse rales are the loudest of the three. They will be heard over the trachea and bronchi. Coarse rales have a gurgling, bubbling quality. They may change in intensity with coughing. Coarse rales usually represent extremely thickened secretions. This type of rale is

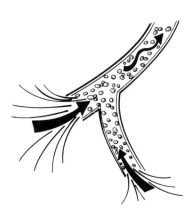

FIGURE 8.13. Air traveling through moisture.

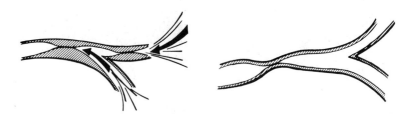

FIGURE 8.14. Air traveling through narrowed lumen.

often equated with the "death rattle" of critically ill or comatose patients.

Rhonchi are adventitious sounds that are the result of air passing through vessels that are narrowed or defective which is shown in Fig. 8.14. The alteration of the vessel contour by either internal or external compression creates these abnormal sounds. Rhonchi are due to the presence of exudate, inflammation, asthma, emphysema, or a solid mass. Rhonchi are more easily heard during expiration, although they may be audible during both phases. Rhonchi are characteristically alternated with coughing, especially if there are secretions in the airways in addition to a change in the vessel contour.

There are two types of rhonchi: *sibilant and sonorous.* Sibilant rhonchi are musical, high-pitched, and wheezy in nature. Sonorous rhonchi are lower-pitched and like snoring.[5]

The third adventitious breath sound is the friction rub. It is typically found in the anterior thorax and is discussed in the following section on that part of the chest (p. 171).

One other abnormality that can affect what the examiner hears in the chest is the loudness of the breath sounds. It has already been said that the normal aging process can cause a decrease in breath sounds. This decrease can also be produced by the existence of emphysema, obstruction, pneumothorax, pleural thickening, or any fluid in the pleural space. Although the sounds may be diminished, one may still be able to hear adventitious breath sounds. The sensations palpated with vocal fremitus can be auscultated, too. This is not usually done for screening purposes, but is implemented when pathology is suspected.

The stethoscope is placed in the same places as when listening for breath sounds. The patient is then asked to repeat certain words. The choice of sounds selected varies according to what is being evaluated. The words will be the loudest at the upper and middle lobes along the spinal column.

There are three abnormal voice sounds: *bronchophony, egophony,* and *whispered pectoriloquy.* Bronchophony is increased voice resonance, with the increase primarily in intensity and to some degree in clarity. For this test the patient is asked to repeat "99." The nurse listens over the designated areas. The exact syllables may not be distinct. Often accompanying bronchophony are increased fremitus, a dull percussion note, rales, and bronchial breathing. This combination of positive findings over a specific area probably indicates a consolidation.

Egophony is an increased version of bronchophony. The major difference is in the bleating quality of the voice sounds. The patient is asked to say a word with the end syllable having an "ee" sound to it, such as "Tennessee." The noise heard through the stethoscope will be an "a", so that "Tennessee" will sound like "Tennessā." This is most often heard in pulmonary consolidation.

Whispered pectoriloquy indicates a clear interpretation of what the examiner hears through the stethoscope when the patient whispers. The words will sound distinct, clearly like whispers to the examiner as she listens through the stethoscope. This is the most obvious of the three tests and it always indicates consolidation.

Examination of the Anterior Thorax*

*Unless otherwise indicated, the exam is the same as posterior thorax.

Inspection
  Skin*
  Thoracic contour*
  Rate and rhythm of breathing*

Palpation
  Lesions*
  Tenderness*
  Thoracic expanse — The thumbs of the examiner's hands are placed along the costal margins, while the rest of the hand lies on the lateral aspects of the rib cage. The rest of the procedure is identical to measuring the thoracic expanse on the posterior aspect.

  Vocal fremitus — The procedure is the same as for the posterior thorax. However, in a woman with breast tissue, fremitus will only be palpable in certain areas.

  Pleural friction rubs — This is a pathologic condition in which the pleural surfaces rub over one another. The sensation is that of two pieces of leather rubbing together. A friction rub is most easily palpated in the anterolateral chest. The mapped boundaries of decreased fremitus, increased fremitus, or a friction rub should be recorded specifically.

Percussion
  General orientation — The procedure is the same as for the posterior chest. The area around the heart and liver will produce a dull note. The gastric air bubble (see abdomen, p. 235) will be tympanic.

Auscultation
  Normal breath sounds*
  Adventitious breath sounds*
  Friction rub — This is the same as with palpation, except the rubbing sensation is heard, not felt.

  Voice sounds*

There are various acute and chronic conditions that affect the respiratory system. Chart 8.5 describes some of the more common respiratory illnesses in terms of the etiology and subjective and objective data.

CHART 8.5

Common Conditions of the Respiratory System

Condition	Age	Etiology	Subjective (Symptoms That May Be Present)	Objective (Signs That May Appear)
Croup	6 months–5 years	Usually viral (can be spasmodic and bacterial)	Barky cough—worse at night Hoarse Afebrile or low grade temp. Difficult breathing URI† symptoms may precede More comfortable sitting	Barky, nonproductive cough Hoarse ± Afebrile or low-grade temp.* Labored breathing Inspiratory stridor
Bronchial asthma	Pediatric	Usually allergic (can be infectious, exertional, or from environmental irritants or stress)	Known history of allergy or family history of allergy Cough SOB† Dyspnea Wheezing Abdominal or chest pain associated with labored breathing	Prolonged expiratory phase Expiratory wheezes SOB and tachypnea Hyperresonance in lungs Rales Intercostal retracting Use of respiratory accessory muscles ↑ A–P diameter Rhinorrhea Eczema
	Adult	(See Etiology, Pediatric above)	Recurrent eczema, etc. (See Subjective, Pediatric above)	(See Objective, Pediatric above)
Pneumonia	Any age	Viral, mycoplasmic (common in school-age children, adolescents, and young adults)	Insidious onset Malaise, fever (low grade) Headache, myalgia Cough after 2–3 days of symptoms; usually nonproductive or small amount Chest soreness on inspiration	Low grade temp. Nasal rhinorrhea Mild to moderate red throat Minimally red ear drums Cervical lymphadenopathy Fine to medium rales Rhonchi and/or wheezes over involved area
		Bacterial	Preceded by URI symptoms Shaking chills Elevated temp. Chest pain Cough, productive, "rust-colored" sputum Malaise, weakness, anorexia, myalgias	Elevated temp, rapid pulse and respiration Tenderness with palpation over involved area Warm, moist skin Shallow, labored breathing Possible cyanosis Dullness to percussion Possible bronchial breathing Fremitus, normal or ↑

Condition	Age	Etiology	Subjective (Symptoms That May Be Present)	Objectives (Signs That May Appear)
				Voice sounds (auscultated), normal or ↑ Crackling rales Possible friction rub
Bronchitis (acute)	Any age	Usually viral (may be bacterial)	Cough, productive, less than 1 tablespoon, mucopurulent Substernal chest pain Labored breathing URI symptoms preceding and associated	Temp. ↑ 101 Malaise, rhinorrhea Normal or resonant percussion note Rhonchi, wheezing, or both Normal or prolonged breath sounds Normal voice sounds and fremitus
Bronchitis (chronic)	±50	Diagnosis made on subjective data: productive cough at some time of the day for 3 months of the year for 2 or more consecutive years	Smoker for years Dusty occupation Productive cough— sputum on arising and produced again 1–2 times during day Mild dyspnea	Normal rate of respiration No distress at rest May be cyanotic Resonant percussion note Coarse rhonchi Wheezing Normal voice sounds and fremitus Normal or prolonged expiration
Emphysema	±60	Unknown	↑ Dyspnea with ↓ activity Minimal cough SOB History of chronic bronchitis, dusty occupation, smoking	SOB Rapid and shallow respiration Barrel-shaped chest Hyperresonant percussion note ↓ Breath sounds ↓ Voice sounds and fremitus Possible wheezes at the end of respiration
Congestive heart failure	Adult	Myocardial deterioration, often due to ASHD† and hypertension	Dyspnea with exertion Rapid, shallow breathing SOB Paroxysmal nocturnal dyspnea Orthopnea Ankle edema Nocturia	SOB Pallor Moist, clammy skin S_3-gallop rhythm Tachypnea Bilatral rales, especially in lower lobes Neck vein distension Bilateral dependent edema in the lower extremities

*A high fever may indicate epiglottitis.
†URI, upper respiratory infection; SOB, shortness of breath; ASHD, arteriosclerotic heart disease.

REFERENCES

1. Wasserman, H. *Ethnic pigmentation: Historical, physiological and clinical aspects.* Amsterdam: Excerpta Medica, 1974.
2. Selmanowitz, V. & Krivo, J. Pigmentary demarcation lines: Comparison of Negroes with Japanese. *British Journal of Dermatology*, 1975, *93*, 371–377.
3. Yeatman, G., Shaw, C., Barlow, M., Bartlett, G. Pseudobattering in Vietnamese children. *Pediatrics*, 1976, *58*, 616–618.
4. Bates, B. *A guide to physical examination* (2nd ed.). New York: Lippincott, 1979, p. 126.
5. Prior J., Silberstein J. *Physical diagnosis: The history and examination of the patient* (4th ed.). St. Louis: Mosby, 1973, p. 199.

EXAMPLE OF A RECORDED HISTORY AND PHYSICAL

Subjective:

Chief Complaint: "My baby has been wheezing for about 2 hours."

HPI: The mother of this 2-year-old states that the baby is in "fair health." He has a 12-month history of this problem. The first episode occurred one day when he went to the baby sitter's and they had a new dog. Baby's mother was called home from work and found the child breathing "fast and hard" and could hear "gurgling" when he "breathed out." She took him to the emergency ward and they gave him "a shot to help him breathe." A prescription was given for "Theophylline Elixir," 1 teaspoon every 6 hours for his wheezing. "The doctor told me he has asthma." The mother states she uses the medicine once a month when "his breath gets short."

Today he was brought in because the same hard breathing started and 1 teaspoon of the medication did not help. The mother noticed his "rib cage moving funny" and he got "very pale. His wheezing was worse than usual." He had a new terry cloth outfit on and was playing outside in the grass. There was no nasal flaring; no runny nose or previous cold; no animals around; and no new soaps, foods, or linens. There has not been any allergy testing, but dogs and cats do bring on symptoms. No foods bother the patient.

His father had a history of asthma as a child. His mother states that the problem is "frightening and seems to be getting worse."

Objective: T. 99° F (rectal); P. 146 (radial); R. 52; B.P. 90/54 (sitting)

Skin: Pale and diaphoretic. No cyanosis of lips, hands, feet, earlobes. No rashes or lesions.

Nose: No rhinorrhea or nasal flaring.

Chest: Intercostal retractions and use of accessory muscles to breathe. Respirations are rapid and shallow. Bilateral hyperresonance over lung fields. Expiratory wheezes audible in both lungs—middle lobes. Prolonged expiratory phase. No rales. No change in fremitus or voice sounds.

9

The Cardiac and Peripheral Vascular System

"The heart is the physiologic pump of the body." Such a sterile, technical statement! In truth and in legend, it is much more. Artists and philosophers have for centuries devoted much of their writing to the heart; it was even viewed by some to be the soul. The heart is often personified and seems to possess its own essence. Anyone reading this chapter has experienced and voiced the expressions, "a heartful of love," "a broken heart," etc.

This chapter deals with the examination of the cardiac and peripheral vascular system. The heart is the unquestioned star. It should be pictured as a unique instrument expressing and reflecting the integrity of its holistic system. It will function inadequately when one of its arteries is occluded. The "heavy" heart of the unhappy, tense, or depressed person has just as important an effect on the whole system of the person.

HISTORY

The cardiac history of the child is elicited to identify children with congenital heart defects. Approximately, 8 to 10 per 1,000 live-born children have congenital cardiac disorders.[1] Some of these defects are detectable at birth or in early infancy and others are not evident until later childhood. Identifiable defects are referred for medical evaluation.

Symptoms of congenital heart disease in children include anorexia, falling asleep after drinking a few ounces of milk, continuous squatting, sleeping in the knee–chest position, decreased exercise tolerance, cyanosis, dyspnea, delayed development, and frequent respiratory infections. It is particularly important to help the parent recall information related to exercise and behavior. The following questions may be helpful in prompting the parent's memory:

1. Does the child play as long as the other children or does he sometimes come home without being called?
2. Does he squat in the middle of play?
3. Does he run easily and go up and down stairs without difficulty?
4. Does he seem to play with the same energy as his siblings do?
5. Does he seem to be growing as fast as his siblings?

Additional data to obtain from the parent include any previous history of mumps, group A β-hemolytic streptococcal infections, rheumatic fever, or maternal rubella during pregnancy.

Pertinent family history is important for all age groups. It is presented here to conclude the history for the child and to introduce necessary information for the adult.

The family history should include information on incidence of heart disease (including age of occurrence), high cholesterol levels, type II hyperlipoproteinemia (familial hypercholesterolemia), high blood pressure, stroke, obesity, congenital heart disease in siblings or other family member, and rheumatic fever.[1]

The goal of the adult cardiovascular history is to detect underlying cardiac disease and to identify cardiac risk factors. Symptoms to be reviewed that indicate cardiovascular disease include: dyspnea, orthopnea, paroxysmal nocturnal dyspnea, edema, cough, hemoptysis, chest pain, wheezing, palpitations, syncope, claudication, fatigue, and a history of hypertension. Of significance is a past history of heart murmur, rheumatic fever, heart failure, heart attack, or varicosities, with or without thrombophlebitis. The examiner should be alert to a history of diseases that involve the heart, including diabetes, obesity, lung disease, endocrine and metabolic disorders, and syphilis.

Data collected regarding the patient's habits and lifestyle can point to potential risk factors. The nurse should inquire about the patient's smoking, alcohol use, eating, and exercise patterns. She should identify areas of stress and anxiety in the patient's work and family relationships. It is also important to determine the patient's perception of his psychological well-being and satisfaction with self.

The cardiac history for the elderly includes what has already been presented for the younger adult. In viewing the elderly client, it is helpful to bear in mind that his system has aged. An evaluation of this client is directed toward compensation, stability, and maintenance of lifestyle and daily patterns of behavior.

Cardiovascular disease is one of the chief hazards to life for those over 50. Frequently, the patient will have already experienced stress or damage to the cardiovascular system. The history then will be concerned with symptoms indicating change or increased damage. Particular symptoms to watch for are increased respiratory effort, fatigue, and edema of the extremities. It is important to determine if these symptoms represent a change or are relatively stable. A change is often expressed by the patient as an inability to maintain his daily routine.

ANATOMY AND PHYSIOLOGY

The Heart

The heart is examined through the anterior chest wall. Figure 9.1 depicts the heart and its location in the chest. The heart is located in the center of the chest, under the sternum, and somewhat to the left of the midline. The upper portion is called the base and the tip is the apex. The apex is about 8 cm to the left of the sternum, at the level of the fifth intercostal space, in the midclavicular line. The heart almost appears to lie on its side. It is divided into four chambers—the right and left atria and the right and left ventricles. Most of the heart accessible to examination is the *right ventricle*. The left ventricle presents a much smaller surface to the examiner. It projects a tip that rests at the apex. The *left ventricle* is of critical importance, as it forms the *left border* of the heart and *produces* the *apical impulse* or *point of maximum impulse* (PMI). The *right border* of the heart is formed by the *right atrium*. Neither the right nor the left atrium is directly accessible to examination.

The Cardiac Cycle. Blood flows from one chamber to the other through valves (Fig. 9.2). The triscupid valve is located between the right atrium and the right ventricle and controls the flow of blood between the two. The corresponding valve on the left is the mitral valve, which controls blood flow from the left atrium to the left ventricle. Because of their positions, these valves are also called atrioventricular valves.

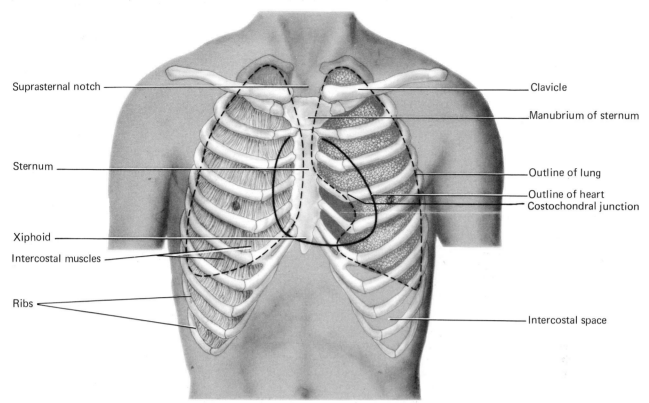

Suprasternal notch

Clavicle

Manubrium of sternum

Sternum

Outline of lung

Outline of heart
Costochondral junction

Xiphoid

Intercostal muscles

Ribs

Intercostal space

FIGURE 9.1. The thorax: thoracic cage and position of organs within it. (From Heagarty, M., Glass, G., King, H., & Manly, M. *Child health: Basics for primary care.* New York: Appleton–Century–Crofts, 1980, p. 138).

Blood leaves the left ventricle to enter the aorta via the aortic valve. Similarly, blood passes to the pulmonary artery from the right ventricle via the pulmonic valve. The pulmonic and aortic valves have a half-moon appearance and for this reason are often called the semilunar valves.

Closure of the valves is responsible for the first and second heart sounds. In order to adequately explain heart function and sounds, it is necessary to begin with a description of pressure within each chamber and the role the varying pressures play in valve closure. Events in the cardiac cycle are described as they occur in the left side of the heart. This is done for three reasons:

1. The left side of the heart carries the greatest workload.
2. It is therefore often the first to become deficient.
3. The whole process is easier to understand if it is explained in this manner.

Blood flows into the left atrium from the pulmonary veins. As the left atrium fills with blood, its pressure eventually becomes greater than the pressure in the left ventricle. When that happens, the mitral valve opens, the left atrium contracts, and the blood is pumped into the left ventricle. As the pressure builds in the left ventricle, the mitral valve closes. *Closure of the mitral valve is responsible for the first heart sound.* The pressure in the left ventricle continues to rise. When the pressure in the left ventricle exceeds the pressure in the aorta, the aortic valve opens and blood is ejected

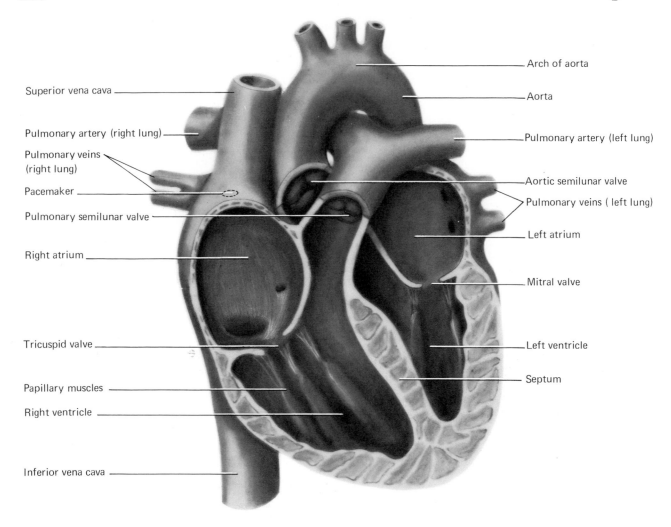

Superior vena cava

Pulmonary artery (right lung)

Pulmonary veins
(right lung)

Pacemaker

Pulmonary semilunar valve

Right atrium

Tricuspid valve

Papillary muscles

Right ventricle

Inferior vena cava

Arch of aorta

Aorta

Pulmonary artery (left lung)

Aortic semilunar valve

Pulmonary veins (left lung)

Left atrium

Mitral valve

Left ventricle

Septum

FIGURE 9.2. The heart and great vessels. (From Heagarty, M., Glass, G., King, H., & Manly, M. *Child health: Basics for primary care.* New York: Appleton–Century–Crofts, 1980, p. 144).

into the aorta. As the pressure in the aorta builds, the aortic valve closes to prevent regurgitation of blood back into the left ventricle. *Closure of the aortic valve is responsible for the second heart sound.*

Events on the right side of the heart occur in a similar manner, but at much lower pressures. *The manner in which myocardial depolarization occurs and the effects of respiration on heart sounds cause events on the right side of the heart to occur slightly later than those on the left.* This is an important fact to remember and will be helpful later in the chapter in determining pathologic sounds.

Heart sounds are given names. S_1 refers to the first heart sound—i.e., closure of the mitral and tricuspid valves. S_2 refers to the second heart sound—i.e., closure of the aortic and pulmonic valves. There are two additional S sounds which may or may not be normal. S_3 *(third heart sound)* is the sound made by the flow of blood from the left atrium to the left ventricle. It is a normal sound when heard in children and young adults. S_4 *(fourth heart sound)* is the sound that marks atrial contraction. This sound is termed an atrial gallop and can be normal.* It is more often related to increased resistance to ventricular filling following atrial contraction and is produced by cardiac pathology.

*"Normal," as used here, means "non-pathologic" rather than "usual."

Systole and Diastole. Flow of blood through the heart has been discussed and related to varying pressures in the chambers of the heart. The first and second heart sounds have been explained. Figure 9.3 depicts these events occurring in a circle as S_1 and S_2 follow each other in a continuous repetitive sequence.

Now that S_1 and S_2 have been explained, they can be related to systole and diastole. *Systole is the period of time occurring between S_1 and S_2.* The circle can then be depicted as in Figure 9.4.

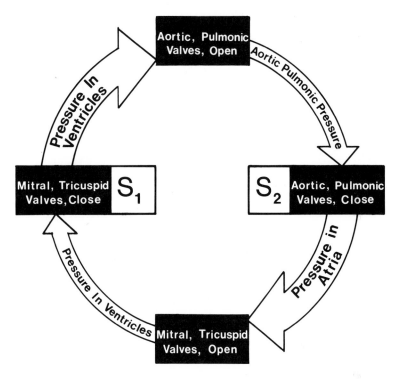

FIGURE 9.3. Events occurring in the cardiac cycle.

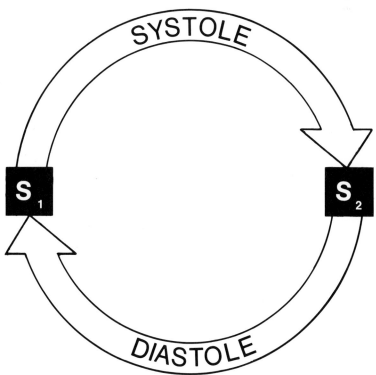

FIGURE 9.4. Diagram depicting systole and diastole in relation to the first cand second heart sounds.

It is important to remember that systole and diastole are periods of time and that particular events occur during each period. Normally, the ventricles contract during systole and relax during diastole. The pressure curve is therefore highest in systole, as the pressure in the ventricle rises to a peak of 120 mm/Hg. Pressure falls to almost zero in diastole as the ventricle relaxes. Late in diastole there is a small rise in pressure represented by the extra volume of blood sent into the ventricles by atrial contraction. Figure 9.5 depicts these relationships.

Location of Heart Sounds. Figure 9.6 depicts the point at which sound is best heard as compared to the location of the valve responsible for the sound.

From Figure 9.6 it is easy to see that the *sound is not heard directly over the valve producing it.* The most obvious theory to explain this occurrence is that the valve closes with force, the blood is ejected forward, and the sound is heard along the trajectory of the ejected blood. Thus:

1. Closure of the *mitral* valve is heard in the left fifth intercostal space just medial to the midclavicular line.
2. Closure of the *tricuspid* valve is heard in the left fifth intercostal space close to the sternum.
3. Closure of the *aortic valve* is heard in the right second intercostal space close to the sternum.
4. Closure of the *pulmonic valve* is heard in the left second intercostal space close to the sternum.

Note the inclusion of Erb's point in Figure 9.6. This area is

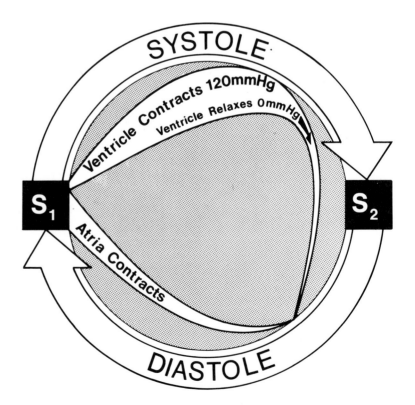

FIGURE 9.5. Pressure changes within the heart during systole and diastole.

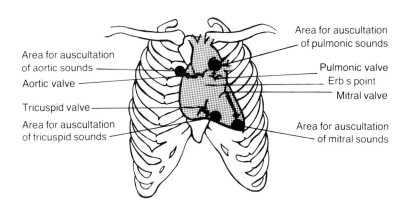

Area for auscultation of pulmonic sounds

Area for auscultation of aortic sounds

Pulmonic valve

Aortic valve

Erb's point

Mitral valve

Tricuspid valve

Area for auscultation of tricuspid sounds

Area for auscultation of mitral sounds

FIGURE 9.6. Anatomic position of the valves compared to areas of auscultation for those valves.

included because murmurs of aortic and pulmonic origin can often be heard in this area. It is located in the third intercostal space close to the sternum.

S_1 and S_2 are audible all over the precordium. Figure 9.6, however, helps in understanding why *S_2 is loudest at the base and S_1 is loudest at the apex.* This knowledge is important and will help during auscultation as the examiner attempts to place abnormal sounds heard within systole and diastole.

Variations in Heart Sounds

First Heart Sound. Pressure is greatest on the left side of the heart; therefore sounds produced by the left side of the heart are longer and louder. Events on the left side slightly precede those on the right. Usually both components of S_1 are heard as one sound, but they are sometimes heard with a slight split. This can be normal but is not heard as frequently as the splitting of S_2 sounds. Such a split is obvious in the tricuspid area. Pathologically, the tricuspid sound is more pronounced with pulmonary hypertension. Although the mitral sound is usually loudest, it may be unduly exaggerated with mitral stenosis. However, a very stenotic mitral valve that moves very little may produce a muffled sound. If the mitral sound is increased, it will be heard in the mitral area.

A louder S_1 with or without splitting may be produced extracardially by the increased metabolic states in exercise, fever, thyrotoxicosis, and anemia.

Second Heart Sound. The ejection time of the right ventricle is slightly longer than the left; therefore the pulmonic valve closes slightly after the aortic. This normal variation is increased during inspiration because of the decreased intrathoracic pressure which facilitates an increase in venous return to the right side of the heart. This further delays pulmonic valve closure and produces what is known as a *physiologic splitting* of S_2. That is to say, the splitting of S_2 varies with respiration, is increased with inspiration, and decreases or disappears (the split disappears, not S_2) with expiration. The splitting is most evident in the pulmonic area.

S_2 is further divided according to the two sounds responsible for it. Thus A_2 refers to the portion of S_2 produced by the closure of the aortic valve, while P_2 represents the closure of the pulmonic valve. It is not unusual to see just "A_2" or "P_2" written when an author wishes to discuss one of the components of S_2.

Abnormal splitting of S_2 occurs with essential hypertension in which the aortic sound becomes very loud and most pronounced in the aortic area. S_2 is abnormally increased in the pulmonic area with pulmonary hypertension and congestive heart failure.

The normally split S_2 may be varied abnormally with a widened, fixed, or paradoxic splitting. A widened splitting is associated with right bundle branch block (delayed pulmonic valve closure). Atrial septal defects produce a fixed splitting of S_2, which means that the split does not vary with respiration. Paradoxic splitting, a reversal of normal splitting (splitting of S_2 is normally increased with inspiration), occurs with left bundle branch block.

Third Heart Sound. As previously described, S_3 is produced by the blood flowing from the atria to the ventricles in early diastole. It is a normal sound in children and young adults. In the older person, an S_3 may signify myocardial failure. S_3's closeness to S_2 produces a triple sound like a galloping horse and is sometimes called a ventricular gallop. *The sound of S_3 is best heard at the apex with the bell of the stethoscope, with the patient lying in the left-lateral decubitus position.*

Fourth Heart Sound. S_4 immediately precedes S_1 and is heard in late diastole. It is marked by atrial contraction and can normally be heard in a young person with a thin chest wall. It is, however, less often a normal sound than S_3. Pathologically, S_4 results from an increased resistance to filling of the ventricles and is associated with hypertensive cardiovascular disease, coronary artery disease, or aortic stenosis. An S_4 may also be associated with hyperthyroidism or anemia.

Because S_4 falls so closely in diastole to S_1, the sound produced is a triple sound again, akin to a galloping horse; thus its additional title of *presystolic* or *atrial gallop*. As with S_3, *S_4 is best heard at the apex with the bell of the stethoscope.* Figure 9.7 depicts S_3 and S_4 as they are related to the cardiac cycle.

Abnormal Extra Heart Sounds. There are two basic abnormal extra heart sounds: the ejection clicks heard in systole and the opening snaps heard in diastole. Both clicks and snaps are caused by diseased heart valves.

Of the clicks in systole, the *aortic click* is the most common. *It is heard at the base and apex and does not vary with respiration.* Pulmonic clicks are loudest in the pulmonic area and vary with respiration, increasing with expiration and decreasing with inspiration. Both these clicks are heard in early systole. Less common are mid- and late-systolic clicks which are associated with a ballooning mitral valve with a coexistent murmur.

Opening snaps are very early diastolic sounds. They are most often related to a stenotic mitral valve, and rarely to a stenotic tricuspid valve. *Mitral snaps are usually heard inside the apex with diffuse radiation toward the lower-left sternal border.* Snaps are not affected by respiration. Figure 9.8 depicts the occurrence of S_3, S_4, clicks, and snaps in the cardiac cycle and displays where they are best heard.

Pericardial Friction Rubs. When the pericardial sac becomes inflamed, the surfaces rub together, producing a scraping sound much like two ballons being rubbed together. It is a distinct, unforgettable

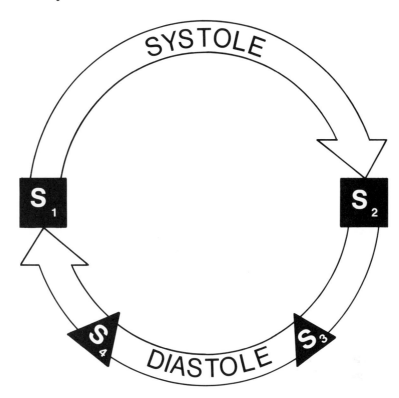

FIGURE 9.7. Occurrence of S_3 and S_4 in the cardiac cycle.

sound, not easily confused with heart sounds or murmurs, which does not vary with respiration and is best heard at the apex and sternum.

Murmurs. Murmurs are "whooshing" sounds occurring in various stages of systole or diastole. They are related to one of three factors:

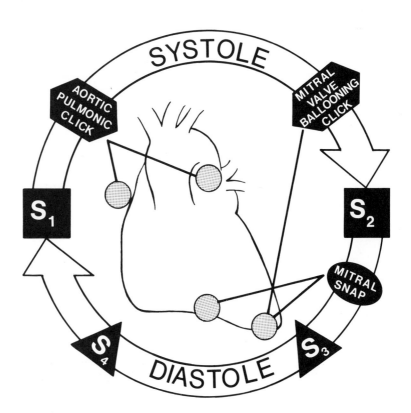

FIGURE 9.8. Occurrence of S_3, S_4, clicks, and snaps in the cardiac cycle, with auscultatory areas included.

(1) an increased rate of blood flow, (2) a forced forward flow through an incompetent valve, or (3) a back flow through an incompetent valve, a septal defect, or patent ductus arteriosus.

There are eight characteristics of murmurs. These eight are critical to commit to memory as they are always included in a written objective description. More important, however, if a murmur can be described according to the eight characteristics, it can lead the examiner, step by step, to the most probable cause of the murmur. It is not unusual for the student to be unsure of what she hears. After methodically working through all eight characteristics, however, the light often dawns. The examiner can distinguish functional from abnormal murmurs and have a very good idea of the cause of the abnormality. The eight characteristics of murmurs are:

1. Timing
2. Frequency or pitch
3. Location
4. Intensity
5. Radiation
6. Quality
7. Effect of respiration
8. Effect of position

Timing. Murmurs are described according to the cardiac cycle in which they are heard. They are, therefore, systolic or diastolic murmurs. In addition, they are described according to the period of time they are heard in the cycle—i.e., early, mid, late, or holo or pan (heard throughout the cycle). For example, a systolic murmur might be: (1) early systolic, (2) midsystolic, (3) late systolic, or (4) holosystolic or pansystolic.

Frequency or Pitch. Frequency or pitch varies from high to medium to low.

Location. The point at which the murmur is the loudest is described in terms of location over the particular cardiac area (e.g., aortic area) or particular interspaces and in terms of centimeters from the midsternal, midclavicular, or axillary line.

Intensity. Loudness of the murmur is described according to a scale varying from I (softest) to VI (loudest).

Grade I: Very faint, heard only after the listener has listened carefully.
Grade II: Quiet, but heard immediately with the stethoscope.
Grade III: Moderately loud, not associated with a thrill (a thrill is a fine vibration palpated with the ball of the hand).
Grade IV: Loud, may be associated with a thrill.
Grade V: Very loud, may be heard with the stethoscope partly off the chest; associated with a thrill.
Grade VI: May be heard with the stethoscope off the chest; associated with a thrill.

The intensity of the murmur is written as a Roman numeral fraction. For example, if the listener hears a Grade II murmur it is written as Gr II/VI. The numerator represents the existing murmur and the denominator represents the maximum possible grades.

Loudness of the murmur is also described according to the pattern of intensity. Words are borrowed from music to describe the varying intensity. The most frequently used terms are crescendo (building to a climax) and decrescendo (starting at a climax and dropping off). *It should be remembered that the crescendo or decrescendo intensity will occur in one of the cardiac cycles.* It is helpful to picture this variation in intensity as being like the vibrations of a tuning fork or to picture what such variations might look like on a tracing from an echocardiogram. A systolic crescendo murmur, for example, would look like the tracing in Figure 9.9. A decrescendo murmur would then look like Figure 9.10.

As in music, there are variations in this theme. Murmurs can be crescendo–decrescendo (also known as diamond-shaped). The crescendo–decrescendo murmur would look like the tracing in Figure 9.11. Finally, murmurs can have a consistent intensity that is heard throughout systole or diastole. The term for this type of murmur is pansystolic of holosystolic. The pansystolic murmur would look like Figure 9.12. Similar variations occur and can be described in diastole.

Radiation. It is important to describe where the murmur is loudest, but the murmur must also be described in terms of radiation of the sound. The examiner should indicate whether or not the murmur radiates into the neck over the carotid arteries (unilaterally or bilaterally), down the left sternal border, or to the axillary line.

Quality. Descriptive terms should be used to give the murmur a character. Examples of such terms are: musical, blowing, harsh, and rumbling.

Effect of Respiration. The examiner should note whether the murmur increases, decreases, or disappears with inspiration or expiration.

Effect of Position. The examiner should determine whether the murmur increases, decreases, or disappears when the patient is in the sitting or supine position. Aortic sounds are increased when the patient is in the sitting position, leaning forward, and mitral sounds are accentuated when the patient is supine and lying on his left side.

Innocent and Functional Murmurs. Not all murmurs are pathologic. It is estimated that 30 to 50 percent of infants and young children have innocent murmurs (no demonstrable pathology). There are several theories that explain this phenomenon, but the most plausible is that the chest wall is thinner and the sounds have higher pitches in children.

The term "functional" is sometimes used interchangeably with "innocent" to describe murmurs. Generally, however, innocent murmurs refer to those found in childhood. Functional murmurs occur in the abscence of structural changes in the heart and disappear when the causative factor is remedied. The following paragraph gives examples of functional murmurs.

Pregnant women after the eighth week of pregnancy have an increasing circulating blood volume. It is, therefore, not abnormal to detect a murmur in the second and especially the third trimesters. Fever and acute infections will also sometimes produce murmurs that resolve with the infection.

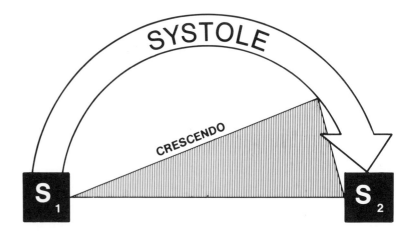

FIGURE 9.9. The crescendo murmur.

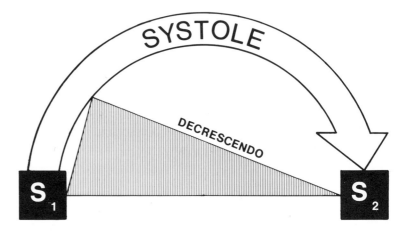

FIGURE 9.10. The decrescendo murmur.

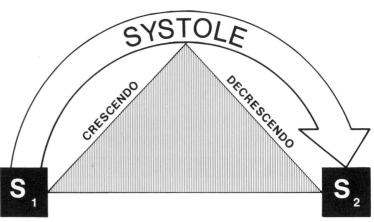

FIGURE 9.11. The diamond-shaped or crescendo–decrescendo murmur.

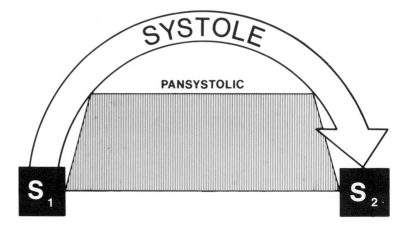

FIGURE 9.12. The holosystolic or pansystolic murmur.

Innocent and functional murmurs have particular characteristics in common that help to distinguish them from abnormal sounds. They are:

1. Usually systolic, except for the venous hum.
2. Usually of short duration.
3. Usually loudest at the lower-left sternal border or at the second- or third-left intercostal space.
4. Varying in loudness and presence from visit to visit.
5. Usually soft (no more than Grade II/VI and localized).
6. Rarely transmitted.
7. Of varying loudness with changes in position.
8. Heard best in the recumbent position, during expiration, and after exercise, except for the venous hum.
9. Associated with normal heart sounds.
10. Accompanied by normal pulses, respiratory rate, and blood pressure.[2]

The venous hum was mentioned twice in the list above. Venous hums are normal, murmur-like sounds that are often confused with abnormalities. They are produced by blood flow through the jugular veins. They are heard under the clavicles, in the neck, and to the right and left of the sternal border. The murmur that is produced is low-pitched, ranges as high as Grade III–IV/VI and is continuous throughout the cardiac cycle. It may vary with respiration and disappear in the supine position. It can be eliminated by tilting or rotating the head, occluding the veins in the neck with the examiner's thumb, or performing the Valsalva maneuver. The Valsalva maneuver is performed by asking the patient to exhale forcibly while holding his mouth and nose closed. It increases intrathoracic pressure and impedes venous return to the heart.

The Peripheral Vascular System

Arteries and Pulses. Pressure changes in the left ventricle as it contracts are transmitted as pressure waves to the root of the aorta. These pressure waves are then transmitted to the peripheral arteries, where they can be palpated as pulses. The pressure waves of the arteries travel much faster than the circulating blood within them. It takes the red blood cell about 2½ seconds to go from the left ventricle to the dorsalis pedis area, whereas the pressure transmitted by the contraction of the left ventricle will be palpated over the dorsalis pedis pulse in considerably less than ½ second. The arteries expand and contract in rhythm as they transmit pressure waves. All arteries exhibit a pulse throughout, but these pulses are normally palpated only when the artery is close to the skin and overlying a bone. Arterial pulses are evaluated according to five characteristics:

1. Condition of the wall
2. Rate and rhythm
3. Quality or amplitude
4. Type or contour
5. Equality

Condition of the Wall. This is checked first because other characteristics will be affected if the condition of the wall is altered. The arterial wall is normally elastic. Abnormally, it may be described as thickened, hard, rigid, beaded, inelastic, or calcified.

Rate and Rhythm. Rate is termed normal, rapid, or slow. The definition of the rapid and slow pulse varies, but a rate above 100 is generally agreed to be rapid (tachycardia), and a rate below 60 is termed slow (bradycardia).

Rhythm is described as regular or irregular. An irregular pulse is caused by a cardiac arrhythmia. The physiology of arrhythmias is beyond the scope of this book, but the most frequent causes are atrial fibrillation; atrial flutter, with varying heart block; second degree heart block, with varying dropped beats; sinus irregularity; and premature beats. An irregularity in pulse will be palpated in the peripheral arteries as missed beats. That is to say that the actual heart rate will not be palpated peripherally because of the irregularity. The difference between peripheral arterial rate and actual heart rate is termed *pulse deficit.*

Quality or Amplitude. Arterial pressure waves can be depicted graphically. As the pressure is transmitted, it produces a wave that reaches its peak as the ventricle contracts in systole and falls to its low point as the ventricle relaxes in diastole. Pulse quality or amplitude is the extent of the divergence between systolic and diastolic pressure waves. On a graph the normal amplitude would appear as it does in Figure 9.13.

Amplitude of the pulse is regularly described as strong or weak. The strong pulse appears in Figure 9.14. The weak pulse is depicted in Figure 9.15.

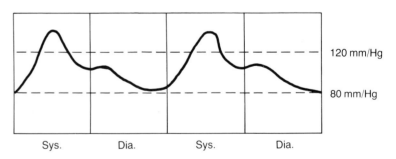

FIGURE 9.13. Amplitude of the normal pulse.

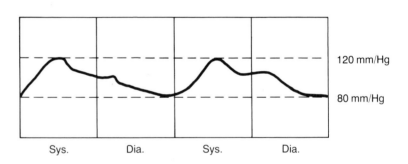

FIGURE 9.14. Amplitude of the strong pulse.

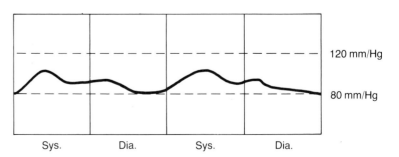

FIGURE 9.15. Amplitude of the weak pulse.

Strong pulses are most often associated with increased cardiac output. Frequent causes are stress, fear, fever, and increased physical activity. A weak pulse will have two basic causes: (1) partial occlusion of an artery (the weak pulse will be palpated distally to the occlusion), and (2) any abnormality reducing cardiac output, such as endocardial lesions, myocardial disease, pericardial disease, or shock.

In addition to defining pulses as weak or strong, they are given a rating on a scale of 0 to 4:

0: No pulses.
1: Pulse is thready, weak, and difficult to palpate; it may fade in and out and is easily obliterated with pressure.
2: Pulse is difficult to palpate and may be obliterated with pressure, so light palpation is necessary; once located, it is stronger than 1.
3: Pulse is easily palpable, does not fade in and out, and is not easily obliterated by pressure; *this is considered to be the normal pulse.*
4: Pulse is strong or bounding, easily palpated, and not obliterated with pressure; in some cases, such as aortic regurgitation, it may be considered pathologic.[3]

There are two abnormalities associated with pulse amplitude that are worthy of mention. *Pulsus alterans* is an alteration of a weak and strong beat, as in Figure 9.16. It occurs with abnormal heart function, particularly left ventricular heart failure. *Pulsus paradoxus* is a change in amplitude with respiration. Amplitude is decreased with inspiration and returns to full amplitude in expiration, as in Figure 9.17. Pulsus paradoxus occurs when one of the following conditions exists:

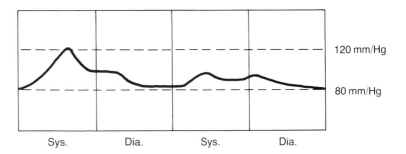

FIGURE 9.16. Pulsus alterans.

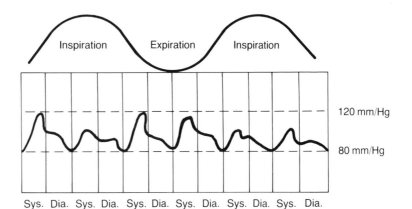

FIGURE 9.17. Pulsus paradoxus.

1. Impairment of return of venous blood to the right ventricle during inspiration (pericardial effusion, constrictive pericarditis).
2. Gross exaggeration of diaphragmatic and rib cage movements during inspiration (tracheal obstruction, asthma, emphysema).
3. Normal forced expiration.

Type or Contour. Contour or type of pulse is defined as the speed of the rise of the pressure wave in systole, the duration of the summit, and the speed with which the wave falls back to the diastolic level. There are three variations in contour from the normal pulse.

Plateau pulse occurs with endocardial lesions and is manifested by a decreased amplitude, a slower rise in systole, a longer summit, and a more gradual fall in diastole. It is classically associated with aortic stenosis and appears on a graph as shown in Figure 9.18.

A *waterhammer pulse* is felt as a knock-like sensation and is characterized by increased amplitude, a rapid rise in systole, a high momentary peak, and a sudden fall in diastole. It is classically associated with aortic insufficiency and appears on a graph as shown in Figure 9.19.

Pulsus bisferiens was created just to confuse us all and is a combination of aortic stenosis and aortic insufficiency. The resultant wave is a combination of a rather rapid rise to a summit with a double impulse at the summit and a weak falling off to the diastolic level. This appears in Figure 9.20.

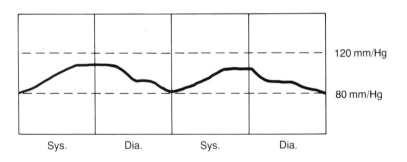

FIGURE 9.18. Plateau pulse.

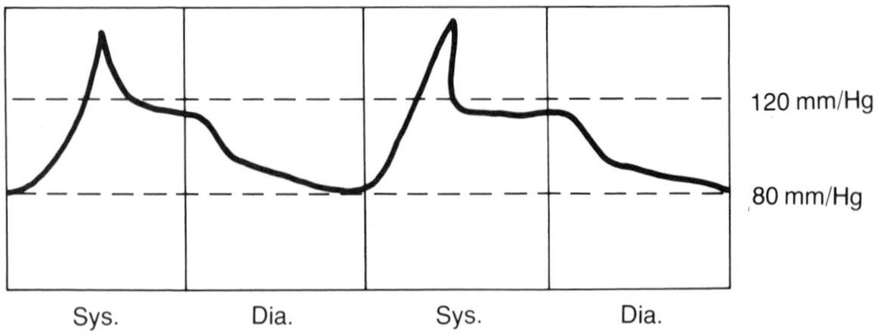

FIGURE 9.19. Waterhammer pulse.

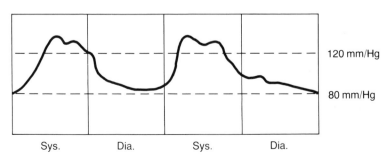

FIGURE 9.20. Pulsus bisferiens.

Equality. All of the pulses are compared to each other for equality and symmetry. Inequality is related either to an abnormally placed artery or to an obstruction.

Veins and Pulses. Venous pulses and waves are evaluated at the external and internal jugular veins. Pressure in the venous system is significantly lower than in the arterial. Extent of venous pressure is dependent upon the relative force with which the left ventricle contracts. Pressure is also affected by blood volume, the ability of the right atrium to receive venous blood and pass it to the right ventricle, and the right ventricle's subsequent ability to eject blood into the pulmonary system. When any of these variables are altered, venous pressure will be affected—it will fall when blood volume or left ventricular force decreases and it will rise when blood flow to the right atrium is impeded. *Congestive heart failure is the most frequent cause of increased venous pressure.*

Figure 9.21 depicts the location of the external and internal jugular veins. The external jugular veins are the most superficial and most visible and lie above the clavicle close to the insertion of the sternocleidomastoid muscles. Visualization of the internal jugular veins is more difficult, as they lie deep to the sternocleidomastoid and are quite close to the carotid arteries. Visible pulses from the internal jugular veins are seen in the surrounding soft tissues. Measurement of internal jugular pressure is more accurate than measurement of external jugular pressure.

The internal jugular pulse is composed primarily of two waves, *a* and *v*, that give information on right atrial pressure. The *a* wave is produced by atrial contraction and has a quick rise and fall. The *v* wave occurs during ventricular contraction but is produced by a build-up of pressure in the right atrium. It rises slowly and falls rapidly after the fall of the carotid pulse. The descent of the *v* wave is what is actually noted, and this is sometimes referred to as the *y* descent. Figure 9.22 depicts the relationship of the *a* and *v* waves

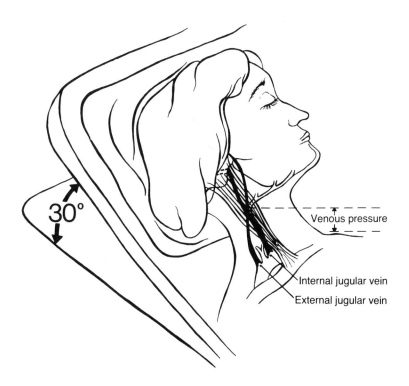

FIGURE 9.21. Location of the external and internal jugular veins.

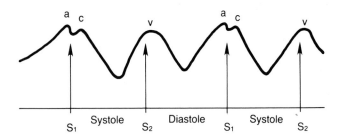

FIGURE 9.22. Pulse waves of the internal jugular pulse.

and the y descent to the cardiac cycle. The c represents a reflection of the carotid artery. The a wave amplitude is increased in patients with tricuspid stenosis, pulmonary stenosis, or pulmonary hypertension. The v wave amplitude is increased with an incompetent tricuspid valve.

PHYSICAL ASSESSMENT

Assessment of the cardiac and peripheral vascular system includes:

1. Blood pressure
2. Peripheral pulses
3. Examination for phlebitis
4. The heart
5. Great vessels of the neck

Necessary equipment includes a sphygmomanometer, a stethoscope with a bell and a diaphragm, a penlight, and a centimeter ruler. The blood pressure is usually taken at the onset of a complete physical exam and the peripheral pulses are integrated with examination of the skin and musculoskeletal system. The great vessels of the neck may be checked at the time of examination of the thyroid and lymph nodes of the neck. Examination of the heart follows examination of the lungs.

Blood Pressure

To obtain an accurate blood pressure reading, it is important to obtain an appropriately-sized cuff. The cuff should not be more than 20 percent wider than the diameter of the patient's limb and should be long enough to completely encircle it. A bag that is too narrow or short will produce readings that are falsely high. A large cuff will result in falsely low readings. If the patient is very obese, it may be necessary to use a thigh cuff on his arm.

In an initial screening, the blood pressure is taken in three positions (lying, sitting, and standing) and in the left and right arms and in one leg. The thigh blood pressure is equal to that in the arm before 1 year of age. After the first year, systolic pressure is slightly higher in the lower extremities because larger muscle masses in the thighs produce an increased resistance to compression of the artery. If the pressure in the thighs is lower than the arms, *coarctation of the aorta* should be suspected.

To take the blood pressure, the patient should be in a relaxed position with his arm flexed. If the blood pressure is taken in only one arm, the same arm should be used each time, as the pressure will normally vary 10 to 15 mm between the right and left arm. The nurse should wrap the cuff around the arm so that it is 2 to 3 cm above the antecubital area. She should then palpate the brachial artery and place the diaphragm of the stethoscope over it in the antecubital area and below but not underneath the cuff. The next step is to inflate the cuff 30 to 40 mm Hg above the level at which the radial pulse disappears and then slowly deflate the cuff. The tappings and murmurs heard while taking the blood pressure are called Korotkoff sounds. Three sounds are read and recorded. The first sound, a sudden tapping, is the systolic blood pressure. The next reading is at the point where the sounds become muffled. The third reading is where the sounds disappear. There is a debate as to whether the diastolic pressure is indicated by the muffling or the disappearing sound. Both should be recorded for accuracy.

Information on hypertension and cardiovascular disease has led to an increased effort to monitor blood pressure in children. Cuffs are available for infants and small children. Because hypertension is more frequent in Blacks and appears in this population at considerably earlier ages, particular attention must be given to obtaining the blood pressures of Black patients. Chart 9.1 depicts normal values of blood pressure for various age groups.

In infants and young children, however, the blood pressure may be difficult to hear due to the smallness of the extremity and poor cooperation. The blood pressure can be estimated by use of the flush technique. The child's arm is elevated to drain the blood from it. The cuff is applied and an ace bandage is wrapped from the fingers to the antecubital space. The examiner then inflates the cuff and removes the bandage. The arm is lowered to the child's side as the cuff is gradually deflated. The point where the arm flushes is recorded as the median between the systolic and diastolic pressure.

There are variations in blood pressure due to age, exercise, pain, crying, emotional upset, and some drugs (i.e., estrogens and antihistamines). Before a blood pressure is considered elevated it should be taken on several different days, at several different times of day, and in different environments (i.e., home, school, work). The nurse should note the difference between the systolic and diastolic recordings. This is called the pulse pressure and is normally 30 to 40 mm Hg. A widened pulse pressure can be due to both systolic and diastolic hypertension, aortic regurgitation, patent ductus ar-

CHART 9.1.

Normal Blood Pressure Values

Age	Systolic		Diastolic	
	50th PER-CENTILE (mm Hg)	95th PER-CENTILE (mm Hg)	50th PER-CENTILE (mm Hg)	95th PER-CENTILE (mm Hg)
Birth–6 months	80	110	45	60
3 years	95	112	64	80
5 years	97	115	65	84
10 years	110	130	70	92
15 years	116	138	70	95
Adults	120	140	80	90–95

From Rudolph, A. M. (Ed.). *Pediatrics* (16th ed.). New York: Appleton–Century–Crofts, 1977, p. 1485.

teriosus, AV fistulas, coarctation of the aorta, and emotional stress. A narrowed pulse pressure can be found with tachycardia, severe aortic stenosis, pericardial effusion, and ascites.

In addition to a lowered blood pressure, the patient should be examined for other manifestations of hypotension. These include a decreased mental status, agitation and lethargy, tachycardia, tachypnea, dilated pupils, orthostatic changes, and pallor.

Peripheral Pulses

Palpable arteries of the body include the temporal, external carotid, brachial, radial, ulnar, abdominal aorta, femoral, popliteal, dorsalis pedis, and posterior tibial. Palpation of the carotid artery is discussed along with the great vessels of the neck and palpation of the abdominal aorta is covered in the examination of the abdomen. The peripheral pulses are taken with the patient in the supine position, using the index and middle fingers. The pulses are palpated bilaterally for condition of the wall, rate and rhythm, quality or amplitude, type or contour, and equality. Condition of the wall is evaluated by flattening the artery with digital compression and rolling the vessel back and forth. Pulses are auscultated in the carotid and abdominal aortic area for bruits.

Pulse Rate. Pulse rate varies normally with age and exercise. In addition, normal average rates vary by race. Black newborns have higher heart rate levels during sleep than white newborns.[4] Chart 9.2 includes a list of normal pulses for the various age ranges.

Tachycardia is an increased heart rate occurring in a variety of instances, including exercise, excitement, fever, anemia, hyperthyroidism, and heart disease. Bradycardia is a slow heart rate, which can be normal in athletes.

Palpation of the Pulses. Figure 9.23 depicts the areas for palpation of the arterial pulses.

Temporal Pulse. This pulse overlies the temporal bone and is palpated anterior to the ear. The temporal artery is the only palpable artery of the head and is normally tortuous. It should always be palpated when headache is a complaint.

Brachial Pulse. This pulse is palpated in the groove between the biceps and the triceps muscles. The brachial pulses are usually palpated only when arterial insufficiency is suspected. Just below the elbow the brachial artery branches into the radial and ulnar arteries.

Radial Pulse. The radial artery extends down to the radial side of the forearm to the wrist. The radial pulse is the most commonly palpated and is located on the flexor surface of the wrist laterally.

Ulnar Pulse. The ulnar artery extends down the ulnar side of the forearm and wrist. It then divides into two branches, which anastomose with branches of the radial artery to form the arterial arches of the hand. The ulnar pulse is found on the flexor surface of the wrist medially. It is usually palpated only when arterial insufficiency is suspected.

CHART 9.2.

Normal Pulse Rates

Age	Pulse Rate
Newborn	70–170
11 months	80–160
2 years	80–130
4 years	80–120
6 years	75–115
8 years	70–110
10 years	70–110
Adult	60–100

Adapted from Vaughn, V. C. & McKay, R. J. (Eds.). *Nelson textbook of pediatrics* (10th ed.). Philadelphia: Saunders, 1975, p. 1003.

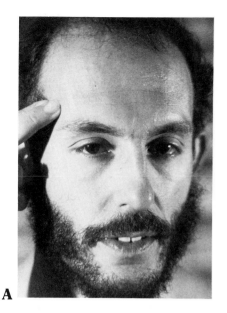

A

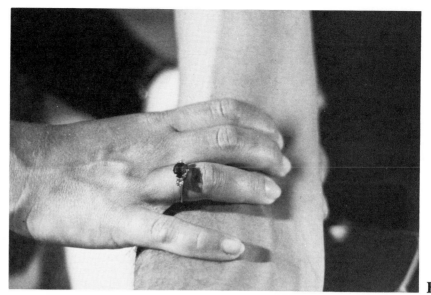

B

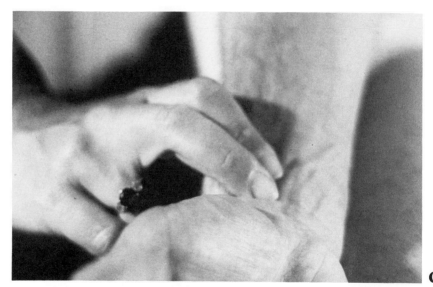

C

FIGURE 9.23. (A–H) Palpating the arterial pulses: (A) The temporal pulse. (B) The brachial pulse. (C) The radial pulse. (D) The ulnar pulse. (continued on p. 198)

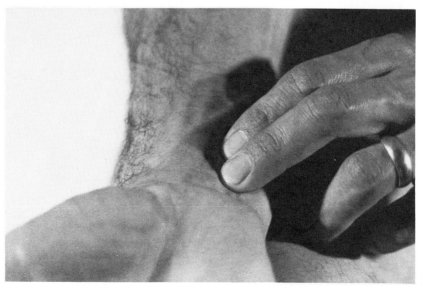

D

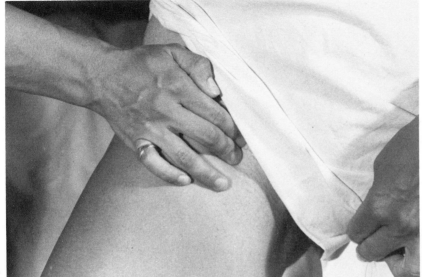

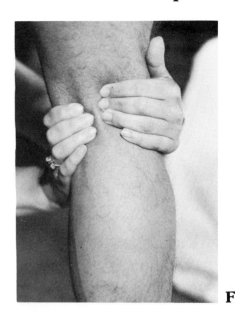

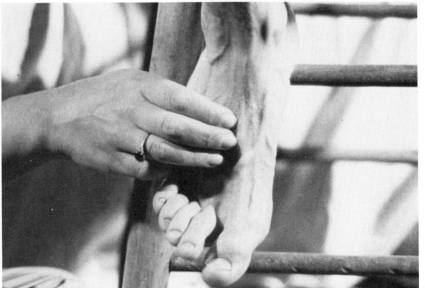

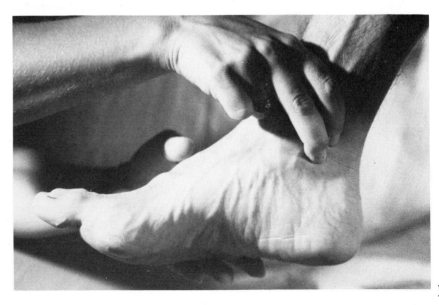

FIGURE 9.23. (E) The femoral pulse. (F) The popliteal pulse. (G) The posterior tibial pulse. (H) The dorsalis pedis pulse.

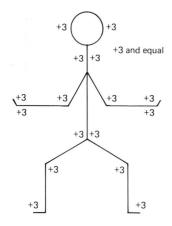

FIGURE 9.24. A stick figure used to record location of arterial pulses.

Femoral Pulse. The femoral artery arises at the level of the inguinal ligament and extends downward through the thigh. The femoral pulse is palpable at the inguinal ligament midway between the anterior-superior iliac spine and the pubic tubercle. It is especially important to identify this pulse in infants and children. Its absence or diminution in relation to the radial pulse may indicate coarctation of the aorta.

Popliteal Pulse. The popliteal artery is a continuation of the femoral artery and is located behind the knee. To palpate the popliteal pulse, the patient should be asked to slightly flex his knee. The examiner then places the fingertips of both hands deeply into the popliteal fossa. This is often a difficult pulse to locate.

Posterior Tibial Pulse. The posterior tibial artery reaches down the posterior aspect of the leg around the medial malleolus to the side of the foot. The posterior tibial pulse is palpable behind and below the medial malleolus. It may also be congenitally absent.

Dorsalis Pedis Pulse. This pulse is felt in the groove between the first two tendons on the medial side of the dorsum of the foot. It is congenitally absent in approximately 10 percent of the population. The criteria for estimating pulses have already been described. (After palpating the pulses, it is sometimes helpful to draw a figure that depicts at once the relative equality of the pulses. A stick figure is used, as displayed in Figure 9.24.)

Examination for Phlebitis

Examining for the presence of phlebitis is included in the peripheral vascular exam. Signs of phlebitis include redness, edema, and tenderness over the inflamed vein. The calves are inspected for redness and swelling. Because redness and swelling may not be apparent in highly pigmented patients, palpation is crucial. The calves are palpated to detect firmness or tension of the muscles and to detect edema over the dorsum of the foot. They are pushed from side to side to test for tenderness. In the presence of deep phlebitis of the leg, forceful dorsiflexion of the leg produces pain in the calf muscles. This is called a positive *Homans' sign.*

The Heart

Examination of the heart includes inspection, palpation, and auscultation. Percussion of the cardiac borders is not the most accurate technique for determining the size of the heart, but it is a technique that was used in the past. Now it is rarely used. Inspection and palpation give much of the information obtained from percussion, so it is imperative to develop these skills.

Inspection and Palpation. The techniques of inspection and palpation will be described together because they have a close relationship. For example, a movement observed over the precordium can often also be palpated. For adequate inspection and palpation of the anterior chest wall, the patient should be supine with his head elevated 30° to 45°. To observe pulsations that are visible on the chest, light must come from the side, so that rays are tangential to the skin. The examiner should observe from the patient's right side.

The entire precordium is inspected for visible cardiac impulses. In a systematic manner the examiner inspects and palpates the aortic area, the pulmonic area, the right ventricular area, and the left ventricular or apical area. Figure 9.25 depicts the areas on the chest wall to be closely inspected and palpated.

The entire precordium is palpated, using the palmar surface of the hand at the base of the fingers. This area is the most sensitive to vibrations. When a pulsation is identified by either inspection or palpation, its exact timing in relation to the cardiac cycle is determined. This is done by simultaneously auscultating or palpating the carotid artery to locate the pulse in either systole or diastole.

Examination of the aortic area involves assessment of the function of the aortic valve. Normally, the aortic area is quiet to palpation. The presence of valvular aortic stenosis will often produce a thrill. A *thrill* is a palpable vibration caused by blood flowing through a narrowed opening. In patients with hypertension the accentuated valve closure can be palpated as a thrill.

The pulmonary artery and valve are assessed in two areas. The first area is immediately to the left of the sternum in the second intercostal space and the second area is in the third intercostal space, just to the left of the sternum (Erb's point). In the presence of pulmonic valve stenosis, it is possible to palpate a thrill. There is also accentuated pulsation in this area due to the abnormally sharp closure of the pulmonic valve in pulmonary hypertension. These thrills and pulsations should be timed in relation to the cardiac cycle.

The right ventricular area is observed and palpated for any general lift or heave, and for thrills. Normally, the right ventricle is not strong enough to produce a visible impulse. *Lifts or heaves* occur with *right ventricular hypertrophy*. A *systolic thrill* is associated with a ventricular septal defect. This is a congenital problem resulting in the mixing of blood from the two ventricles. When there is increased cardiac output, as seen with anxiety, anemia, fever, pregnancy, or hyperthyroidism, slight outward pulsations may be observed to the left of the sternum.

The apical impulse (PMI) is assessed in the apical or left ventricular area. Using the tips of the fingers, the impulse can only be palpated in a small area less than 2 cm in diameter. The amplitude of the impulse is normally light or absent and the impulse normally lasts no longer than half the duration of systole. The impulse will be longer and more forceful in amplitude than normal with left ventricular hypertrophy and will last longer throughout systole.

Once the impulse is located, it is described in terms of location, size, character of impulse, and distance from the sternal border. In adults, the apical impulse is palpated in the fifth intercostal space in the midclavicular line. In children under 7 years of age, it is located in the fourth intercostal space. The impulse may normally be located lateral to the midclavicular line in association with a high diaphragm in pregnancy. It will be *abnormally displaced to the left and down with left ventricular hypertrophy.*

Figure 9.26 depicts the examination of the epigastric area. The palm of the hand is placed on the epigastric area. The examiner then slides the fingers under the rib cage to the left of the base of the sternum. The fingers are immediately under the right ventricle, and

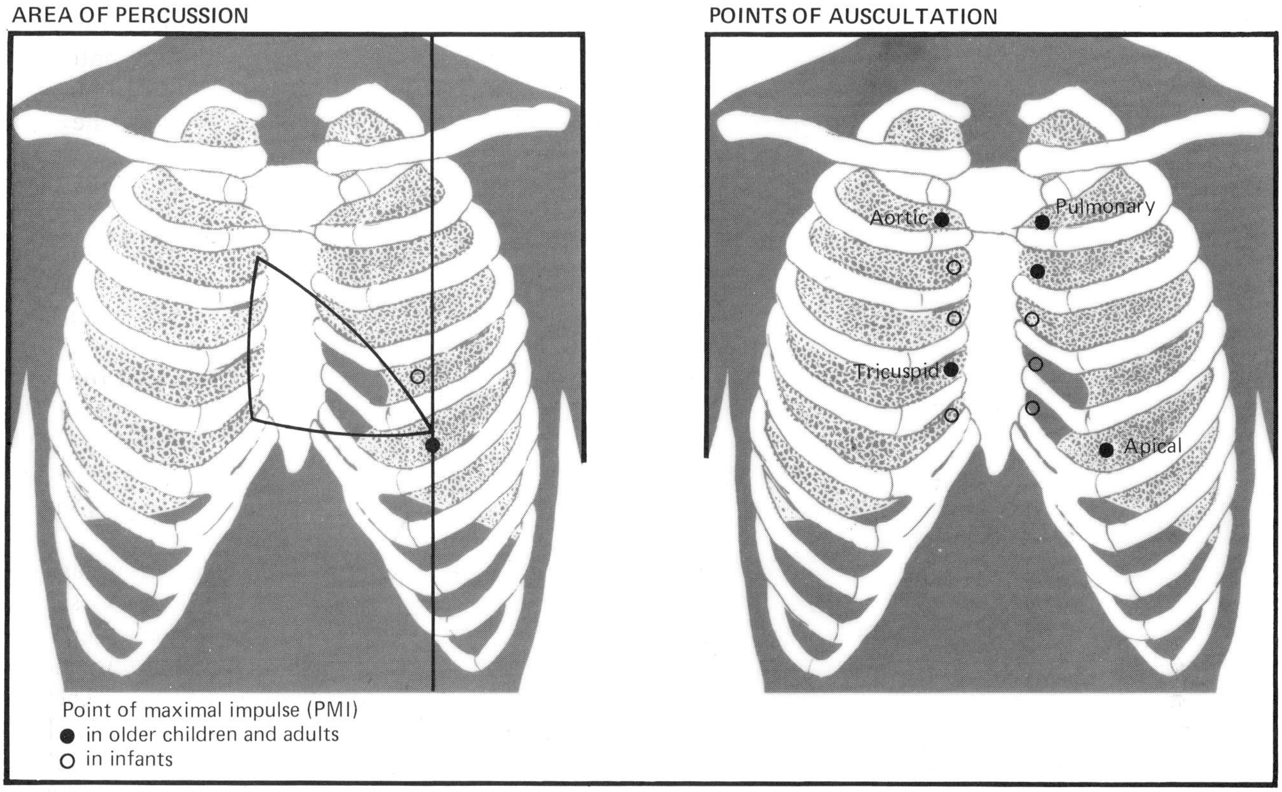

AREA OF PERCUSSION

POINTS OF AUSCULTATION

Aortic

Pulmonary

Tricuspid

Apical

Point of maximal impulse (PMI)
● in older children and adults
○ in infants

FIGURE 9.25. Points of palpation (left) and auscultation (right). (From Heagarty, M., Glass, G., King, H., & Manly, M. *Child health: Basics for primary care.* New York: Appleton–Century–Crofts, 1980, p. 144).

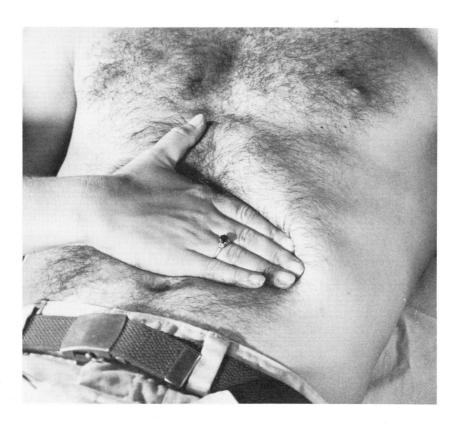

FIGURE 9.26. Palpation of the epigastric area.

under the palm of the hand is the pulse of the abdominal aorta. An increased amplitude of the abdominal aortic pulse may indicate the presence of an aortic aneurysm or aortic regurgitation. However, epigastric pulsation can occur following exertion.

Auscultation. To auscultate the heart, the examiner needs a stethoscope with a diaphragm and a bell. The diaphragm detects high-pitched sounds and is pressed snugly against the skin. The bell detects low-pitched sounds and is applied lightly to the skin. If the bell is applied snugly, it will form a diaphragm. The examining room should be free of distracting noises. The patient is examined in the sitting and recumbent positions. The heart sounds of a thin person sound sharp and clear, while those of an obese person are distant and muffled. The entire heart is auscultated first with the diaphragm and then with the bell.

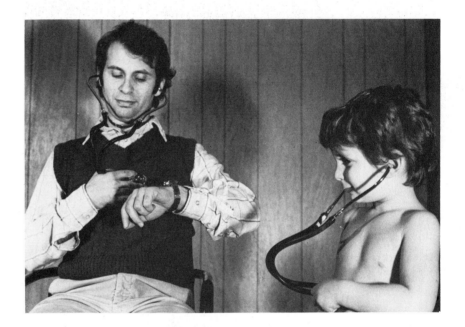

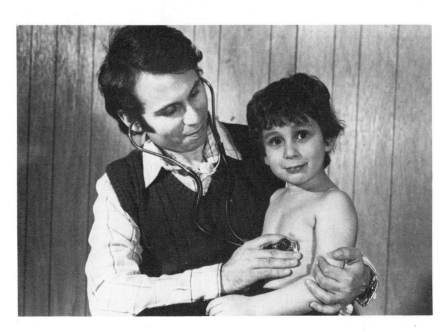

FIGURE 9.27. Allowing the child to become familiar with the equipment creates happy feelings for all concerned.

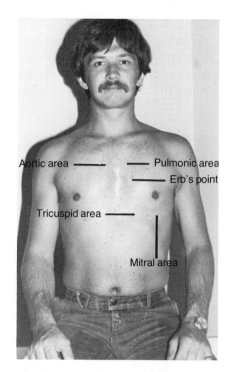

FIGURE 9.28. Anterior view of the chest for palpation and auscultation of the heart.

Aortic area

Pulmonic area

Erb's point

Tricuspid area

Mitral area

Children can be easily frightened by the stethoscope. It is always difficult to auscultate the heart of a crying child. Referring to the stethoscope as a telephone and allowing the child to handle the equipment can facilitate a trusting interaction and afford the examiner the opportunity to listen in a quiet atmosphere (Fig. 9.27).

A systematic approach to auscultation of the heart is essential. The same order used in inspection and palpation is repeated, using the bell and the diaphragm and with the patient in the sitting and supine positions. The examiner starts in the aortic area and proceeds to the pulmonic area, the right ventricular area, and the left ventricular or apical area. The stethoscope moves in a sliding, progressive fashion across and down the sternum and out to the axillary area. Figure 9.28 depicts the areas of auscultation. This can be compared with Figure 9.29, which shows the examiner auscultating the chest.

The examiner must be familiar with the events of the cardiac cycle. *She must identify the rate, rhythm, heart sounds, and extra sounds in systole and diastole.* While auscultating the heart, she should concentrate on each event, blocking out the other events. To identify S_1, she must palpate the carotid artery while auscultating. S_1 just precedes the carotid impulse and is synchronous with the onset of the apical impulse. As mentioned earlier, S_1 is normally more intense than S_2 at the apex. An increased intensity of S_1 may accompany exercise, anemia, hyperthyroidism, and mitral stenosis. A diminished S_1 is present in first degree heart block and in mitral regurgitation. If S_1 varies in intensity, there may be complete heart block. Splitting of S_1 is heard best in approximately the fifth intercostal space along the left sternal border. If the split is wide or heard in an area other than the tricuspid area, the patient should be referred.

Next, the examiner should concentrate on the second sound, noting its intensity and splitting. Normally, S_2 is louder than S_1 at the base. If there is an increase in the pulmonic component (P_2) of S_2, pulmonary hypertension should be considered. Arterial hypertension may produce an increase in the aortic component of S_2.

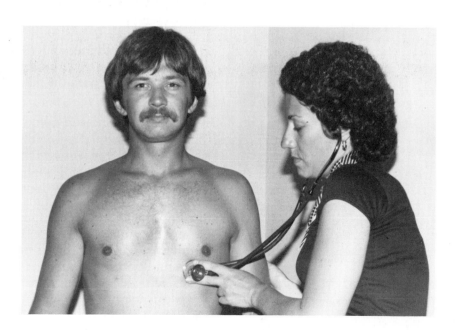

FIGURE 9.29. Examiner auscultating the chest.

Splitting is best heard in the pulmonic area. If the sound is split, it is described in terms of its degree of splitting and its relationship to inspiration and expiration. As mentioned previously, S_2 is normally more apparent during inspiration and diminishes or disappears during expiration. If the split is wide, fixed, or paradoxical, the patient should be referred.

Extra Sounds. Once S_1 and S_2 have been identified, the examiner listens for extra sounds in systole and diastole. The extra sound to listen for in systole is an ejection click due to the opening of a diseased semilunar valve. Sounds to listen for in diastole are an opening snap, S_3, and S_4. The opening snap is the first sound heard in diastole, occurring close to S_2. It is due to the opening of a diseased atrioventricular valve.

S_3 can be differentiated from the opening snap because it occurs slightly later in diastole. S_4 is heard just before S_1 in late diastole, producing a presystolic gallop.

Sounds that can be heard in systole and diastole are venous hums, pericardial friction rubs, and murmurs. As the final portion of auscultation, the examiner listens for murmurs. Murmurs are described according to the eight characteristics presented earlier. For the student, however, a helpful hint is worthy of note here. As she listens in each area, she should concentrate first on identifying heart sounds. Her thinking should then proceed as follows:

Q. Do I hear S_1 and S_2?
A. Yes.
Q. Which is loudest?
A. S_1 (then I must be listening at the apex).
Q. Do I hear another sound?
A. Yes.
Q. Is it heard in systole or diastole?
Q. Is it crescendo, descrescendo, diamond-shaped or pan?
Q. Is it high- or low-pitched?
Q. What grade is it?
Q. Is it harsh, musical, blowing, or rumbling?
Q. Does it increase, decrease, or show no change with respiration?
Q. Does it radiate, and to where—up the sternal border, into the neck, or to the axillary line?
Q. Is it louder with the patient sitting up or lying down?

In this manner she can come very close to identifying murmurs. There are two additional methods that are helpful if abnormalities are suspected of being of aortic or mitral origin.

Aortic murmurs, especially those of aortic regurgitation, are best auscultated with the patient sitting up and leaning forward. The patient is asked to exhale and hold his breath. The examiner auscultates with the diaphragm of the stethoscope and listens in the aortic area and down the left sternal border. Figure 9.30 depicts the examiner auscultating in this manner.

S_3 and mitral murmurs are best elicited with the patient lying on his left side. The examiner auscultates with the bell of the stethoscope in the apical area.

Chart 9.3 depicts the signs of abnormal heart sounds.

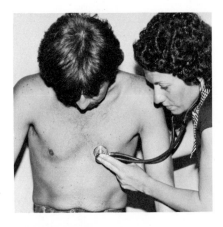

FIGURE 9.30. The patient leans forward as the examiner listens for an aortic murmur.

CHART 9.3.

Systolic and Diastolic Murmur

Type of Murmur	Diagnosis	Auscultation	Other Physical Examination
Systolic Murmurs: Left Second Interspace	Innocent murmur	Murmur variable with respiration	Likely in normal thin chest, straight spine, or pectus excavatum
	Physiologic murmurs	Disappear with treatment of primary condition	Signs of thyrotoxicosis, anemia, fever, etc.
	Atrial septal defect	S_2—wide, fixed split S_1—split, accentuated tricuspid closure sound Middiastolic rumble at lower-left sternal border	Right ventricular lift Pulmonary artery lift
	Pulmonary stenosis	Ejection click S_2 split, P_2 delayed and soft	Thrill Right ventricular lift Venous *a* wave prominent
	Partial anomalous pulmonary venous return	S_2 accentuated Not fixed split	
	Idiopathic dilatation of pulmonary artery	Ejection click	
Systolic Murmurs-Right Second Interspace	Aortic stenosis	Early systolic murmur transmitted to neck Rarely may be maximal at apex S_2(A_2) soft with rigid valve Ejection click with mobile valve	Left ventricular lift Slow-rising pulse Narrow pulse pressure Systolic thrill S_4 gallop Paradoxical splitting of S_2
	Aortic regurgitation	Decrescendo diastolic murmur Early systolic murmur Middiastolic murmur at apex (Austin Flint)	Wide pulse pressure Fast-rising pulse Left ventricular lift
	Mitral regurgitation	Holosystolic murmur, not transmitted to neck, heard better at apex and axilla	Left ventricular lift
	Aortic sclerosis	Short systolic murmur	Age: usually over 50 years Evidence of atherosclerosis
	Bicuspid aortic valve	Short systolic murmur Early decrescendo diastolic murmur Ejection click	Common in youths Associated congenital abnormality, coarctation, ventricular septal defect
	Aortic dilatation or aneurysm	Short systolic murmur Diastolic murmur may be present Tambour S_2 Lift in right second interspace	Signs of syphilis or Marfan's syndrome

(continued on p. 206)

CHART 9.3. (continued)

Type of Murmur	Diagnosis	Auscultation	Other Physical Examination
	Hypertension	Short systolic murmur Loud A_2 S_4 may be present	Hypertension
	Carotid bruit	Systolic murmur heard best over neck and carotids Runs over S_2	Signs of atherosclerosis
Systolic Murmurs: Apex and Left-Lower Sternal Border	Mitral regurgitation (rheumatic) Chronic	Holosystolic usually radiating to axilla S_1 soft S_3 common No change with respiration	Left ventricular lift
	Acute	Crescendo–decrescendo murmur, holosystolic or ending before S_2, radiation to base or axilla S_4	Signs of pulmonary hypertension
	Hypertrophic cardio-myopathy (IHSS)	Crescendo–decrescendo murmur S_4	Rapid, bifid carotid left ventricular heave
	Ventricular septal defect (small)	Holosystolic, lower-left sternal border, high-pitched, harsh	Thrill, lower-left sternal border
	Tricuspid regurgitation	Holosystolic maximum toward sternum, in-crease with inspira-tion, not transmitted to axilla	v Waves in jugular venous pressure Pulsating liver Signs of right ventricu-lar hypertension and congestive failure
	Aortic stenosis (transmitted)	Ejection, early systolic murmur—also heard in right-second interspace	Thrill, right-second interspace
	Mitral valve prolapse	Mid to late systolic murmur, may be pre-ceded by click or clicks	
	Papillary muscle dysfunction	Mid to late pansys-tolic murmur S_4 gallop	Ectopic left ventricular impulse
Diastolic Murmurs: Apex	Mitral stenosis	S_1 snapping OS present Middiastolic rumble Presystolic accentuation S_2 loud	Right ventricular lift
	Mitral regurgitation (diastolic flow murmur)	S_1 soft or absent S_3 present Middiastolic murmur Not usually typical rumble of MS Systolic murmur of mitral regurgitation	Left ventricular lift

CHART 9.3. (continued)

Type of Murmur	Diagnosis	Auscultation	Other Physical Examination
	Flow murmur secondary to increased pulmonary blood flow—e.g., in atrial septal defect, ventricular septal defect, or patent ductus arteriosus	S_1 normal S_2 fixed split in atrial septal defect Murmurs of primary lesion	
	Tricuspid stenosis	Diastolic murmur heard best near sternum Increased by inspiration	Big *a* waves, jugular venous pressure
	Aortic regurgitation (transmitted)	Decrescendo diastolic murmur Lower-left sternal border Onset with S_2	Signs of aortic regurgitation Left ventricular lift
	Aortic regurgitation (Austin Flint)	S_1 normal or soft OS absent Middiastolic rumble Presystolic rumble	Peripheral signs of aortic regurgitation Left ventricular lift
Diastolic Murmurs: Second Interspace Right and Left (Base)	Aortic regurgitation	Murmur descrescendo heard right-second interspace and third-left interspace S_2 may be of decreased intensity, but normal; S_2 does not exclude severe aortic regurgitation	Left ventricular lift Peripheral signs of wide pulse pressure
	Pulmonary regurgitation	$S_2(P_2)$ loud if pulmonary regurgitation secondary to pulmonary hypertension Murmur left-second interspace, not to right of sternum In absence of pulmonary hypertension normal Murmur rough and scratchy crescendo–decrescendo	Right ventricular lift Peripheral signs of aortic regurgitation absent
	Diastolic component of continuous murmur (transmitted)	Characteristic continuous murmur heard elsewhere—e.g., under left clavicle or over neck	

Adapted from Harvey, A. M., et al. *The principles and practices of medicine* (19th ed.). New York: Appleton–Century–Crofts, 1976, pp. 273, 276, 277, 280, and 282.

**Great Vessels
of the Neck**

The great vessels of the neck, including the carotid arteries and jugular veins, are assessed as a part of the cardiac exam. They reflect on the status of the heart. The carotid arteries are examined for the characteristics of their pulsations. The jugular veins are assessed for pulse waves and pulse pressure.

Carotid Arteries. The techniques of examination utilized in the examination of the carotid arteries are inspection, palpation, and auscultation. The arteries are observed for abnormally large and bounding pulses. The pulses are then palpated for rate, rhythm, and character, as are all of the peripheral pulses. Last of all, they are auscultated for bruits indicating local obstruction or transmitted cardiac murmurs.

The patient should be comfortable, with his head and neck elevated on a pillow 15° to 30°. Relaxation of the sternocleidomastoid muscle is facilitated by turning the head toward the side being examined. The patient's clothing about his neck and upper chest is removed so the examiner can easily inspect the area. The arteries are gently palpated by hooking the index and middle finger in the groove at the medial edge of the sternocleidomastoid muscle. Figure 9.31 depicts this maneuver. One side is palpated at a time, taking care to avoid the carotid sinus, which is located at the level of the thyroid cartilage just below the angle of the jaw. Massage of the carotid sinus may produce slowing of the heart rate. The arteries are auscultated with the bell of the stethoscope. The patient is asked to hold his breath as the examiner listens for the presence of bruits (Fig. 9.32).

Jugular Veins. The internal jugular vein gives the best estimate of right heart function. It reflects changes in pressure from the right atrium. The patient is elevated to the level of maximum oscillation in the internal jugular veins. If the venous pressure is greatly elevated, the patient should be examined sitting erect. When the pressure is moderately elevated, the patient should be elevated to

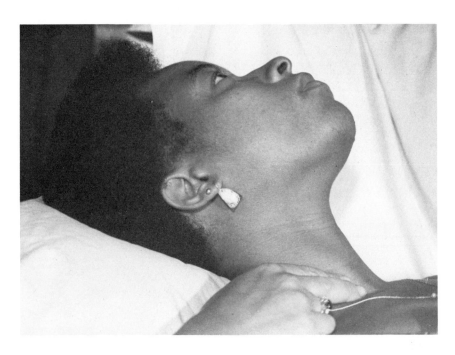

FIGURE 9.31. Palpating the carotid artery.

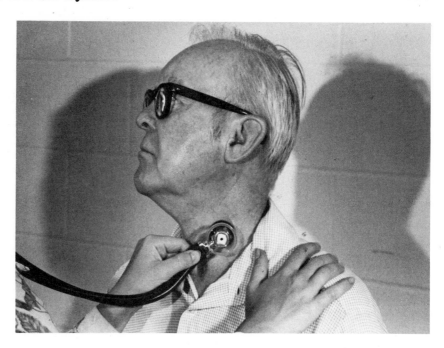

FIGURE 9.32. Auscultating for bruits over the carotid artery.

45° or more. The head and neck should be supported with a pillow to relax the sternocleidomastoid muscle. The examiner then looks tangentially across the sternocleidomastoid muscle, using a penlight to observe the *a* and *v* waves of the internal jugular vein and the *c* wave of the carotid artery. The *a* wave will be almost synchronous with S_1. The *v* wave is almost synchronous with S_2. The internal jugular vein lies very deep in the sternocleidomastoid muscle, so only the pulsations transmitted through the soft tissues are seen. They may be seen in the suprasternal notch, around and behind the acromioclavicular joint, or just behind the sternocleidomastoid muscle. Normally, the pulsations are not observed when the patient is in a sitting position. When the patient is elevated to 45°, the pulsations should not be observed more than 2 cm above the manubrium of the sternum. In most people, the venous pulsations can be observed in the supine position.

To determine the pulsations, the nurse should have the patient move his head away from the side being examined and use the tangential light. The *a* and *v* waves are differentiated from those of the *c* wave of the carotid artery. Chart 9.4 depicts the characteristics that identify the waves.

CHART 9.4.

Differential Characteristics of Jugular and Carotid Pulses

Jugular Pulse	*Carotid Pulse*
Increases with expiration	Not affected by expiration
Three pulse waves	One pulse wave
Changes with position	Does not change with position
Eliminated by light pressure on the vein above the sternal end of the clavicle	Not eliminated by pressure
Rarely palpable	Palpable

From Bates, B. *A guide to physical examination* (2nd ed.). Philadelphia: Lippincott, 1979, p. 182.

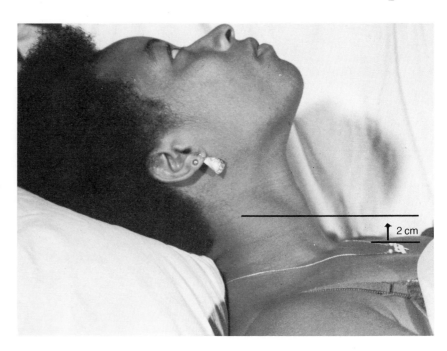

FIGURE 9.33. Measuring the venous pulse pressure.

After identifying the pulse waves, the examiner should measure the pulse pressure. Figure 9.33 depicts this maneuver. This can be done by using either the internal or external jugular veins. The examiner should note the distance between the end of the sternal angle of Louis to the point above which the veins may be distended to the angle of the jaw when the patient is erect. Congestive heart failure is the most frequent cause of abnormally increased venous pressure.

If the presence of congestive heart failure is suspected and cannot be determined by the methods already described, the *hepatojugular reflux* may be employed. Figure 9.34 depicts this maneuver. To perform the maneuver, pressure is applied over the

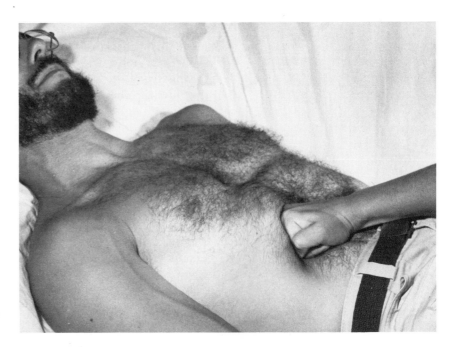

FIGURE 9.34. Elicitation of the hepatojugular reflux.

right-upper abdominal quadrant for 30 to 60 seconds. The examiner watches for an increase in the jugular venous pressure during this maneuver. A rise greater than 1 cm above the previous level is abnormal.

This completes the examination of the cardiac and peripheral vascular systems. As with other chapters, a written example of a chief complaint and subjective and objective information is provided here from a situation involving this system.

REFERENCES

1. Chow, P. M., Durand, M. P., Feldman, M. N., & Mills, M. A. *Handbook of pediatric primary care.* New York: Wiley and Sons, 1979, pp. 581, 582.
2. Caceres, C. H. & Perry, L. W. *The innocent murmur.* Boston: Little, Brown, 1967, pp. 99–100.
3. Miller, K. M. Assessing peripheral perfusion. *American Journal of Nursing.* 1978, *78*, 1674.
4. Schachter, J., Lachin, J., Wimberly, F. Newborn heart rate and blood pressure: Relation to race and to socioeconomic class. *Psychosomatic Medicine,* 1976, *38*, 390–398.

BIBLIOGRAPHY

Fowler, N. O. *Examination of the heart. Part II: Inspection and palpation of venous and arterial pulses.* New York: American Heart Association, 1965.

Hurst, J. W. & Schlant, R. C. *Examination of the heart. Part III: Inspection and palpation of the anterior chest.* New York: American Heart Association, 1965.

Patient assessment: Pulses. *American Journal of Nursing,* January 1979, pp. 115–132.

Sprague, H. B. *Examination of the heart. Part I: History taking.* New York: American Heart Association, 1965.

Tilkian, A. G. & Boudrea–Conover, M. *Understanding heart sounds and murmurs.* Philadelphia: Saunders, 1979.

EXAMPLE OF A RECORDED HISTORY AND PHYSICAL

Subjective:

Chief Complaint: "Shortness of breath for 4 weeks."

HPI: Patient is a 48-year-old male who describes himself as being 5' 9" tall, weighing 150 lb, and feeling well until 4 weeks ago. At that time, he began to exercise and jog because, "I should be in better shape and my wife gave me a jogging outfit for my birthday." Since that time, he has noticed fatigue and increasing shortness of breath during jogging. "It's working the wrong way—instead of running more each day, I'm walking more." Patient feels he has followed instructions carefully and has done proper exercising, gradually increasing walking and running. The weather has averaged 50° F and he does not feel that weather has been a factor. Three of these jogging outings have ended in fits of nonproductive coughing that lasted 2 to 3 minutes. He has noticed a dry cough that is more prevalent at night and thinks it began also within the past few weeks. He has taken no medications or treatment and relieves his shortness of breath by stopping his running. Prior to jogging he was not physically active and took occasional walks in the neighborhood. He does not smoke and drinks about four beers at social events three to four times a month. He has no pain, fever, nausea, or headaches. He had measles and chicken pox as a child and was in the hospital for about 2 weeks when he was 14 for rheumatic fever. He was checked 6 months after discharge by his physician and told he was in good health. Visits to the doctor since then have been only episodic for such conditions as flu or colds. He denies edema of the legs, varicose veins, a history of murmur, increased blood pressure, orthopnea, and palpitations. He has had no other illness or hospitalizations. There is no family history of cardiovascular or respiratory diseases.

Objective:

B.P.:	Left	120/100/80	Right	118/84/86	sitting
		120/104/82		122/86/80	lying
		120/100/80		126/82/84	standing
P. 76				128/90/88	leg/lying
R. 18					

General: 5'9", 142 lb, male in no acute distress. Physical appearance is pleasant. Talks freely and expresses symptoms and feelings clearly.

Lungs: No visible deformities or respiratory irregularity. All lung fields clear of palpable fremitus. No dullness to percussion. Breath sounds clearly audible without adventitious sounds. Expansion of diaphragm equal and symmetrical.

CV and PV:

PULSES. 3 + and equal; elastic, regular rate and rhythm; of normal contour (Fig. 9.24)

cv: No lifts or thrills visible or palpable. No pulsations noted or palpated in the epigastric area. S_2 louder than S_1 at the base. S_1 is louder than S_2 at the apex, but S_2 is unusually loud. In addition, there is a fixed snapping of S_1 and an early diastolic opening snap that does not vary with respiration. There is also a middiastolic rumbling murmur that is low and grade III/VI. It is loudest at the apex and radiates slightly toward the lower-left sternal border. It is best heard with the patient lying on his left side, auscultating with the bell. The PMI is visible and palpable in the 5th ICS, 8 cm from the left sternal border. It is about 1 cm wide and gives a short sound synonomous with that of S_1. *Carotid artery*—no bruits auscultated. *Jugular veins*—external and internal jugular veins are 2 cm above the sternal angle with the head of the bed elevated 30 degrees. The *a* wave is synchronous with S_1, as the *v* wave is with S_2. *Extremities*—no edema of hands or feet. No varicosities or calf tenderness in either leg.

10

The Breast

The breast is a very significant part of the human body—especially for a woman. To the preadolescent female, breast development indicates approaching menarche and womanhood. To the new mother, the breast is a means of feeding her new baby. For all women the breast can be a very sensuous part of their bodies. And most unfortunately, the breast is a common place for disease. Problems can be either acute or neoplastic, including benign and malignant lesions.

It is estimated that 1 out of 13 American women will be diagnosed as having breast cancer. The breast is the leading site of cancer in women and breast cancer is the leading cause of death in women between the ages of 30 and 44 years.[1] With good reason, cancer is a major concern of American women.

Despite this, a Gallup survey showed in 1974 that many women have mistaken beliefs about the disease.[2] A second Gallup survey in 1977 indicated that only 75 percent of the women had done a self breast examination, but only 24 percent said they were doing it on a monthly basis.[3] The monthly breast exam remains one good way to detect underlying disease early, thereby increasing the chances for a good prognosis. Women cannot and should not rely merely on an annual breast check by their health care providers.

HISTORY

*With the exception of the questions pertaining to the menstrual cycle, these questions should be asked of the male patient, too.

The major purposes of the history are to alert the nurse to any symptoms of underlying breast disease and to assess normal developmental changes. The general review of this system for a woman includes the following questions.*

1. Has she ever noticed any breast masses? If so, what did she do about them?
2. Has she ever had any pain or tenderness in her breasts? Does this relate to her menstrual cycle?
3. Has there ever been any discharge from the nipple? Rash on the areola area?

A thorough medication history is essential because some medications can cause a discharge from the nipple. The drugs that may alter hormone balance and cause nipple discharge include oral contraceptives, phenothiazine, digitalis, diuretics, and steroids.[4] In addition, some medications show a relationship to cancer, especially in women who have other risk factors. These drugs include phenothiazine, Rauwolfia alkaloid, and methyldopa.[5] Exogenous estrogens taken for birth control or for the treatment of menopausal symptoms have caused cystic breast changes in some women, but at present there is no association with the development of cancer.

The family history and the patient's past medical history are extremely important in identifying risk factors for breast cancer. There is an increased risk if the patient's mother, sister, aunt, or grandmother developed cancer before menopause.[6] If the patient has a history of cancer in one breast, she is at greater risk of developing cancer in the second breast.[7] Age at menarche, age at menopause, and age at the time of the first pregnancy bear a relationship to increased risk for cancer. There is a higher incidence in the woman who has an early menarche (before 13), as well as in the woman who has a late menopause (after the age of 50). The woman who had her first child after 35 or who has never had children is also at greater risk. A history of fibrocystic disease, especially proliferative fibrocystic disease, is considered a possible risk factor[8]. Ethnic or racial background is also related to incidence of breast cancer. American Caucasian women have a greater chance of getting breast cancer as women from Japan or China.[9]

Of great importance, too, is the history of self breast examination. The examiner should determine what technique the patient uses, as well as when she does the examination in relation to her menstrual cycle.

The normal breast changes in a woman should be investigated. Typical times for physical changes to occur are in young adolescence, pregnancy, and during or after menopause.

With the young adolescent, it is important to inquire about breast development. The young female should be questioned as follows:

1. Has she noticed her breasts changing?
2. When did it begin to happen?
3. What changes did she notice?
4. How does she feel about the changes?

The young adolescent male should be questioned regarding breast development, too. Fifty percent of all teenage boys have enlargement of the breasts (either one or both) during these years. This condition is called *gynecomastia* and is caused by hormonal changes during puberty. It is a normal variance and should resolve without treatment in 1 or 2 years. In the adult male this finding may be associated with liver disease, lung cancer, or other pathology and should be referred for further investigation.

It is essential to discuss breast changes with the pregnant woman. These changes can be quite traumatic if she is not anticipating them. The following questions should be asked:

1. Is there any tingling or tenderness?
2. Are the breasts enlarging?
3. Do the veins appear more prominent?*
4. Are the nipples more erect, or are they inverted? Is the areola darker?*
5. Can a thick, yellowish fluid be extracted from the nipple?*

*These changes occur in the latter phases of pregnancy.

As a woman goes through menopause, she may notice that her breasts are losing their firmness. This is especially evident in the postmenopausal female, whose estrogen levels have decreased. If the estrogen decline was rapid as well as marked, she may notice some shrinkage, too. This will not be prevalent in the overweight patient or in the woman whose breast tissue has changed prior to menopause because of past pregnancies. Regardless, it is important to ask the older woman about size and firmness of the breast tissue.

ANATOMY

The breasts lie on the ventral surface of the thorax directly over the muscles of the chest. Each breast extends from the second rib to the sixth rib and from the sternal border to the axillary line. There are

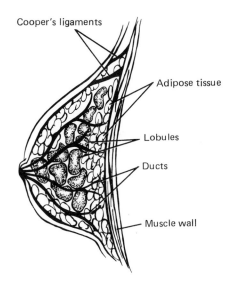

Cooper's ligaments

Adipose tissue

Lobules

Ducts

Muscle wall

FIGURE 10.1. Anatomic structures of the breast.

multiple fibrous bands which begin at the subcutaneous layer of connective tissue immediately beneath the skin of each breast. These bands, called Cooper's ligaments, run deeply through the breast to attach loosely to the fascia over the muscles of the chest wall (Fig. 10.1). When these ligaments become stretched due to lack of good support the breast becomes pendulous.

The breast is a modified sebaceous gland with the largest portion of glandular tissue located in the upper-outer quadrant. There is a portion of breast tissue which extends from this quadrant into the axilla called the tail of Spence (Fig. 10.2). Approximately 50 percent of breast tumors are located in the upper-outer quadrant and the tail of Spence.

The primary components of the breast are the milk-producing glands, a duct system, and a nipple. Each breast contains 10 to 20 separate lobes which consist of many smaller lobules. Within each lobule there are between 10 and 100 milk-producing glands (Fig. 10.1). The duct system drains the lobules and these ducts branch and join each other. There is one terminal duct for each lobe that exits on the surface of the nipple.

The nipple is located slightly below the center of each breast. At the tip of each nipple there are 10 to 20 perforations—the openings of the ducts. The nipple is surrounded by the pigmented areola. Sebaceous glands on the areola present as small, round elevations called Montgomery's tubercles. The remainder of the breast consists of fat, which determines the size of the breast. This is related to heredity and nutritional factors.

In embryonic development there are ridges that extend from the axilla to the groin. These ridges usually disappear, except at the site of the normal breast and nipple. Occasionally this ridge does not atrophy and a woman may have a supernumerary breast or nipple. The most frequent locations are in the axilla and below the normal breast. A supernumerary nipple consists of a small nipple and areola. It is less common for glandular tissue to be present.

There are two normal patterns of venous drainage in the mammary region visible on the anterior chest. In the first or transverse type, the superficial veins radiate laterally from the pectoral venous plexus toward the axillary and costoaxillary regions. In the second type, the veins radiate in a fan-like pattern downward and laterally into the breast from the point where the anterior jugular vein turns beneath the sternocleidomastoid muscle. Classification as to pattern type is determined by the drainage of the mammary region. The pattern is constant, and the only known alterations in pattern are due to breast tumors.[11] Knowledge of the lymph drainage of the breast is important to understanding the spread of cancerous cells. Depending on the location of a lesion in the breast, metastases may occur to the axillary nodes, to the supraclavicular and infraclavicular nodes, or even to the opposite breast.

Most of the lymphatic drainage of the breast is to the nodes of the axilla. There are four lymph node groups in the axilla (Fig. 10.2). The lateral axillary nodes are on the inner aspect of the upper part of the humerus, along the axillary vein. The central axillary nodes are located deep in the apex of the axilla close to the ribs. The subscapular nodes are under the anterior edge of the latissimus dorsi muscle. The pectoral nodes are behind the lateral edge of the pectoralis major.

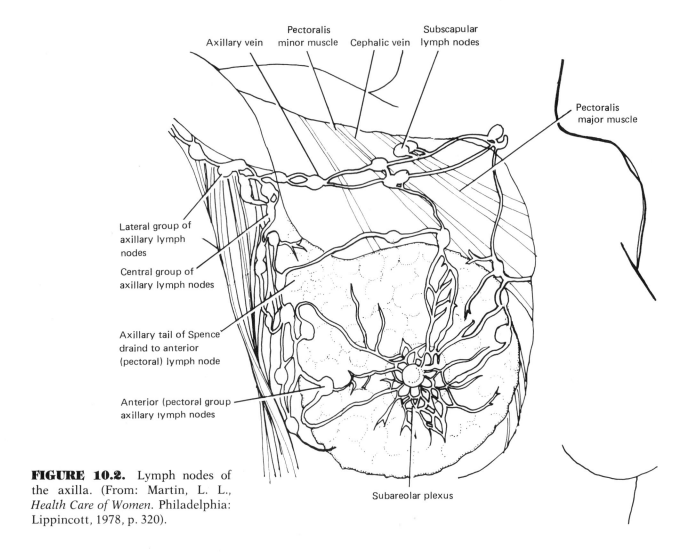

Axillary vein   Pectoralis minor muscle   Cephalic vein   Subscapular lymph nodes

Pectoralis major muscle

Lateral group of axillary lymph nodes

Central group of axillary lymph nodes

Axillary tail of Spence draind to anterior (pectoral) lymph node

Anterior (pectoral group axillary lymph nodes

Subareolar plexus

FIGURE 10.2. Lymph nodes of the axilla. (From: Martin, L. L., *Health Care of Women*. Philadelphia: Lippincott, 1978, p. 320).

Female Breast Development through the Life Span

Neonates, both male and female, are often born with enlarged, firm breasts. The bilateral enlargement is a result of the mother's hormones, which transfer across the placenta. This normal physiologic response usually disappears in 4 to 6 weeks.

No further breast development should occur in young girls until 1 or 2 years prior to menses. About the time a girl reaches 10 years of age, breast buds will have appeared. The nipples darken and there is an enlargement of the areolar diameter. One breast may grow more rapidly than the other. However, by young adulthood the breasts will have reached their full (nonpregnant) size and will be relatively symmetrical. It is not unusual for the normal breasts to be unequal in size.

During pregnancy the breast may enlarge to 2 or 3 times its original size. The changes related to the first trimester will be primarily subjective: tingling and tenderness. Some enlargement occurs, but the real increase in size begins after the second month. The nipples enlarge and the areola becomes darker. Surface veins appear. As pregnancy progresses, colostrum may be expressed from the nipple.

After a woman has had one or more pregnancies and her breast size has increased and decreased one or more times, it is realistic to expect a lessening in the firmness of the breast tissue. In addition, if a woman is overweight, more subcutaneous tissue may form causing enlargement. Both of these changes can cause flabby breast tissue.

As a woman approaches menopause and the estrogen level decreases, the breast may shrink. The firmness may also lessen. Throughout life, alteration of breast tissue takes place, and this can provide clues to physical as well as psychosocial changes.

TECHNIQUES OF EXAMINATION

A good time for the examiner to give instructions for the self breast examination is while she (the examiner) is inspecting and palpating the breasts. Verbal instructions should be supplemented with reading material and the woman's understanding should be evaluated by a return demonstration.

Inspection

The examination of the breast begins with inspection. Good lighting is essential. The patient is seated with her arms relaxed at her sides and her gown lowered to the waist. It is necessary to have the patient properly exposed. The breasts are compared for symmetry. Then each breast, nipple, areola, clavicular area, and axilla is inspected individually. It is not uncommon to notice some difference in the sizes of the two breasts. However, recent increase in the size of one breast may denote inflammation or underlying tumor. There may also be a difference in size due to underlying cystic formation.

The superficial appearance of each breast is examined for redness, edema, an increased superficial vascular pattern, and dimpling or retraction of the skin. Redness of the breast may indicate inflammation or involvement of the superficial lymphatics by a neoplastic process. In edema of the breast, the follicular openings are more pronounced and may denote inflammation or neoplasm. Edema associated with cancer is caused by the mechanical blocking of the lymphatic channels in the skin by cancer cells. The appearance of the skin in this situation is described as being like orange peel or pig skin (Fig. 10.3). The subcutaneous veins over the breast may be visibly dilated, indicating an accessory blood supply to a neoplasm. This should be differentiated from the bilaterally increased vascular pattern seen in pregnancy.

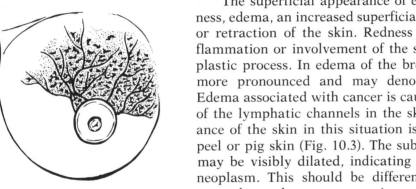

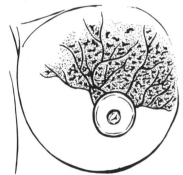

FIGURE 10.3. The orange peel or pigskin appearance of breast cancer.

One of the most important parts of the breast examination is inspecting for dimpling or retraction (Fig. 10.4). When Cooper's ligaments are invaded by cancer they become fibrotic, causing retraction of the skin over the lesion. To bring out the dimpling that may be missed on simple inspection, the client is asked to raise her hands over her head and then press her hands against her hips.[13] If the breasts are very large and pendulous, the woman is asked to stand and lean forward, holding the hands of the examiner. Any maneuver that causes a contraction of the pectoral muscles is a good way to bring out retraction.

The areola and nipple are examined for color, lesions, discharge, and position. In Caucasian patients, the areola and nipple are normally pink, but become brown with pregnancy. In darkly pigmented individuals, the nipple area is usually darker than other skin surfaces, and becomes even darker with pregnancy. Ulceration of one nipple may indicate Paget's disease, which is a malignant condition. If the ulceration is bilateral, it may be due to a dermatologic problem. Eczema-like lesions do occasionally develop in this

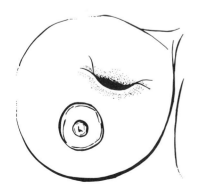

FIGURE 10.4. Dimpling or retraction of the breast.

area.[12] However, any ulceration of the nipple should be viewed with suspicion and the woman should be referred. Discharge from the nipple usually does not indicate any underlying cancer, but is of great concern to patients. A yellowish discharge is normally present during pregnancy. Chronic cystic mastitis is a disease along the ductal system, producing, a discharge that ranges from clear to blue-yellow. Bleeding from the nipple may be due to a benign intraductal papilloma, but it can also be a presenting sign of carcinoma.

The position of the nipples should be carefully noted. The nipples should be pointing in the same direction. Inversion of a nipple is a common variant of the normal and is usually a long-standing feature. Recent development of inversion in a previously erect nipple may be due to retraction and the examiner should suspect a malignancy. Retraction or deviation of the nipples is observed as the woman puts her hands over her head or presses her hands on her hips.

Finally, the clavicular and axillary areas are inspected for swelling and evidence of rash or infection. The nodes located in these areas may become enlarged with cancerous spread. The axillary areas often normally appear swollen during pregnancy and lactation.

Palpation

Palpation includes the axillae, the clavicular areas, and the breasts. The axillae and clavicular areas are palpated while the woman is still sitting. The lymph nodes of the axillae are palpated with the woman's arms at her sides, so that the muscles are relaxed. To facilitate this relaxation, the examiner can support the client's right arm with her left hand and palpates the woman's right axilla with her right hand (Fig. 10.5). The examiner then palpates along the upper humerus, inside the anterior axillary fold, along the thorax between the axillary folds, deep in the posterior axillary fold, and high in the axilla. When palpating high in the axilla, the examiner milks the axillary contents downward. Standing in front of the woman and slightly to the side, the supraclavicular and infraclavicular areas are palpated.

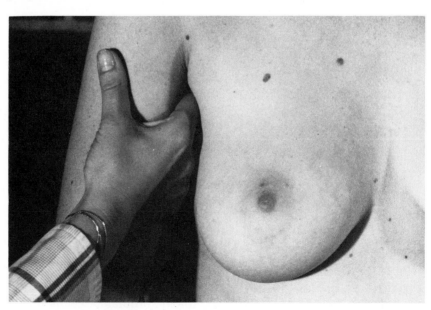

FIGURE 10.5. Palpation of the right axillary lymph nodes.

If the woman has noticed a mass, or if there are any suspicious areas on inspection, the breast should be palpated with the patient in both the sitting and the supine positions. If no problems have been elicited or observed, the breasts need only be palpated with the patient in the supine position. If the breast is large, placing a pillow beneath the woman's shoulder blade on the side to be examined and having her raise her hand behind her neck will stretch the pectoral muscle on that side, shift the breast medially, and thin the breast over the chest wall. This makes palpation easier. If the woman has noted a mass, the examiner should palpate the opposite breast first. This allows for comparison and forces the examiner to consciously examine the normal tissue before zeroing in on an abnormality.

To palpate the breast, the examiner uses the palmar surfaces of the first three fingers in a rotary motion to compress the breast tissue gently against the chest wall. Only one hand should be used while palpating (Fig. 10.6A). When a two-handed technique is used, it is easier to miss breast tissue. One approach is to envision the breast as a wheel. Starting at the nipple, the examiner palpates up the spokes of the wheel (Fig. 10.6B). The tail of Spence should be palpated as a separate unit. The examiner should then palpate the nipple, noting elasticity, and compress the nipple between her thumb and index finger, noting any discharge.

The bimanual technique should be used if the woman's breasts are very large, making it difficult to distribute the tissue evenly over the chest wall. This method is best implemented with the woman in a sitting position. The breast is palpated between the palmar surfaces of the fingers of both hands while the hands are gently and slowly rotated.

Normal breasts vary greatly in their feel to palpation. They differ according to the age of the woman. where she is in her menstrual cycle, the amount of subcutaneous fatty tissue, and the presence or absence of pregnancy.[16] In older women, breasts are commonly stringy and nodular while those of younger women have a softer, more homogenous feel. Just prior to menstruation, the breasts become engorged, lobular, and sensitive. When the breasts are very large they may be more difficult to palpate and more time must be taken. During pregnancy, the breasts are firmer and larger and the lobulations become more distinct.

The best time for a self breast exam differs according to the following factors. A menstruating woman should do the exam on the last day of her menstrual period every month. At this time she should not have the breast swelling and tenderness that comes with the increase in estrogen levels later in the cycle. The woman who has had a hysterectomy and is still premenopausal should examine her breasts each month after breast tenderness and swelling are gone. The postmenopausal woman should also check her breasts at the same time every month. It might be suggested that she use the date of her birth as a reminder. For example, if she was born on 6/16, she should check her breasts on the 16th of every month. A pregnant woman is not immune to cancer and must continue with her monthly breast exam.

If a mass is located on palpation, it is described in terms of location, size, contour, consistency, tenderness, mobility, and discreteness. The location of the mass is described according to the quadrant in which it is palpated. The size can be described in terms of centimeters or by comparison to the sizes of such common items

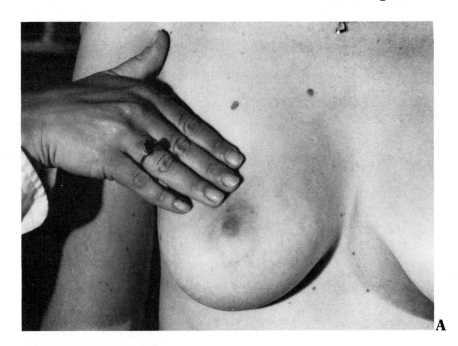

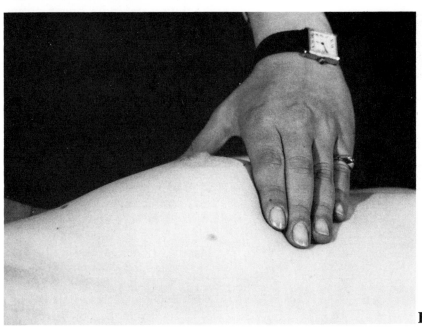

FIGURE 10.6. Palpating the breast.

as peas and walnuts. "Contour" is a description of the surface as either irregular or regular. It is essential to know if the mass is fixed to the chest wall or if it is freely mobile. The margins of the mass are described as being discrete or difficult to find.

There are some typical characteristics of the various masses found in a breast. In cystic disease, the mass is mobile, often tender, and round, and has a well delineated border. A benign neoplasm is mobile, usually nontender, and round, and has a well delineated border. A cancerous mass is irregular, is not clearly delineated from surrounding tissues, may be fixed to the skin or underlying tissue, and is usually nontender. These descriptions are only generalizations, and any mass that is palpated must be referred for further evaluation.

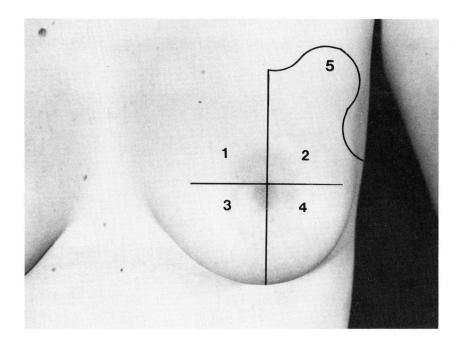

FIGURE 10.7. Breast quadrants.

To adequately describe what is seen on inspection and felt on palpation, the breast is divided into four quadrants and the tail of Spence. The quadrants are the upper-inner, upper-outer, lower-inner and lower-outer (Fig. 10.7). An alternate method of localizing findings on the breast is to describe their locations in terms of time zones on a clock and give the distance in centimeters from the nipple. For example, a lesion may be located at 1 o'clock, 2 cm from the nipple. A picture of the breast should accompany the written description.

COMMON NONMALIGNANT CONDITIONS

Not all breast disease is malignant. The majority of women with signs and symptoms of breast disease do not have neoplasms. The most common benign conditions include:

Fibrocystic disease: This most commonly occurs in women between the ages of 30 and 55. The cause is not known. An estrogen-related factor is believed to exist because the disease is less prevalent and regresses after menopause. The signs are multiple cysts, usually bilateral. The cysts are movable and well defined and may be either soft or hard. They can be tender or painless. These cysts change with the menstrual cycle. They get larger and more tender premenstrually. Diagnosis is confirmed by aspiration or biopsy.

Fibroadenoma (adenofibroma): This is a tumor of the breast which occurs in women under 30. The mass is firm, nontender, movable, and well defined. It appears suddenly and can become very large. A biopsy should be done for confirmation of diagnosis. Fibroadenomas should be excised.

Mastitis: This is an inflammatory condition of the breast. Its intensity and involvement can vary. Mastitis is particularly common in the nursing mother. Symptoms include elevated temperature (often up to 103° or 104°F), chills, lethargy, and muscle aches. The breast will be erythematous, hard, and painful with palpation. The most common etiology is *Staphylococcus aureus.* Appropriate referral is necessary. Antibiotics and warm, moist packs applied to the involved breast comprise the usual treatment. Nursing should be continued.

REFERENCES

1. 1979 Cancer Facts and Figures. New York: American Cancer Society, Inc., 1978
2. 1976 Cancer Facts and Figures. New York: American Cancer Society, Inc., 1975.
3. 1979 Cancer Facts and Figures. New York: American Cancer Society, Inc., 1978.
4. "Round Table: Developing Cancer Risk Factor Profiles." *Patient Care* 10.2 (1 February, 1976): pp. 65–84.
5. Anthony, C. "Risk Factors Associated with Breast Cancer," *Nurse Practitioner*, July–August, 1978, pp. 31–32.
6. 1976 Cancer Facts and Figures. New York: American Cancer Society, Inc., 1975.
7. 1976 Cancer Facts and Figures. New York: American Cancer Society, Inc., 1975.
8. "Round Table: Odds and Options in Breast Cancer Risks." *Patient Care*, 9.7, (1 April, 1975) pp. 20–57.
9. Rhodes, G., Glober, G., & Stemmermann, G. A review of some tumors of interest for demographic study in Hawaii. *Hawaii Medical Journal*, 1974, *33*, 283–284.
11. Spuhler, J. Genetics of three normal morphological variations: Patterns of superficial veins of the anterior thorax, peroneus tertius muscle, and number of villate papillae. *Cold Spring Harbour Symposia on Quantitative Biology*, 1950, *15*, 175–189.
12. Greenhill, J.P. Office Gynecology. Chicago: YearBook Medical Publishers, Inc.

EXAMPLE OF A RECORDED HISTORY AND PHYSICAL

Subjective:

Chief Complaint (Reason for Visit): "I felt a lump in my breast yesterday."

HPI: This 24-year-old female considers herself to be in excellent health. Yesterday, when she was taking a shower, she noticed a nonpainful lump "about the size of a peach pit" in her right breast. She says it feels "hard and round, and it moves easily." She has not noticed any changes in her skin or discharge from her nipple. She does a self breast exam every 2 months or so. She has never had anything like this before. Her last menstrual period began 1 week ago (10/23). There is no family history of breast cancer or any other breast disease. She is seeking consultation today because, "I'm afraid that I have cancer."

Objective: T. 98.6 F; P. 74 radial; R. 14; B.P. 126/74 (sitting).

Breast: No evidence of lesions, moles, rashes, redness, or discharge in either breast. Bilateral symmetry on inspection. No dimpling. Right breast: A nontender, round, hard, well defined, movable mass about 2.5 cm in the RUQ at about 11 o'clock, 3 cm from the nipple. No other lumps or tender areas. Left breast: No tenderness or masses palpable. Breast tissue soft throughout.

Lymph nodes: No enlargement or tenderness of the axillary or supra clavicular nodes bilaterally.

11

The Abdomen

The evaluation of the abdomen can be uncomplicated if there are no problems, or it can be extremely involved and time-consuming if concerns are present. There are a multitude of assessments to consider when a patient has abdominal complaints. These range from mild viral infections to emotional stresses to malignant disease.

The physical examination is relatively simple and straight forward. If the nurse is a good investigator, much of the work can be done during the history. Thus the completeness and quality of the history may be more revealing than the findings of the physical exam of the abdomen.

HISTORY

For the general review of this system, areas to be covered include:

1. Pain (see discussion that follows)
2. Bowel habits
    a. Times per week normal for patient
    b. Character of stool: color, consistency, amount
    c. Pain with bowel movements
    d. Hemorrhoids
3. Constipation
    a. What is meant by the word "constipation?"
    b. How often does it occur?
    c. What treatment is used?
4. Diarrhea (see questions for constipation)
5. Change in appetite: recent increase or decrease
6. Thirst: recent increase or decrease
7. Food intolerances
    a. What are they?
    b. How do they manifest themselves?
    c. What treatment is used to remedy them?
8. Heartburn (see questions for constipation)
9. Belching
10. Flatulence
11. Previous problems, evaluations, diagnoses, treatment. Describe.
12. Previous history of jaundice?

If a positive response is given to the question of abdominal pain, then a thorough pain history must be elicited. If it is done well, many causative factors can be eliminated. It is necessary to question the patient about:

Sequence and chronology: Is it always there or does it come and go? Is it related to eating? Does it happen before or after meals? Has it ever happened before? Describe.

Onset: When did it begin?

Location: Where is the pain? Can it be pointed to with one finger or is it more spread out? Does it move around? From where to where?

Quality: Describe the pain. Is it sharp? Dull? Stabbing? Nagging? Aching?

Intensity: Does it peak? When? Is it the same all the time?

Frequency: How often does it occur?

Associated phenomena: Nausea? Vomiting? Diarrhea? Constipation? Flatulence? Belching? Fever? Rectal bleeding? Blood or

*A more complete review of related systems may be indicated.

mucus in stools? Hemetemesis? Difficulty swallowing? Frequent urination, burning, itching?* Vaginal or penile discharge?* Menstrual irregularities, changes, or irregular bleeding?*

Aggravating factors: Foods? Medications? Position? Activities? Stress (occupational, environmental, or people-related)? Eating, drinking, and smoking habits?

Alleviating factors: Treatment used? Hot water bottle? Heating pad? Medications? Rest? Change in position? Relief of stress?

Miscellaneous: Exposure to anyone with the same kind of symptoms? Foods eaten in the last 24 hours? Where (restaurants, picnics, etc.)? Recent change in job, school, home environment? Allergies (or past history of lactose intolerance)?

There are nine major sites to check in the localization of abdominal pain:[1]

1. Esophageal: Midline retrosternal with radiation to the back at the level of the lesion.
2. Gastric: Epigastric; radiation occasionally to the back, particularly the left subscapular area.
3. Duodenal: Epigastric; radiation to the back, particularly the right subscapular area.
4. Gallbladder: RUQ or epigastric; radiation to right subscapular or midback areas.
5. Pancreatic: Epigastric; radiation to midback or left lumbar areas.
6. Small Intestine: Periumbilical.
7. Appendicular: Periumbilical, migrating to RLQ.
8. Colonic: Hypogastrium, RLQ or LLQ; sigmoid pain may radiate to the sacral region.
9. Rectal: Deep pelvic location.

Sometimes a guide such as this may be helpful in locating causes. Use this chart only as a guide—it is not absolute by any means.

ANATOMY

Because the abdominal region has many underlying organs, the area is divided by two systems of imaginary landmarks (Fig. 11.1). This region has certain boundaries and these should be described, too, in order to help clarify the imaginary landmarks. The *xiphoid process* is the superior boundary of the abdominal region. The *symphysis pubis* lies directly below the xiphoid and is the inferior marking. With these parameters in mind, it is easy to divide the abdomen into four quadrants. Specific organs lie in each designated region (Chart 11.1).

The other imaginary method of dividing up the abdomen resembles a tic-tac-toe board. This nine-region division has smaller sections and is most helpful for describing midline findings. The terms *epigastric*, *umbilical*, and *hypograstric* are most frequently adopted from this particular method. The *kidneys* are not often described within the two imaginary systems, but are referred to as being in the *costovertebral* region. This landmark is named for the meeting of the spinal cord and the twelfth rib.

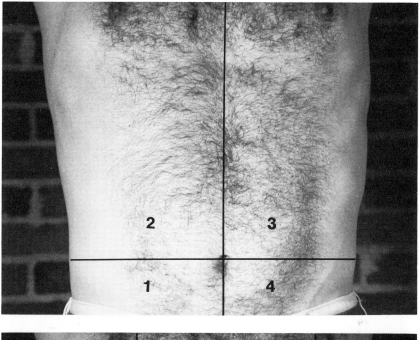

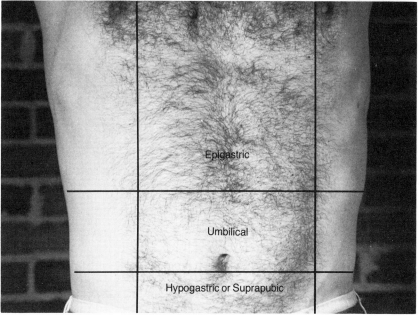

FIGURE 11.1. Imaginary landmarks of the abdomen. A: Four quadrants: (1) Right lower quadrant (RLQ), (2) Right upper quadrant (RUQ), (3) Left upper quadrant (LUQ), (4) Left lower quadrant (LLQ). B: Nine region division.

The organs of the abdominal region are involved in many systems of the body. The specific organs of the gastrointestinal system that lie in this area are the *stomach*, the *pancreas*, the *liver* and *gallbladder*, and the *small* and *large intestine* (Fig. 11.2). The stomach begins at the end of the *esophagus* and extends to the beginning of the small intestine. The *cardiac sphincter* is at the esophageal entrance and the *pyloric sphincter* is at the duodenal entrance. The stomach is an organ for the motility of food, hydrochloric acid secretion, and the enzymatic digestion of foods.

The pancreas lies behind the stomach. It contains the endocrine hormones insulin and glucagon. Exocrine hormones and pancreatic enzymes are also located there.

CHART 11.1

Organs in the Abdomen

Right-upper Quadrant	*Left-upper Quadrant*
Liver	Left lobe of liver
Gall bladder	Stomach
Pancreas	Spleen
Right adrenal gland	Upper lobe of left kidney
Upper lobe of right kidney	Pancreas
Hepatic flexure of colon	Left adrenal
Section of ascending colon	Splenic flexure of colon
Section of transverse colon	Section of transverse colon
	Section of descending colon

Right-lower Quadrant	*Left-lower Quadrant*
Cecum	Lower portion of left kidney
Appendix	Sigmoid colon
Right ovary	Left ovary
Right fallopian tube	Left fallopian tube
Right ureter	Left ureter
Right spermatic cord	Left spermatic cord
Section of ascending colon	Section of descending colon

Midline

Bladder
Uterus

From Malasanos, L., Barkauskas, V., Moss, M., Stoltenberg–Allen, K. *Health assessment.* St. Louis: Mosby, 1977, p. 240.

The liver lies under the diaphragm and extends across the right upper quadrant and left-upper quadrant. It secretes bile, which aides in the digestion of fat. Liver cells function in iron metabolism, plasma protein production, detoxification of plasma substances, metabolism of hemoglobin breakdown products, and in other capacities. The liver is essential to life.

The storehouse for bile is the gallbladder, which lies behind the liver. This organ is not essential to life and can be removed without permanently damaging the digestive system.

The small intestine is made up of three branches and is responsible for the most absorption in the gastrointestinal tract. The three components making up the 18 feet of the small intestine are the *duodenum*, the *jejunum*, and the *ileum* (Fig. 11.2). Located on the wall of the small intestine are villi, which control the small intestinal absorption of carbohydrate, protein, and fat.

The large intestine is different than the small intestine. There are no villi and it is a much wider organ. The large intestine has three branches. They are the *ascending colon*, the *descending colon*, and the *transverse colon* (Fig. 11.3). The function of the large intestine mainly concerns the absorption of water and the storage of feces.

Portions of the reproductive system also lie in the abdominal region. In the female these include the *uterus*, the *right* and *left ovaries*, and the *fallopian tubes*. In the male the *left* and *right ureters* and the *left* and *right spermatic cords* are found in the abdomen.

Somewhat accessible to examination in the abdomen are the *kidneys*. Although they belong to the urinary system, they are

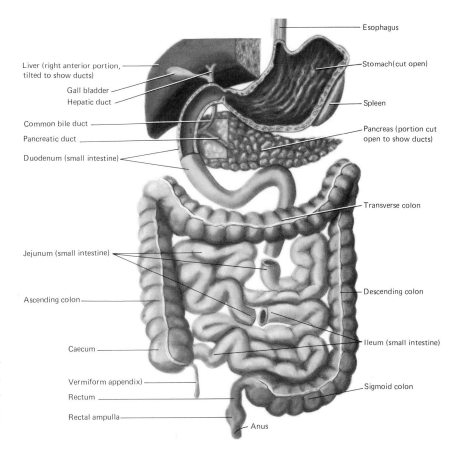

Esophagus

Liver (right anterior portion, tilted to show ducts)

Stomach(cut open)

Gall bladder

Hepatic duct

Spleen

Common bile duct

Pancreatic duct

Pancreas (portion cut open to show ducts)

Duodenum (small intestine)

Transverse colon

Jejunum (small intestine)

Descending colon

Ascending colon

Caecum

Ileum (small intestine)

Vermiform appendix)

Rectum

Sigmoid colon

Rectal ampulla

Anus

FIGURE 11.2. The gastrointestinal system. (From Heagarty, M., Glass, G., King, H., & Manly, M. *Child health: Basics for primary care.* New York: Appleton–Century–Crofts, 1980, p. 156).

examined as parts of the abdomen. They lie behind the muscles of the posterior abdominal wall. The upper borders reach the diaphragm at about T_{12}. The lower borders are located in the area of L_3. The right kidney is usually lower than the left due to liver placement.

The *adrenals*, which lie directly on top of the kidneys, are parts, of the endocrine system, but are discussed along with the abdominal

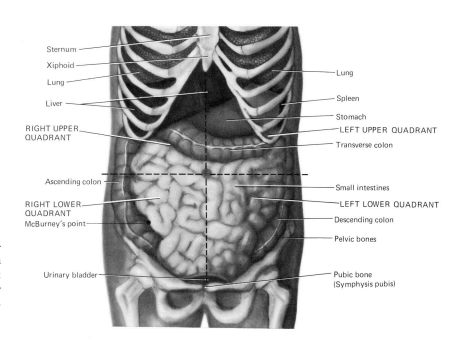

Sternum

Xiphoid

Lung

Lung

Liver

Spleen

RIGHT UPPER QUADRANT

Stomach

LEFT UPPER QUADRANT

Transverse colon

Ascending colon

Small intestines

RIGHT LOWER QUADRANT

LEFT LOWER QUADRANT

McBurney's point

Descending colon

Pelvic bones

Urinary bladder

Pubic bone (Symphysis pubis)

FIGURE 11.3. The gastrointestinal system: the abdomen. (From Heagarty, M., Glass, G., King, H., & Manly, M. *Child health: Basics for primary care.* New York: Appleton–Century–Crofts, 1980, p. 156).

anatomy. These small but extremely potent glands have a major role in the production of the corticosteroids, epinephrine, and norepinephrine.

PHYSICAL ASSESSMENT

All four techniques of examination are used to perform the abdominal exam. However, this is one system in which the order is different. As always, inspection begins the examination. In this case, auscultation follows inspection. The abdomen is auscultated for bowel sounds. If percussion and palpation precede auscultation, then the bowel sounds will be falsely stimulated.

Among the items required for the abdominal exam are a relaxed patient with an empty bladder, good lighting, a stethoscope, a marking pen, and a ruler (tape measure).

The patient should be as relaxed as possible. Any stress or fear will tighten up the abdominal muscles and make the exam more difficult. Some hints to help the patient and the examiner are as follows.

1. The examiner should place a pillow under the patient's knees.
2. She should have him place his arms at his sides or across his chest.
3. She should converse with the patient during the exam.
4. She should watch his face, not his abdomen, because any distress signs will appear on the face.
5. She should palpate with the patient's hand under her own if the patient is ticklish, gradually easing his hand away.
6. She should examine the tender areas under suspicion last.

Inspection

When inspecting the abdomen, the examiner observes shape, symmetry, skin and movement. The shape is usually described as flat, round, protruding, or sunken. A sunken abdomen is often the result of dehydration. A protruding belly may have several causes: pregnancy, distension, obesity, or a tumor. Rounded "tummies" can be noted in infants, toddlers, and young children. Extreme roundness in a young child may well indicate malnutrition (if this is being considered, a comprehensive diet history should be elicited). A flat abdomen is usually the result of appropriate weight and muscle tone. In our society this is a highly valued commodity.

An abdomen is normally symmetrical. Asymmetry can occur as a result of pregnancy or other masses, a hernia, obstruction, or fluid.

The skin is inspected carefully. If a scar or scars exist, several features about it should be noted: where it is exactly (from what point to what point), how long and wide it is (exact measurements are appropriate), and when and how it occured (old scars are silver or skin-toned, while new scars are pinker in color). It is helpful to draw a picture of the abdomen with the placement of the scar when recording the data. *Striae* are stretch marks, which can result from a rapid weight gain, as in pregnancy, or a large weight loss. Red striae indicate recency. As with scars, silver striae show age. Purple striae may indicate Cushing's disease and can often be found on people who have a long history of cortisone usage.

The skin should also be inspected for lesions, moles, and rashes of any type. The location, color, and size of these should be recorded. If a mole is changing color and/or size, it is important to know at what rate that is occurring. If a record is made of the location, color, and measurements, then future comparisons can be made. This is especially important when a malignancy is suspected.

The *umbilicus* is observed for its position, shape, redness, irritation, discharge, and the presence of hernias. An *umbilical hernia* is one that protrudes through the umbilicus. In infants, in whom such hernias occur most often, this defect may be the result of inadequate closing of the abdominal wall. Large umbilical hernias that can be seen during inspection may be larger than 6 cm. The visibility may be magnified by the child's crying or straining. Umbilical hernias in adults are not very common. The cases that do occur are seen primarily in the obese and in pregnant women.

In the newborn, the remains of the mother's umbilical cord on the baby's umbilicus are present for the first 2 weeks of the baby's life. At around that time the stub should slough off. This is a common site of infection for the newborn. The cord and umbilicus should, therefore, be observed for erythema, swelling, discharge, and odor. Any or all of these signs may include infection and call for a referral.

Movement in the abdomen occurs with respiration, peristalsis, and pulsations. Abdominal breathing can be observed while inspecting the abdomen. Men are much better abdominal breathers than women. Most women employ only their thoracic muscles and the result is superficial breathing techniques. Men, on the other hand, use both thoracic and abdominal breathing muscles. Using both sets of muscles provides for the most efficient air exchange.

Pulsation from the aorta may be observed in the epigastric area. This pulsation is most likely to be seen in thin adults or children. Peristalsis may or may not be visible. It too, is most evident in thinner people. To see peristalsis the examiner's eyes should be level with the patient's abdomen and she should be watching across the abdomen for a wave-like movement.

Auscultation

As mentioned previously, the abdomen is auscultated before it is percussed or palpated. The purpose of auscultating this area is to listen for active bowel sounds. One must hear this irregular, tinkly noise in all four quadrants. Such noises normally occur every 5 to 20 seconds. Bowel sounds are described with the terms *hypoactive*, *hyperactive*, and *audible*. Before concluding that they are inaudible, one must listen for 3 to 5 minutes. The examiner can flick the abdominal wall with her fingers to stimulate intestinal movement.

Absence of bowel sounds means decreased intestinal motility. One reason may be a paralytic ileus, which occurs post operatively or as a result of such electrolyte disorders as low potassium. Other causes could be gangrenous bowel or appendicitis. Any obvious decrease in bowel sounds warrants immediate attention.

Increased bowel sounds, or *borborygmi*, can be the result of laxative ingestion or of anything else that might increase gastric motility. Increased bowel sounds, along with flatulence, abdominal cramping, and diarrhea, are common symptoms among lactase-deficient individuals who consume a sufficient quantity of milk. Most of the world's peoples (except those from Northern Europe) become lactase deficient in late childhood.[2,3] Gastroenteritis will also often cause an increase in bowel sounds, among other objective findings.

The abdomen is also auscultated for bruits. A bruit is an abnormal flow sound (see Chap. 9) likely to be heard over the abdominal aorta or renal arteries (in the flank areas). It can rarely be heard over the liver; when it can it usually indicates malignant disease of the liver.

The friction rub is another abnormal sound that can be heard in the abdomen. This is a grating sound that resembles two pieces of leather riding over one another. Such sounds are most commonly heard over the liver or spleen and are related to infection or malignancy.

Percussion

Percussion of the abdomen is utilized to detect the presence of fluid, air, or solid tissue. This technique is also used to outline the borders of the liver and of the spleen and to assess the fullness of the bladder. A tympanic percussion note is heard throughout the air-filled areas of the abdomen. The solid areas give a duller sound.

The abdomen is percussed in an organized and thorough manner. Percussion may elicit a painful response over tender areas. If it is possible to determine where the tenderness is from the history, then the examiner should avoid percussing and palpating the tender area until the end of the abdominal exam. Evincing pain early in the exam might cause the patient to guard, which will make the evaluation more difficult.

General Orientation. The examiner percusses over all four quadrants, including the flank region. Any areas that are full to percussion are noted. This fullness may indicate stool, other masses, or an increase in fluid. Tenderness may be elicited as well.

Percussion of the Liver Borders. This is not a difficult procedure if the examiner can picture the underlying organs (Fig. 11.3). The liver can be percussed along the right midclavicular line and the midsternal line. The midclavicular (MCL) measurement alone is an acceptable estimate if there are no related problems. When in doubt, the measurement at the midsternal line should be used, too.

It is helpful to remember that the lower border of the liver normally lies just above the right costal margin and the upper border sits approximately between the fifth and seventh intercostal spaces along the midclavicular line. (Fig. 11.4)

The examiner should begin by percussing upward at the level of the umbilicus along the right MCL. Tympany will predominate here. Somewhere around the costal margin, the tympanic note will change to one of dullness. The point at which the change in percussion notes occurs is the lower edge of the liver. (Note: percussion over a rib will also sound dull.) This point should be marked with a pen.

Next the examiner percusses down from the right nipple along the MCL from lung resonance to the first note of dullness. Once again, if a rib is not being percussed, the point of dullness denotes the upper border of the liver. The examiner should mark this point and measure the span. The average width of the liver at the MCL is 6 to 12 cm in the adult.

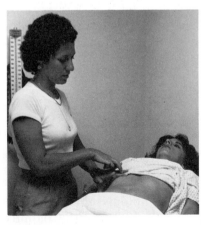

FIGURE 11.4. Percussing the liver.

In measuring the span at the midsternal line, the same procedure is followed. The average span along the midsternal line is 4 to 8 cm. These distances may be greater in men and taller people.

Accuracy may be obscured if dullness exists due to right pleural effusion or a consolidation in the right lung. Excess air in the colon may increase the tympanic area in the right-upper quadrant and also distort correct measurements of the lower border. Liver displacement can occur as a result of pregnancy, abdominal or flank tumors, or ascites. These conditions, too, will affect the measurement of the liver span.

Percussion of the Spleen. The spleen can be percussed most easily if it is enlarged (as in mononucleosis). However, a slight change in the percussion note can be heard over the normal spleen somewhere between the sixth and tenth ribs close to the left midaxillary line (Fig. 11.3). As with the liver, the note will change from tympany to a duller tone.

Percussion of the Stomach. The tympanic sound of the gastric air bubble is elicited in the left anterior rib cage.

Palpation

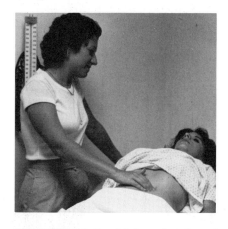

FIGURE 11.5. Light palpation of the abdomen.

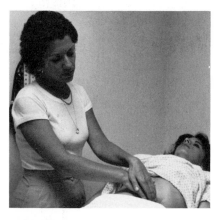

FIGURE 11.6. Deep palpation of the abdomen.

Palpation is used to detect tenderness, to outline abdominal organs, and to determine the presence of masses or distension. Two types of palpation are performed: *light* and *deep*. Light palpation is utilized to assess superficial pain, organs, and masses. Deep palpation is used to distinguish inferior organs or to elicit deep pain. In either method the examiner should always observe the patient's face, not his abdomen, while palpating. It is important to remember that pain will be evinced by a change in facial expression or by muscle guarding.

For light palpation, the palmar surfaces of the fingertips are used (Fig. 11.5). The examiner depresses her hand lightly and systematically over the entire abdomen (if the patient is ticklish, the examiner should slide the patient's hand under her own). The examiner feels for tenderness, muscle tone, abdominal stiffening, or masses. If a sensitive area is discovered, she should postpone examining it until the end, as done with percussion.

Sometimes malingering is suspected. In this case, while auscultating the four quadrants for bowel sounds, the examiner should apply some light pressure to the diaphragm of the stethoscope. If a painful response has been elicited during light palpation, then the same response should occur during the application of pressure over that spot. This maneuver mimics light palpation.

Next, deep palpation is begun. Once again, all four quadrants are surveyed thoroughly and systematically. The patient must be as relaxed as possible for this portion of the exam, which may cause considerable discomfort. Deep abdominal breathing will help the patient to relax. Here, too, tender areas should be palpated last.

The same portion of the examiner's hand is used for deep palpation as for light palpation. However, this time much more pressure is applied. In fact, many examiners use two hands. In this method, one hand is superimposed on the other and the top hand is used to exert pressure (Fig. 11.6). This bimanual approach is thought to allow for deeper palpation and better delineation of organs and masses. As with any mass that is discovered, the examiner should note its size, location, mobility, contour, consistency, and tenderness.

When a painful area is discovered, a test for rebound tenderness needs to be done. The examiner depresses her hand deeply into the involved area and then lets go quickly. If the pain is increased with the release of the hand, as opposed to increasing with the deep palpation, the test is positive. This tests for peritoneal inflammation and is commonly used to aid in the diagnosis of appendicitis. If the history indicates that peritoneal inflammation is a possibility, and if among the objective findings is right-lower quadrant rebound tenderness, then proper referral is needed quickly.

In children under 6 months of age, it is not unusual to palpate an umbilical hernia. This may or may not have been seen on inspection. This type of hernia can be felt by pressing down inwardly with one finger on the umbilicus. If a fingertip can be admitted, a small hernia is present. They will often resolve spontaneously without treatment by 1 year of age, especially if they are small. An average size ranges from 1 to 5 cm. Appropriate referral is indicated for an exceptionally large hernia or one that does not disappear.

Specific Organs that Undergo Deep Palpation

The Liver. Palpation of the liver is used to detect enlargement and tenderness. There are two commonly used methods. In both methods, the examiner should be standing on the patient's right side.

In the first approach, the examiner's left hand is placed on the posterior thorax at about the 11th or 12th rib (Fig. 11.7). She then pushes upward with that hand to brace the upcoming anterior palpation. The right hand is placed at about a 45° angle to the right of the rectus muscle along the rib cage. The procedure is explained to the patient and he is told that he might experience some discomfort or queasiness when his liver edge is felt. The patient is then asked to inspire deeply (inspiration causes the liver edge to descend). When the patient inhales, the examiner slides the lateral portion of her hand (or the fingertips) under the costal margin (Fig. 11.7). If the patient breathes deeply and the examiner applies enough pressure, the liver edge will whisk by her hand during the patient's inspiration. The liver edge as it slides by will give a firm, blunt sensation to the examiner's hand under the ribcage. It may be necessary to ask the patient to take two or three deep breaths before the liver edge can be palpated. It is important for the examiner not to retract any pressure, but to continue to palpate deeper as the patient inspires again. Some livers are harder to palpate than others. This is especially true of obese, tense, or very physicially fit people.

The second method uses the same basic principles. This approach involves the superimposition of the examiner's left hand over the right hand along the right costal margin (Fig. 11.8). This method gives the examiner more anterior pressure, but the posterior pressure is lost. Either method is acceptable. The method chosen should provide the most accurate information.

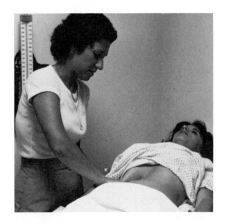

FIGURE 11.7. Palpation of the liver, with the examiner's left hand on the posterior thorax.

The Spleen. The spleen should not be palpable in a healthy adult, but it can occasionally be felt in a small child. Palpation of the spleen follows liver palpation. The examiner reaches across the

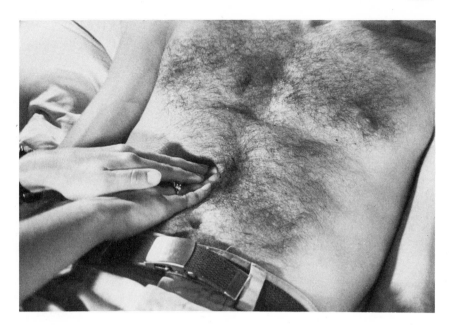

FIGURE 11.8. Palpation of the liver, with superimposition of the hands.

patient's abdomen and places her hand on the left posterior thorax (Fig. 11.9). The patient is asked to roll slightly to the right to facilitate the exam. The right hand is then placed below the left costal margin. Sliding the fingertips under the rib cage is the easiest way to reach the spleen. Short fingernails are a must!! The patient should again be asked to inspire; the spleen will descend as did the liver edge. If the spleen can be felt at all, it will be during inspiration.

The Kidneys. It is almost impossible to palpate the normal kidneys except in a child or a very thin adult. However, the right kidney is more likely to be felt. Picturing the kidneys anatomically helps to understand the approach to palpation (Fig. 11.3) The kidneys lie along the midaxillary line lateral to the rectus muscle. The goal of palpation is for the examiner to feel the lower pole of the kidney between her palpating hands (Fig. 11.10).

The examiner places her hand along the inferior edge of the costal margin on the right anterior abdominal area. The other hand is placed on the posterior thorax at about the same place. The patient is asked to inspire and the examiner pushes her hands together. The kidney will descend with inspiration and the pole will be felt between the hands. The procedure is repeated for the other kidney.

Costovertebral Angle Tenderness. CVA tenderness occurs when there is inflammation of the kidney(s). A light blow is delivered in the posterior flank area over each kidney. If pain is elicited, then there is a good chance that inflammation exists. The recorded note should read, "CVA tenderness over the left kidney."

The Aorta. This tube-like structure is palpated to the left of the umbilicus in the epigastric area. The examiner rolls her fingertips horizontally over this area while applying pressure. The aortic pulsation will be felt once the aorta is located.

It is important to remember that the accuracy of these findings depends on the patient's relaxation, cooperation, and trust in the

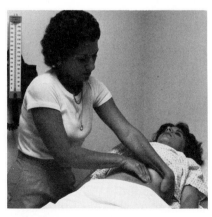

FIGURE 11.9. Palpation of the spleen.

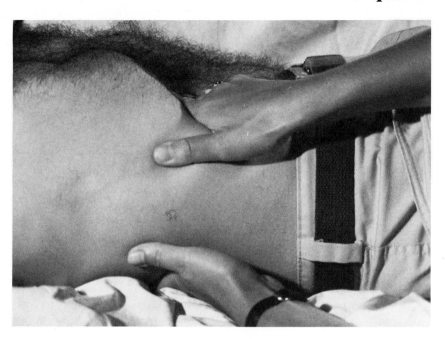

FIGURE 11.10. Palpation of the kidneys.

examiner. Therefore, as with any procedure, a thorough explanation of the procedure as well as telling the patient when he may experience discomfort are essential.

REFERENCES

1. Judge, R. D. & Zuidema, G. D. *Methods of clinical examination: A physiological approach* (3rd ed.). Boston: Little, Brown, 1974, p. 208.
2. McCracken, R. Lactase deficiency. *Current Anthropology*, 1971, *12*, 479–517.
3. Tripp–Reimer, T. & Pollack, R. Lactase deficiency. *Nursing 77*, 1977, 7, 82–85.

EXAMPLE OF A RECORDED HISTORY AND PHYSICAL

Subjective:

Chief Complaint: "I've had a stomach ache for 4 days."

HPI: This 54-year-old female considers herself to be in "basically good health except for the usual flus, colds, etc." In the last few months, she has had intermittent episodes of "burning, gnawing" epigastric and left-upper quadrant pain. This happened the first time 4 months ago, shortly after her mother passed away. She had "waves of this pain for a couple of days at a time." It would appear between meals and get worse over a period of 15 minutes, "then I'd take a Rolaid and it would go away. Eating doesn't seem to make it worse or better. I wouldn't be bothered again for several days. It seems to be happening weekly now for the last 6 weeks. This week the pain lasted 4 days instead of the usual 2."

She notices some mild nausea associated with the pain, but not enough to have a decreased appetite. There is no radiation of the pain, vomiting, change in bowel habits, diarrhea, constipation, heartburn, belching, flatulence, food allergies, fever, rectal bleeding, or mucus in stools.

She has a large amount of formed brown stool every other day. Her bowel habits have not changed in frequency or character. She has no food intolerances but cannot "eat a lot at one time or I get the pain." She tries to eat "a balanced diet—a lot of fruit and vegetables. I never fry or eat greasy foods." She drinks a mixed drink or two on a weekend night on an irregular basis. She smokes 1 ppd of True filters and has been smoking for 15 years.

Patient considers herself under some stress presently. Since her mother died, there is "a lot of business I must attend to. We were very close, and I miss her a lot." Patient is a secretary for a project that will end next month, "and then I'll be out of work." She feels she gets a lot of support from her family and "my husband tells me not to worry about finding another job."

She is taking no medicines other than an occasional aspirin (10 grains 1 or 2 times/month) and a Rolaid or two when the pain is "bad." She has not found changing positions helpful. She has not tried eating dairy products when she has the pain.

She has never had any abdominal pain prior to the onset of this and has not sought treatment until today. Her mother died of "cancer of the colon". She was 80. No other family history of abdominal disorders. Patient can still go to work with the pain, but is "frightened, as my mother had the same symptoms 2 years ago."

Objective: T. 98.4°F orally; P. 86 radial; R. 18; B.P. 146/86 sitting.

Abdomen: Round abdomen, loose mucle tone, symmetrical. No scars, lesions, moles, rashes. Peristalsis not visible. Bowel sounds audible in all quadrants. Abdomen soft and nontender throughout, except in the epigastric area. Some guarding with deep palpation. No rebound tenderness or masses. LIVER: 8 cm span at MCL. Nontender. SPLEEN: Not palpable. Nontender. AORTA: pulsations palpable. No tenderness. No bruits. CVA: No tenderness.

12

The Female Genitalia

Examination of the genital area is viewed with hesitation by many women. The adolescent girl may approach her first examination with a fear of the unknown. The same may be true for the young pregnant woman who has heard unpleasant stories from friends or relatives about their experiences with childbirth. Very modest women (e.g., many of Mexican–American descent) may hesitate to have a pelvic examination. If great concern for modesty is apparent, efforts should be made for a female to conduct the examination. Commonly, once a woman is past her childbearing years, she will stop coming for routine pelvic examinations. Many of the concerns felt by women can be identified during the gynecologic history that is taken prior to the physical examination. The nurse's attitude can make a great deal of difference in how the woman views the pelvic exam. The best approach is to have a calm, reassuring, and attentive manner. Once rapport is established, the nurse may be able to dispel much of the anxiety.

HISTORY

The essentials of the gynecologic health history are some demographic facts, the menstrual pattern, the obstetric history, the contraceptive history, the genitourinary history, and the sexual history. Demographic data relevant to this system are the woman's age, marital status, number of children, and their ages. These data help to direct questions appropriate to the woman's place in the life cycle.

The menstrual history is nonthreatening to most women, so this is a good place to begin the interview. The patient will usually answer the questions directly without embarrassment. The menstrual history includes the age at menarche, age at menopause, and a description of the woman's menstrual pattern.

Most girls experience their first menses *(menarche)* between 12 and 14 years of age. Generally, Blacks and Asians tend to reach pubertal maturity more rapidly than do Caucasians.[1] A young girl and her mother may become concerned if menarche does not occur within this normal range. In this case, the examiner should gain information about the presence of other secondary sex characteristics and the mother's menstrual history. The mother's age at menarche may be relevant, although it has not been established that there is an inherited tendency. Consultation should be sought if there is any question of a hormonal problem or if the girl has not experienced menarche before 16 years of age. If menses has been established, the examiner should inquire into the circumstances of the onset of menses. The girl should be asked how she was prepared for its occurrence and how she reacted to the onset.

Menopause refers to the cessation of monthly menses. The perimenopausal period is the time around the menopause when hormonal shifts take place in the woman. This time period commonly takes place between the ages of 40 and 55. If the woman is in the perimenopausal period, the nurse should identify symptoms that may be related specifically to this time in her life. The most common problems are related to vasomotor instability, including hot flashes, numbness and tingling, headaches, and heart palpitations. The patient should be asked if she is undergoing estrogen therapy or any other treatment to alleviate these symptoms. Inquiry should be made about her attitude toward menopause. The nurse should ask if she welcomed it or experienced it as a loss.

Information necessary for determining a woman's menstrual pattern includes date of the first day of the last menstrual period, number of days between the first day of each period, amount and duration of bleeding, any associated discomforts (e.g., breast tenderness, bloating, cramping, moodiness), amenorrhea, and intermenstrual spotting or bleeding. A common and often normal finding obtained from this information is menstrual irregularity. Although this can be experienced at any time during the childbearing years, irregularity is most frequently a problem in the young woman first beginning her cycles and again in the woman approaching menopause. Usually menstruation is irregular and the girl is unable to conceive for 1 to 2 years after the menarche. Often all that is needed is reassurance. Slowing of flow, irregularity, and skipped periods can be associated with the menopause. In both cases, the examiner should not overlook the possibility of pregnancy.

In obtaining the obstetric history, the nurse is interested in knowing the woman's *gravity* and *parity*. Gravity is the number of pregnancies, regardless of outcome, and parity is the number of births with a fetal size compatible with extrauterine life. Abortions are listed separately. Each pregnancy is explored in relation to the type of delivery, duration of the pregnancy, birth weight, condition of the infant, and complications of the pregnancy or postpartum period. It is important to ask adolescents and young women if their mothers took hormones during pregnancy. There is an increased incidence of vaginal and cervical adenocarcinoma in daughters of women who took *diethylstilbestrol* (DES) while pregnant.[2] Additional checkups and medical supervision are required in this high-risk group.

The current and past contraceptive practices of every woman of childbearing age should be elicted. The nurse should be sure to include adolescents and women who are perimenopausal. Ironically, it is during these time periods that women are often most lax and pregnancy is least desired. The nurse should inquire about the present method of birth control and identify any problems the patient may be experiencing. She should determine if the patient and her partner are presently satisfied with their choice of birth control. The nurse should also ask about the methods the patient has used in the past and her reasons for discontinuing these methods. This information may also be elicited during the sexual history. The importance lies not in where the data are collected, but in the fact that they are collected. This is a good time to inquire about the patient's (and her partner's) plans for future pregnancies.

During each visit, symptoms related to the presence of a genitourinary problem are reviewed. Symptoms indicating a vaginal or bladder infection include vaginal itching, vaginal discharge, frequency, urgency, dribbling, pain on urination, and hematuria. A woman with poor vaginal support may complain of *stress incontinence* (loss of small amounts of urine with laughing or coughing). *Dyspareunia* (painful intercourse) is usually caused by a lack of vaginal lubrication. This may result from inadequate stimulation during foreplay, but it is also commonly experienced during the hormonal changes of menopause. The lower estrogen levels at this time result in atrophy of the vaginal mucosa, causing painful intercourse and increased susceptibility to infections. The past history of this system includes a history of any venereal disease, urinary tract infection, and vaginal infection. If the patient has a positive history of any of these, she should be asked about when they occurred, the symptoms she had, the treatment she received, and follow-up care.

Once the woman has discussed the above information, she may be at ease and comfortable enough to discuss her sexual history. The goal of this portion of the history is to identify her feelings about her sexuality and detect any problems (see section on the sexual history in Chap. 1). Use of the developmental approach will help facilitate the discussion and gather data appropriate to her stage in the life cycle.

ANATOMY

The anatomy of the female genitalia and the rectum are covered here.

Female Genitalia

The external female genitalia consist of the *mons pubis, labia majora, labia minora, clitoris,* and *vestibule* (Fig. 12.1). In front of the symphysis pubis lies a rounded pad of fat called the mons pubis. At puberty this becomes covered with hair. The labia majora are two folds of skin and fat that extend backward from the mons pubis toward the rectum. The skin of the labia majora contains hair follicles, sweat glands, and sebaceous glands. The labia minora are reddish folds of stratified squamous epithelium located between the labia majora. These folds are soft and devoid of hair follicles and sweat glands. Anteriorly, the labia minora meet to form the *prepuce* that partially covers the clitoris. The clitoris is composed of erectile tissue similar to that of the penis. Posteriorly, the labia minora are connected by a slight transverse fold called the *fourchette.* The *perineum* extends from the *introitus* (vaginal orifice) to the *anus.*

The vestibule is the cleft between the labia minora and behind the clitoris. The vagina and the *urethra* open into this area. The urethra is located on the anterior surface of the vagina about 2.54 cm behind the clitoris. The *Skene's glands* are located just posterior to either side of the urethral opening. The *Bartholin's glands* are situated in the floor of the vestibule, one on either side of the vaginal orifice.

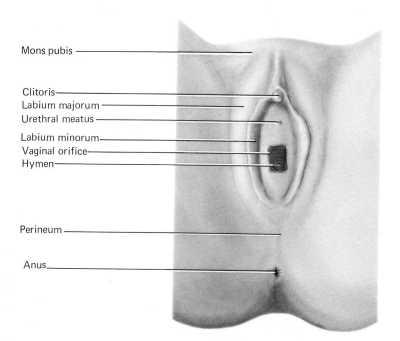

FIGURE 12.1. External female genitalia. (From Heagarty, M., Glass, G., King, H., & Manly, M. *Child health: Basics for primary care.* New York: Appleton–Century–Crofts, 1980, p. 162).

Mons pubis

Clitoris

Labium majorum

Urethral meatus

Labium minorum

Vaginal orifice

Hymen

Perineum

Anus

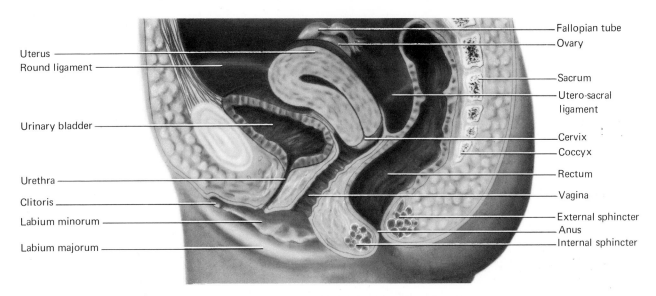

Uterus

Round ligament

Urinary bladder

Urethra

Clitoris

Labium minorum

Labium majorum

Fallopian tube

Ovary

Sacrum

Utero-sacral ligament

Cervix

Coccyx

Rectum

Vagina

External sphincter

Anus

Internal sphincter

FIGURE 12.2. Internal structure of the female genitalia. (From Heagarty, M., Glass, G., King, H., & Manly, M. *Child health: Basics for primary care.* New York: Appleton–Century–Crofts, 1980, p. 162).

The internal female genitalia consist of the *vagina, cervix, uterus, ovaries,* and *uterine tubes* (Fig. 12.2). The vagina is a muscular tube measuring 8 to 10 cms in length. The vagina is covered by a mucous membrane which lies in transverse folds called *rugae*. The upper end of the vagina is attached to the cervix. There are recesses of the vagina behind, at both sides of, and in front of the cervix. These are called the *posterior fornix,* the *lateral fornices,* and the *anterior fornix*.

The uterus is a muscular organ that communicates with the vagina below and the uterine tubes above. The upper portion of the uterus is called the *body* and the lower portion the cervix. The upper portion of the uterus between the uterine tubes is referred to as the *fundus*. The cervix projects into the vagina, where it forms lips that surround the *os*. The uterine cavity reaches into the vagina through the cervical os.

The *ovaries* are almond-shaped structures about 3 cm in length. They are located on either side of the uterus, below the uterine tubes. The two uterine tubes (*fallopian tubes*) are approximately 10 cm long. They each penetrate the uterine wall and open into the uterine cavity. The free end is in intimate contact with the ovary. This is called the *fimbriated end* due to finger-like projections, or *fimbriae*.

The levator ani and the *coccygeus* are the muscles of the pelvic floor that support the uterus. The levator ani is a paired muscle arising from the pubis and extending backward toward the midline. The urethra, vagina, and anal canal pass through this muscle. On contraction it raises the pelvic floor. The coccygei are two small muscles that extend from the spines of the ischium and insert on the sacrum and coccyx. When contracted they pull the coccyx forward.

The Anus and Rectum

The anal canal extends from the anus to the rectum and is about 4 cm in length. Strong sphincter muscles guard the anal opening.

The voluntary external sphincter is a cylinder of skeletal muscle that helps close the anus. In the upper part of the anal canal is the involuntary internal sphincter. The rectum extends from the *anal canal* to the *sigmoid colon*. It ascends from the tip of the coccyx along the coccyx to the hollow of the sacrum. In the lumen of the rectum are three folds called *valves of Houston*. These folds support the fecal mass held in the rectum. The lowest one, which projects posteriorly, can sometimes be felt. Through the anterior wall of the rectum it is possible to palpate the male prostate, the female cervix, and, in some instances, the female uterus.

PHYSICAL ASSESSMENT

Prior to the onset of the pelvic examination, the patient should be asked if she has douched within the last 24 hours or if she is menstruating. Both conditions may require postponement of the examination. Douching can interfere with accurate evaluation of vaginal secretions, smears, and cultures. Menstruation may result in an inaccurate Papanicolaou smear.

All necessary equipment should be set up in the room. It is very inconsiderate of the examiner to have to leave the patient for forgotten equipment in the middle of the examination. The equipment needed includes a good light source, drapes, vaginal specula (three sizes available), slides for vaginal and pap smears, culture media for gonorrhea, cytology fixative, 10 percent potassium hydroxide solution, saline solution, sterile swabs, Ayre spatula, cotton balls, lubricant, and gloves.

The genital area is not devoid of bacteria, so it is not necessary to use sterile technique for a routine pelvic examination. The goal is to have a working area with a minimal number of microorganisms and to prevent spread of infection to other patients. This is achieved by use of clean technique. The examiner is using clean technique when she washes her hands with warm, soapy water between examinations and uses clean rubber gloves. Each patient should be draped with a freshly laundered sheet. Metal specula are washed in a disinfectant solution and plastic specula are discarded at the completion of the examination. When a procedure is performed, such as the insertion of an intrauterine device, sterile technique is a necessity.

Patient explanation before beginning the pelvic examination is important to allay fears and to obtain the patient's cooperation. The instruments should be shown to the patient while explaining the procedure. The placement of mobiles or clever signs over the examination table can help promote relaxation. The patient is encouraged to take slow breaths in and out through her mouth while fixing her stare on the mobile.

The patient is asked to empty her bladder and then lie on the examining table in the lithotomy position. A drape placed over the patient's abdomen preserves modesty and still allows the examiner to assess her face during the examination. The patient is asked to place her hands across her chest to relax her abdominal muscles and to begin her deep breathing. The examination proceeds from the external examination to the speculum examination and finally to the bimanual examination, which includes the rectovaginal exam. The nurse explains each phase as she moves along.

External Examination

It is recommended that the nurse glove both hands for the examination. This will allow her to completely assess the genitalia and prevent the spread of infection to herself and to other patients.

To begin the examination, the nurse places one hand on the woman's inner thigh and moves her hand toward the perineum. This eliminates the startle reaction usually obtained when the perineum is touched directly. The external genitalia are then systematically inspected, including the pubic hair, labia majora, labia minora, clitoris, urethra, and anus.

The hair distribution is assessed for distribution and quantity. The distribution is normally triangular, with the base near the upper border of the pubic bone and the sides running posteriorly, covering the outer surfaces of the labia majora. The quantity of hair varies with age. It presents approximately 1 year before menarche. It is thick and kinky during the menstruating years, becoming sparse and straighter after the menopause. The skin is inspected for lesions that may indicate the presence of pubic lice, infected hair follicles, venereal warts, or lesions of herpes.

The labia majora differ with age and parity. They are scaphoid in a child, plump and well formed in the menstruating woman, and thin in the postmenopausal woman. In the nulligravida, the labia majora cover the labia minora. After childbirth the labia minora become more prominent between the now separated labia majora.

The clitoris is examined for size and lesions. The prepuce may need to be retracted for clear visualization. It is normally not longer than several centimeters. True enlargement of the clitoris is obvious. This is a common location for the chancre of syphilis in a young woman and cancerous lesions in the older woman. The urethra is examined externally for signs of inflammation.

The buttocks must be spread to inspect the anus. It is inspected for the presence of external hemorrhoids and lesions. At this time the perineum is checked for the presence of an episiotomy scar.

Palpation of the external genitalia includes palpation of the Skene's and Bartholin's glands and assessment of the support of the vaginal outlet. The Skene's glands are palpated by inserting the index finger palm side up into the introitus approximately 2.54 cms (Fig. 12.3). The urethra is then milked from the bladder neck down. If any discharge is present it should be cultured for gonorrhea (see p. 254).

The Bartholin's glands are not palpable except in infection. The index finger is now moved to the posterior end of the introitus and the thumb is placed outside the posterior part of the labia majora (Fig. 12.3). The examiner palpates between the index finger and the thumb for swelling and tenderness, one side at a time.

To assess the support of the vaginal outlet the patient is asked to bear down. Bulging observed on the anterior wall of the vaginal outlet indicates the presence of a *cystocele*. A cystocele is a prolapse of the anterior wall of the vagina and the bladder into the vagina. A *rectocele* is a prolapse of the posterior wall of the vagina and the rectum into the vagina. This is identified by a bulging on the posterior wall of the vagina. Another sign of weak vaginal support is stress incontinence as the woman bears down. Next, two fingers are inserted into the vagina and the fourchette is depressed to check resistance. Strong resistance indicates that the perineal body is intact. The patient is then asked to contract her pelvic muscles around the examiner's fingers. If she had difficulty knowing which

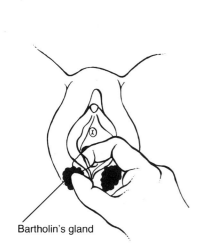

FIGURE 12.3. Palpation of Skene's and Bartholin's glands.

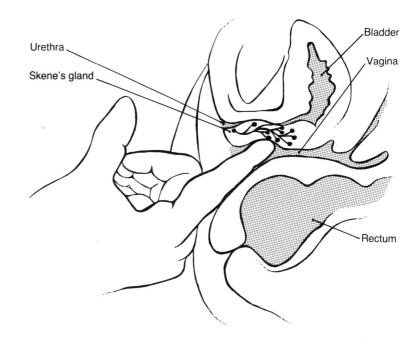

muscles to contract she should be asked to pretend she is holding her urine back. The examiner should feel pressure if the muscles are intact.

The Speculum Examination

The examiner should be sure that the speculum is of the correct size. This involves a rather rough estimate, based primarily on the patient's sexual and obstetrical history. If the woman is virginal, the smallest size of speculum is used. A medium speculum can be used comfortably with most sexually active women. A medium to large speculum is used with women who have had children. The nurse is encouraged to practice opening and closing the blades prior to insertion of the speculum. It is uncomfortable for both the patient and the examiner if the examiner does not know how to remove the blades once inserted.

Specula can be either plastic or metal. The metal speculum should be warmed either by running warm water over the blades or placing it on a heating pad. Running water over the plastic speculum will facilitate insertion. Lubricant should not be used on the blades if any smears or cultures are to be taken, as this will contaminate the results.

If the woman has never had a vaginal examination before, it is recommended that the examiner insert two fingers into the vagina and explore the introitus prior to insertion of the speculum. This is to make sure that there are no abnormalities in the vagina. This is also a good practice in general to help locate the cervix and give a clue as to where to direct the speculum.

Prior to introduction of the instrument, the patient is asked to bear down. The examiner then admits her two fingers into the vagina approximately 5 cms and spreads open the vagina with pressure on the posterior wall. The speculum, with the blades firmly together, is inserted obliquely over these two fingers (Fig. 12.4). This is to avoid contact with the sensitive urethra on the anterior vaginal wall. The fingers are then removed. Once in the vagina, the blades

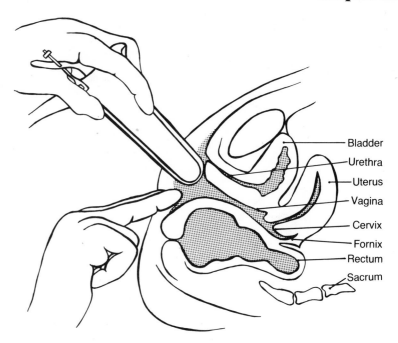

Bladder
Urethra
Uterus
Vagina
Cervix
Fornix
Rectum
Sacrum

FIGURE 12.4. Insertion of the speculum.

are turned parallel to the table for 2.54 cms and then directed at a 45° angle into the vagina. When a firm structure is reached, the instrument is opened and the cervix should be observable between the blades of the speculum. If it is not seen, the blades should be closed and directed either upward or downward to locate the cervix in the anterior or posterior position. Once the cervix is identified the speculum is secured in place.

The *cervix* is inspected for *shape of the os, color, lesions,* and *discharge.* The nulliparous os is small and either round or oval. After childbirth the cervical os presents with a slit-like appearance. The cervix is usually pink in color, but after menopause is normally pale. The cervix has a bluish appearance in early pregnancy called *Chadwick's sign.*

Three of the more common changes on the surface of the cervix are *erosions, eversions,* and *Nabothian cysts* (Fig. 12.5). An erosion presents as a beefy red, irregular area around the cervical os that bleeds easily on touch. This is not easily distinguished from a cancerous lesion and requires further assessment. An eversion is present when the lining of the cervical canal pouts out. It appears red, symmetrical, and smooth. An eversion can be due to a previous laceration or can be a variation within normal limits. Nabothian cysts are small elevations on the cervix. They are typically round, smooth, and white. They are due to obstruction or occlusion of the mucosal folds of the cervix and can be associated with chronic cervicitis.

The characteristics of the cervical discharge are observed. Normal cervical discharge varies with the menstrual cycle. Following menstruation, estrogen levels are low, so there is little discharge. Several days before ovulation the discharge becomes a cloudy yellow and is sticky. The discharge at ovulation is highly lubricative, with the consistency of egg white. This discharge, which can be heavy, persists for 1 to 3 days after ovulation. As the progesterone levels increase, the mucus becomes cloudy and sticky. Then im-

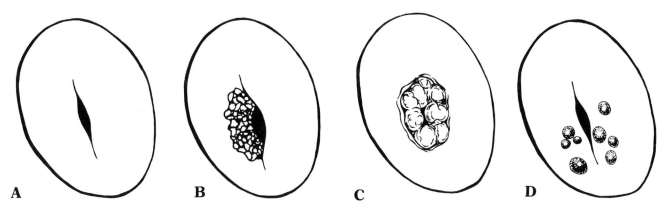

FIGURE 12.5. The cervices: (A) normal cervix, (B) eroded cervix, (C) everted cervix; (D) Nabothian cysts.

mediately prior to menstruation the discharge becomes clear and watery.

Abnormal discharges are often signs of an infectious process. The three most common types of vaginal infections are *Trichomonas vaginalis, Candida albicans,* and *Haemophilus vaginalis. Trichomonas vaginalis* produces a greenish yellow, bubbly or foamy, profuse discharge with an offensive odor. In addition, red spots may be observed on the cervix and vaginal walls. Discharge from *Candida albicans* may be thin, but is characteristically thick, white, and curdy. This discharge may cling to the walls of the vagina, giving the appearance of cottage cheese. *Haemophilus vaginalis* has a gray discharge with little or no odor. Correct identification of the specific type of discharge is not possible by observation alone. When there is suspicion of a vaginitis, vaginal smears should be obtained (see p. 254).

After the cervix is inspected, a gonorrhea culture is obtained and a Papanicolaou smear is taken. Then the blades of the speculum are unlocked and held open with the thumb. As the speculum is withdrawn, the blades are rotated to observe the walls of the vagina. The vagina is inspected for color, discharge, rugations, and lesions. The vagina is normally pink in color and becomes pale in the postmenopausal woman. When the vagina is inflamed, the walls are markedly reddened and often coated with discharge. Many folds or rugae are present in the vaginal walls of a premenopausal woman. The walls become very thin and smooth in the postmenopausal woman.

Bimanual Examination

The bimanual exam includes palpation of the vagina, cervix, uterus, adnexa (including the ovaries and fallopian tubes), and the rectum. This exam is to be done in a systematic fashion, working from the exterior to the interior. The hands remain gloved and lubricant is applied to the index and middle finger of the examining hand. These two fingers are inserted into the vagina. At the same time the thumb is hyperextended and the ring and little fingers are flexed into the palm (Fig. 12.6). The surfaces of the hand should remain perpendicular to the floor. The vaginal wall is palpated for any nodularity or tenderness. The cervix is located and described in terms of

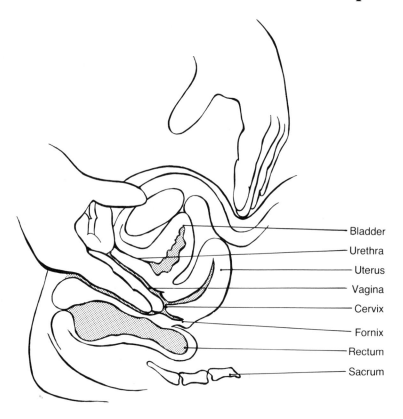

Bladder
Urethra
Uterus
Vagina
Cervix
Fornix
Rectum
Sacrum

FIGURE 12.6. Bimanual examination.

position, consistency, mobility, and patency of the os. The position of the cervix is determined by the direction in which the os is pointing. If the os is directed toward the anterior wall of the vagina, the cervix is in the *anterior position*. The cervix is in a *midline position* when the os is pointed toward the vaginal outlet. The os is directed toward the posterior wall of the vagina when the cervix is in the *posterior position*. The consistency of the cervix is normally firm—like the tip of the nose. During pregnancy the cervix softens and feels like the lips of the mouth (*Goodell's sign*). In the presence of a tumor the cervix becomes very hard. As the index finger is swept around the cervix, the cervix normally feels smooth, but if Nabothian cysts are present they may be palpated as small, round elevations.

Mobility of the cervix is determined by holding the cervix between the index and middle finger and moving it laterally and medially. Normally the cervix is freely moveable and this movement causes no discomfort. If there is malignancy or scarring due to chronic pelvic inflammatory disease, the cervix will be fixed in one position. In the presence of acute pelvic inflammatory disease, the patient will experience so much discomfort she will literally reach for the ceiling when her cervix is moved. This is called a positive *Chandlier's sign*. The examination may have to be discontinued at this point because the woman will be too uncomfortable to allow adequate palpation of the pelvic organs.

The index finger is placed at the cervical os to check for patency. Normally the os is 3 to 5 mm in diameter. If the examiner is able to admit the tip of her finger, something may have recently passed through the os, such as the contents of an abortion.

The uterus is palpated by placing the free hand on the abdomen halfway between the umbilicus and the symphysis pubis (Fig. 12.6).

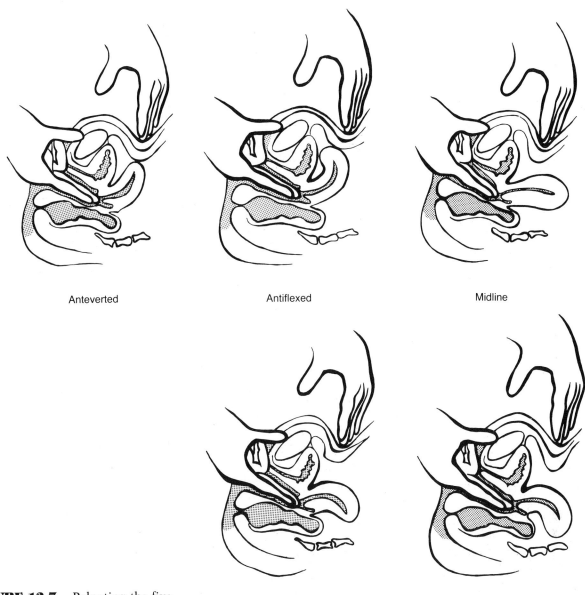

Anteverted

Antiflexed

Midline

Retroverted

Retroflexed

FIGURE 12.7. Palpating the five positions of the uterus.

The examiner simultaneously locates the vaginal fingers in the anterior vaginal fornix. The abdominal hand is moved slowly toward the pubis until the uterus is trapped between the two hands. If the uterus is not felt, the vaginal fingers are placed in the posterior fornix and the examiner again attempts to trap it between the two hands. When neither of these two methods is successful, the middle finger is placed in the rectum, leaving the index finger in the vagina. The uterus may be palpated in the posterior position through the rectal wall. The uterus is described in terms of its position, size, regularity, consistency, and mobility.

The five positions of the uterus are *anteverted, anteflexed, midposition, retroverted,* and *retroflexed* (Fig. 12.7). When the os of the cervix is pointed posteriorly and the uterus is palpated between the abdominal hand and the vaginal hand located in the anterior vaginal fornix, the uterus is *anteverted.* If the cervix is pointed anteriorly and the uterus is palpated between the abdominal hand and the vaginal hand located in the anterior vaginal fornix, the uterus is *anteflexed.* The uterus is in a *midline position* when the cervix is midline and the uterus is palpated by the abdominal and vaginal hands deep in the abdomen. The uterus is *retroverted* when the cervical os is pointed anteriorly and the uterus is palpated either in the posterior vaginal fornix or through the rectum. The uterus is *retroflexed* when the cervix is directed posteriorly and the uterus is palpated either in the posterior vaginal fornix or through the rectum.

The size of the uterus varies normally in relation to childbearing and the production of estrogen. The uterus is usually about the size of a fist and is located within the pelvic cavity. True enlargement of the uterus in a young woman should make one suspicious of pregnancy. The regularity and consistency of the uterus are determined by walking the fingers of the abdominal hand down the sides of the uterus. The surfaces of the uterus are normally smooth. Irregularities may indicate the presence of fibroids. The normal consistency of the uterus is firm. The uterus softens in pregnancy due to hormonal influence and increased circulation. As early as the fifth week of pregnancy, softness will be noted on the anterior side of the uterus just above the uterocervical junction. This is known as *Ladin's sign.* Around the sixth week of pregnancy the lower uterine segment becomes very compressible. This is *Hegar's sign.* The uterus is normally freely moveable, but may become fixed due to the adhesions of malignancy, chronic pelvic inflammatory disease, or endometriosis.

The adnexa are examined one at a time. First the abdominal hand is placed on the right-lower quadrant and the vaginal hand is placed in the right-lateral fornix. The abdominal hand is maneuvered downward along the iliac crest to trap the right ovary. This procedure is repeated on the left side. The fallopian tube is normally not palpable. The ovaries are assessed for *size, consistency, mobility,* and *tenderness.* If the ovary is palpable, it should be less than 3 to 4 cm long. It is smaller in the postmenopausal woman, and if it is palpable, a tumor should be suspected. Ovaries are usually smooth and quite mobile. Irregularities on the surface of the ovary may suggest malignancy. Anything that may cause adhesions in the pelvic cavity, such as endometriosis, may cause the ovary to become fixed. There is some discomfort normally when the ovary is compressed between the finger tips. Excessive discomfort indicates inflammation or possibly an ectopic pregnancy.

Rectovaginal Examination

The last part of the pelvic exam involves assessment of the rectovaginal area. The examining glove is changed to prevent spread of infection and the new glove is well lubricated to ease insertion. The index finger is introduced into the vagina and the middle finger is slowly moved into the rectum, allowing time for the sphincter to relax (Fig. 12.8).

The lateral, anterior and posterior walls of the rectum are systematically palpated for the presence of tumors and polyps. The anterior wall is called the *rectovaginal septum* and is normally thin, smooth, and pliable. The vaginal finger is kept on the cervix to prevent confusion when palpating through the anterior wall. Here the posterior surface of the uterus may be palpated in the ret-

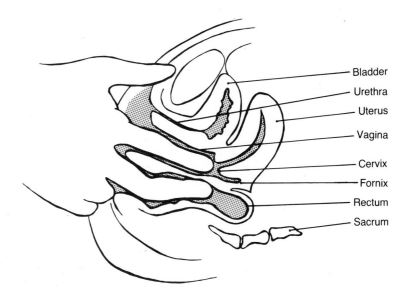

FIGURE 12.8. Rectovaginal examination.

roverted or retroflexed position. The uterosacral ligaments may not be palpable or may be felt as resilient, band-like structures. Any mass not identified as an ovary or the uterus is abnormal. After completing the examination, the nurse should inspect the stool left on the glove. If it is tarry black, it indicates the possible presence of blood in the upper gastrointestinal tract. Regardless of the apparent color of the stool, it should be tested for the presence of blood.

Vaginal Smears and Cultures

The *Papanicolaou smear* (Pap smear) is a simple screening test for cervical cancer. The American Cancer Society recommends that all asymptomatic women age 20 and over, and those under 20 who are sexually active, have a Pap test annually for two negative examinations and then at least every three years until the age of 65. Women who are at risk for developing cancer need more frequent testing. Vaginal discharge is obtained from three sites: the *endocervix, cervix,* and *vaginal pool* (Fig. 12.9). A swab is inserted into the os of the cervix and rotated 360°. The discharge is gently rolled onto the slide in the location marked *E*. The longer end of the Ayre spatula is placed at the squamocolumnar junction and is rotated a full 360°. This discharge is rolled onto the slide in the

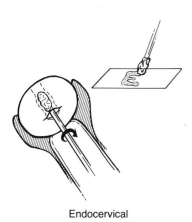

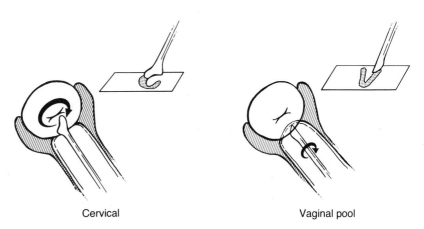

Endocervical   Cervical   Vaginal pool

FIGURE 12.9. Obtaining a Pap smear.

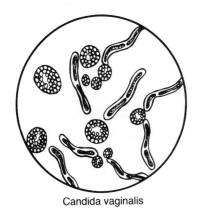

Candida vaginalis

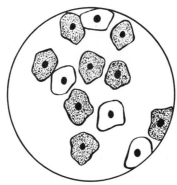

Haemophilus vaginalis
"Clue cells"

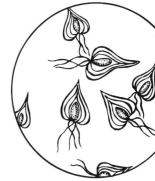

Trichomonads

FIGURE 12.10. Microscopic findings in common vaginal infections.

location marked *C*. Under the cervix, discharge collects on the lower blade of the speculum. This is called the vaginal pool. This discharge is obtained with the handle of the Ayre spatula and placed onto the slide in the location marked *V*.

When a *gonorrhea culture* is indicated, the examiner should be sure to obtain it prior to the Pap smear. If the Pap smear is done first, the necessary discharge may have been removed and the gonorrhea culture returns may be falsely negative.

To obtain the gonorrhea culture, a swab is placed in the cervical canal and rotated 360°. If the history indicates exposure to gonorrhea through oral or rectal intercourse, the specimen is obtained from the appropriate location. The discharge is placed on a Thayer Martin Plate or Transgrow bottle in a *Z* pattern. The Thayer Martin culture is placed upside down in a large jar with a candle. The candle is lit and the cover secured in place. The Transgrow bottle requires the placement of a CO_2 tablet in the plate. Both types of medium are placed in an incubator.

Secretions that look suspicious of a vaginal infection should be obtained from the vaginal pool and placed on a glass slide. To test for *Trichomonas vaginalis* and *Haemophilus vaginalis*, the secretions are mixed with a drop of normal saline and a cover slip is applied. The specimen should be observed immediately under a microscope to identify the spindle-shaped, highly mobile trichomonads. If *Haemophilus vaginalis* is the causative organism, "clue cells" will be seen. These are epithelial cells that appear to be stippled or granulated.[3]

To test for *Candida albicans*, the secretions are mixed with a drop of 10 percent potassium hydroxide (KOH). The specimen is then observed under a microscope to identify the characteristic buds and mycelia. Because of the uncertainty as to which type of vaginal infection may be present, it is best to prepare both a KOH slide and a saline slide and to examine both under the microscope (Fig. 12.10).

REFERENCES

1. Eveleth, P. & Tanner, J. *Worldwide variation in human growth.* Cambridge: Cambridge University Press, 1976.
2. Martin, L. *Health care of women.* Philadelphia: Lippincott, 1978, p. 7.
3. Greenhill, J. B. *Office gynecology.* Chicago: Year Book Medical, 1977, p. 91.
4. American Cancer Society, Inc. *Guidelines for the Cancer-Related Checkup,* New York. Vol. 30 (4), 1980 p. 219.

EXAMPLE OF A RECORDED HISTORY AND PHYSICAL

Subjective:

Chief Complaint (Reason for Visit): Vaginal itching for 3 days.

HPI: This 30-year-old white female considers herself to be in good health. Three days ago she first noticed vaginal itching which has become increasingly worse. It is accompanied by a thick, white, odorless discharge. Her LMP was 10 days ago on March 10th. This was a normal 5 day menses with a moderate flow. She has been on oral contraceptives (Ortho Novum 1/50) for the past 8 years without any known side effects. She is para O, gravida O. She has a satisfying sexual relationship with her husband. She feels that they are both monogamous. She denies urinary frequency, burning, urgency, hematuria, fever, or abdominal pain. No past history of urinary tract infection, venereal disease, or vaginal infections. The family history is negative for diabetes. She finds this problem to be a "nuisance."

Objective:

External Genitalia: Normal female hair distribution, no lesions or rashes. Bartholin's and Skene's glands not palpable.

Urethra: No discharge.

Vaginal: Reddened; thick, white discharge clinging to the walls; no odor.

Cervix: Dark pink to red, no lesions, whitish discharge at os, nulliparous, posterior position, firm, moveable, nontender.

Uterus: Small, smooth, freely moveable, anteverted. No tenderness.

Adnexae: Not palpable. No tenderness.

Rectovaginal: No masses.

13

The Male Genitalia

Our society puts a great deal of emphasis on sexuality. This produces anxieties and concerns particular to the genitourinary system. Parents of newborn boys will have questions regarding the necessity for circumcision. Preadolescent and adolescent boys wonder about their own physical development and often compare themselves to peers. The adult who is sexually active may have times in his life when sexual concerns exist. As men age, the fear of prostatic disease increases, as well as anxiety regarding decreased sexual functioning. For these reasons and more, the nurse should approach the genitourinary history and examination with sensitivity.

HISTORY

The genitourinary history of the male patient differs in accordance with the age of the patient. The infant's history is geared toward identifying parental concerns. Often parents will have questions about the development of their child's genitals which they may be hesitant to mention. The nurse can anticipate these questions by offering reassurance of normal findings while examining the baby.

Toilet training practices should be discussed with all parents of toddlers. The nurse should ascertain the expectations of the parents. Many parents are not aware that physiologically, most children are not ready for toilet training before 18 to 30 months of age.*

Enuresis is involuntary bed wetting during sleep in a child whose age and development indicate that he should have control. It is *primary* enuresis if the child has never established bladder control and *secondary* enuresis if the child has previously established control and later loses it. Complete control of urination should be achieved by 4 to 5 years of age. The parent of the preschool or school-age child should be asked if there is a problem with bed wetting. If there is a positive history, the nurse should determine if it involves primary or secondary enuresis.*

*These questions should be asked of both boys and girls.

Because of the insidiousness of urinary tract infections and the often serious consequences, all children should be asked about related signs and symptoms. These can differ greatly among children and among different age groups. In an infant, failure to thrive, unexplained fevers, lethargy, irritability, vomiting, and diarrhea are common complaints. In a preschooler, anorexia, vomiting, abdominal pain, diarrhea, and enuresis may be the first indications of a problem.*

Obtaining the genitourinary history of an adolescent or adult male can be sensitive for both the female examiner and her patient. The examiner should be comfortable with her own sexuality and view exploration of this system as necessary to understand the patient holistically. Questions should be presented in a matter-of-fact way, using precise terms that are familiar to the patient. Included in the review of the male genitourinary system are questions that may uncover the presence of urinary tract disease, venereal disease, hernias, and prostatic disease. This is an appropriate time to elicit the sexual history (see Chap. 1).

Symptoms of urinary tract infection in the adult are more specific than in the child. Every patient should be asked if he is experiencing painful urination, urgency, hematuria, decreased output or no urine output, backache, lethargy, or abdominal pain. In addition, the examiner should go over the course and treatment of any past urinary tract infection.

Each patient should be asked about symptoms that may indicate the presence of venereal disease. These include lesions or rashes in the genital area, discharge from the urethra, and painful urination. The examiner should ask about any past history of venereal disease and how it was treated. Finally, she should determine the patient's knowledge of venereal disease, including symptoms, prevention, and treatment.

To explore for the presence of hernias, the examiner should ask the patient if he has noticed any swelling in the groin or scrotum that is accentuated with straining, lifting, or coughing. If his occupation requires heavy lifting, he may be at risk for the development of a hernia.

Middle aged and elderly patients should be asked about symptoms that are related to the presence of prostatic disease. These include hesitancy, slow stream, urinary frequency and dribbling, and nocturnia.

The nurse should obtain a family history of kidney problems on all males from infancy through old age. Pertinent information to elicit includes a family history of nephritis, nephrosis, kidney masses, or cancer of the prostate.

ANATOMY

The anatomy of the male genitalia, hernia areas, and prostate will be covered in this section (see Chap. 12 for anatomy of the rectum).

Male Genitalia

The male genitalia include the penis and the scrotum (Fig. 13.1). The penis consists of the *shaft, corona, glans, foreskin,* and *urethra.* The shaft of the penis is formed dorsally by two lateral columns, the *corpora cavernosa,* and ventrally by one column, the *corpus spongiosum,* which contains the urethra. These three columns are bound together by heavy fibrous tissue. At the end of the shaft is the glans penis. The urethra traverses through the glans to its termination point at the tip of the glans. The point where the glans and the shaft meet is called the corona. The prepuce or foreskin is a flap of skin that covers the glans. This is the piece of skin that is removed at the time of circumcision.

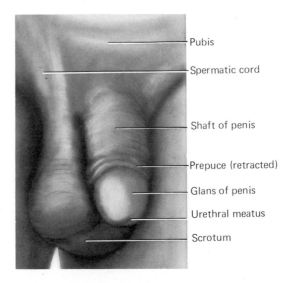

Pubis

Spermatic cord

Shaft of penis

Prepuce (retracted)

Glans of penis

Urethral meatus

Scrotum

FIGURE 13.1. External male genitalia. (From Heagarty, M., Glass, G., King, H., & Manly, M. *Child health: Basics for primary care.* New York: Appleton–Century–Crofts, 1980, p. 164)

The scrotum is a pouch-like sac that is internally separated by a septal fold. Each half contains a *testis* with its *epididymis* and *spermatic cord.* The testis is an oval body about 1.5 inches in length. The testes should be descended by birth. Of those that are undescended, one half descend by the first month and one fourth by the end of the first year. The epididymis is a comma-shaped structure attached to the posterolateral surface of the testis. In approximately 7 percent of men, it is on the anterior surface of the testis. The spermatic cord consists of the *vas deferens, blood vessels, lymphatic vessels,* and *nerves.* The vas deferens passes from the epididymis through the inguinal canal and enters the abdominal cavity, eventually descending into the pelvic cavity.

Hernia Areas

The inguinal ligament goes from the anterior superior iliac spine to the pubic tubercle. Just above the lateral to the pubic tubercle is the *external inguinal ring* of the *inguinal canal.* The inguinal canal, a flattened tunnel between superficial and deep layers of abdominal muscle, extends to the internal ring, which is 1 to 2 cm above the midpoint of the inguinal ligament.

The *femoral canal* is a potential space below the inguinal ligament. It is located medial to the femoral artery and lateral to the pubic tubercle.

There are two types of hernias: *inguinal* and *femoral.* An inguinal hernia can be either *direct* or *indirect* (Fig. 13.2). The direct hernia originates above the inguinal ligament, close to the pubic tubercle and near the external inguinal ring. It emerges directly from behind and through the external ring. The indirect hernia originates above and near the midpoint of the inguinal ligament at the internal inguinal ring. It comes down the canal. A femoral hernia presents on the anterior surface of the thigh just below the inguinal ligament (Fig. 13.2).

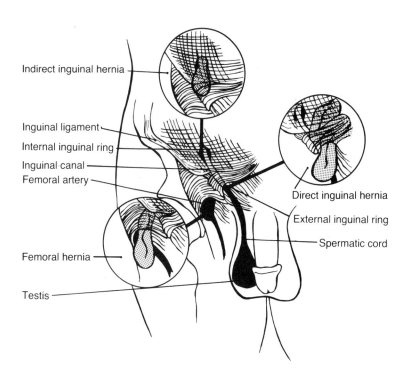

Indirect inguinal hernia

Inguinal ligament
Internal inguinal ring
Inguinal canal
Femoral artery

Direct inguinal hernia
External inguinal ring
Spermatic cord

Femoral hernia

Testis

FIGURE 13.2. Common hernias: femoral, direct inguinal, and indirect inguinal.

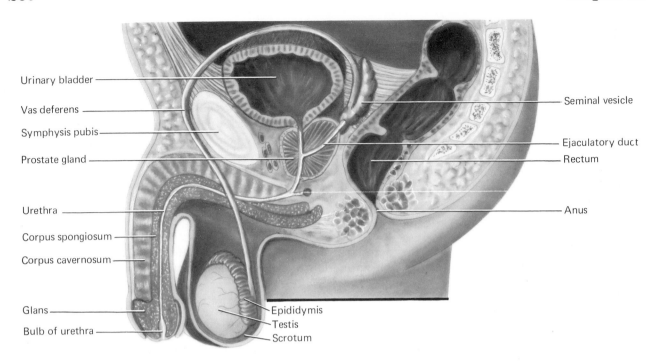

Urinary bladder

Vas deferens

Symphysis pubis

Prostate gland

Urethra

Corpus spongiosum

Corpus cavernosum

Glans

Bulb of urethra

Seminal vesicle

Ejaculatory duct

Rectum

Anus

Epididymis

Testis

Scrotum

FIGURE 13.3. Internal structure of the male genitalia. (From Heagarty, M., Glass, G., King, H., & Manly, M. *Child health: Basics for primary care.* New York: Appleton–Century–Crofts, 1980, p. 164)

The Prostate Gland

The *prostate gland* is a solid, heart-shaped structure about 2.5 cm in length (Fig. 13.3). It lies in the pelvis 2 cm posterior to the symphysis pubis. The posterior surface is in close contact with the rectal wall and is the only portion accessible to palpation. Three lobes comprise the prostate: the *median lobe* and the *right* and *left lateral lobes*. The two lateral lobes are on the posterior surface of the gland and are divided by a *shallow median furrow*. The seminal vesicles extend above and lateral from the prostate (Fig. 13.3).

PHYSICAL ASSESSMENT

It is essential to give patient explanation prior to beginning the examination of the male genitalia, hernia areas, and prostate. The exam should use a systematic approach and should be done quickly, considering the patient's modesty. If further questions arise during the exam, it is best to delay them until the examination is completed and the patient is clothed. These measures help to prevent a potentially embarrassing or uncomfortable situation for the examiner and patient. The examiner should be sure to communicate findings to the patient or his parents. Parents of young children and also adolescent patients need reassurance that all is normal.

The easiest way to begin the exam is with the patient standing and the examiner seated in front of him. The genitalia and groin are exposed for general inspection. This is followed by inspection and palpation of the penis, scrotum, and hernia areas. Finally, the patient turns around and leans over the exam table for the examination of the rectum and prostate. The entire examination of infants and young children can be done in a supine position. The equipment necessary is a glove and lubricant for the rectal and prostate examination and a flashlight to transilluminate a hydrocele or cystocele.

Examination of the Male Genitalia

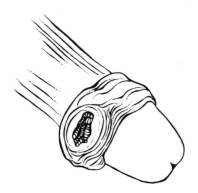

FIGURE 13.4. Syphilitic chancre.

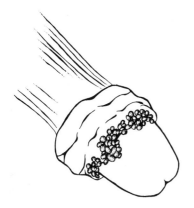

FIGURE 13.5. Condyloma accuminata.

General inspection includes examination of the hair, skin, and groin. Curly pubic hair becomes apparent between 11 and 18 years of age and has a triangular pattern of distribution. The skin over the genital area is inspected for any lesions and the groin is observed for signs of swelling.

The penis is inspected for size, lesions, placement of the urethral opening, and discharge. In infancy, the nonerect penis is 2 to 3 cm, increasing in size between the ages of 10 and 15 years. A mature size of approximately 8 to 10 cm is reached by 16 to 21 years of age. The presence of an infantile penis at adolescence is suggestive of a hormonal problem.

The shaft, prepuce, and glans of the penis are observed for the presence of a *syphilitic chancre, venereal warts, ulcers,* and *nodules.* The *syphilitic chancre* is the primary lesion of syphilis (Fig. 13.4). It appears as an oval, dark red erosion with a smooth, rounded border. It is typically painless and singular. Venereal warts, called *condyloma accuminata,* are small, elongated projections which may be either moist or dry (Fig. 13.5). The syphilitic chancre and condyloma accuminata can be found in children as well as in adults (see Chap. 3). The lesion associated with carcinoma of the penis may be dry and scaly or ulcerated. This is seen more frequently in men who were not circumcised in childhood, and may be masked by the prepuce.

If the prepuce is present, the client should be asked to retract it so that the glans can be observed. It should be easily retractable. A normal exception is in the first 2 to 3 months of life, when the foreskin is normally tight. *Phimosis* is a condition in which the prepuce cannot be retracted. *Paraphimosis* exists when the prepuce is partially retracted and cannot return to normal position. At the time of retraction the external meatus is examined for position and discharge. The meatus should be positioned centrally in the glans. *Hypospadias* is the congenital displacement of the urethral meatus to the inferior (ventral) surface of the penis (Fig. 13.6). *Epispadias* is malpositioning of the meatus on the dorsal surface of the penis (Fig. 13.6). To observe for discharge from the urethra, the examiner should have the patient hold the penis with his thumb and index finger at the base and then milk downward.

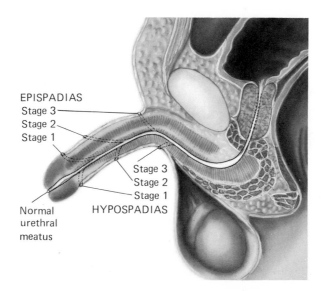

FIGURE 13.6. Abnormalities of urethral meatus. (From Heagarty, M., Glass, G., King, H., & Manly, M. *Child health: Basics for primary care* New York: Appleton–Century–Crofts, 1980, p. 164).

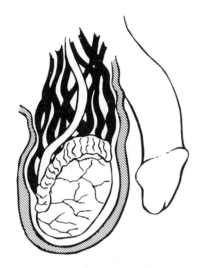

FIGURE 13.7. Varicocele.

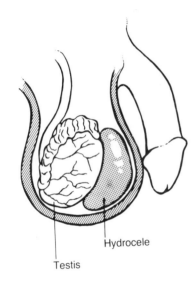

Hydrocele

Testis

FIGURE 13.8. Hydrocele.

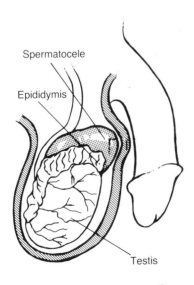

Spermatocele

Epididymis

Testis

FIGURE 13.9. Spermatocele.

If any penile lesions or urethral discharge have been observed on inspection, gloves must be worn while palpating the genitalia. The penis is held between the thumb and first two fingers and gently palpated. The examiner should note any tenderness of lesions and the size of nodules that are present. Some patients have nontender hard plaques just beneath the skin, usually along the dorsum of the penis. These patients often complain of crooked, painful erections. This is known as *Peyronie's disease*, which is a chronic disease of unknown cause.

When inspecting the scrotum, it is essential to lift the sac up to observe the undersurface as well as the anterior surface. The scrotum is inspected for symmetry, size, lesions, and swelling. The left side is lower than the right because of a longer spermatic cord on that side. Size of the scrotum varies considerably among boys at the age of puberty. The scrotum begins to increase in size at the average age of 12 to 13 years and full development is reached at the average age of 18 to 21 years. Size of the scrotum normally changes with temperature. The *dartos muscle* of the scrotum contracts when the scrotum is cold and relaxes when it is warm. Sebaceous cysts are common cutaneous skin lesions found on the scrotum. They are yellow-white in appearance and on palpation are firm and nontender. A taut swelling of the scrotum with pitting edema may be associated with the generalized edema of cardiac or nephrotic disease.

The scrotum is gently palpated between the thumb and first two fingers on both sides simultaneously. The contents of the scrotum, including the testes, epididymis, vas deferens, and spermatic cord, are palpated separately. The testes should be descended into the scrotal sac. If they are not in the scrotum, the examiner should explore for their presence in the inguinal canal or in the abdomen just proximal to the internal inguinal ring. This is done by placing the index finger at the bottom of the scrotum to allow enough skin to invaginate the tissue up to the inguinal ring. Be aware of the cremasteric reflex in boys (see Chap. 15), causing the testes to ascend into the abdomen when the boy is cold or embarrassed. This may cause an apparent undescended testis. The reflex can be eliminated by having the child sit cross-legged on the table. Compression of the testes is normally painful. A very hard testicle or a lump in a portion of the testicle should make the examiner suspicious of cancer.

The epididymis is normally resilient. A hard, enlarged, nontender epididymis may be due to tuberculosis. Acute epididymitis may result from trauma or an adjacent infection. This results in an epididymis that is tender and swollen. Each spermatic cord with its vas deferens is palpated (between the thumb and index finger) along its course, from the epididymis to the external inguinal ring. Any swelling or nodules are noted. A *varicocele* consists of varicose veins of the spermatic cord (Fig. 13.7). It is more common on the left, because the left spermatic vein empties into the left renal vein and is competing for blood from the kidney. The right spermatic vein empties directly into the vena cava. A varicocele feels like a bag of worms and disappears when the patient is supine. If it does not disappear in the supine position, obstruction from malignancy should be suspected.

Any swelling or mass in the scrotum should be evaluated by transillumination. This is done by pulling the scrotal wall tightly over the mass and putting the flashlight in contact with the posterior side of the scrotum. After darkening the room, the examiner shines a beam of light through the mass looking for transmission of light as a red glow. Serous fluid will transilluminate; tissue and blood will not. The examiner is specifically observing for a *hydrocele* or *spermatocele*.

A hydrocele is the most common mass in the scrotum. It is a soft or tense fluid-filled sac either surrounding the testis or located in the spermatic cord (Fig. 13.8). The mass may be due to infection or trauma and can be transilluminated. Hydroceles in infancy result from the accumulation of peritoneal fluid in the scrotal sac. The fluid usually resorbs during the first year. They may be associated with a potential hernia. A *spermatocele* is a cyst of the epididymis just above or behind the testis which can be transilluminated (Fig. 13.9). This mass contains spermatozoa and feels like a third testis.

Examination of the Hernia Areas

When the patient is relaxed, the inguinal and femoral areas are inspected for any obvious bulges that may indicate the presence of a hernia. The patient is then asked to strain down, with the examiner again observing for any masses.

Inguinal hernias are palpated by having the client stand with his ipsilateral leg slightly flexed and the examiner seated in front of him. Using the right index finger for examining the patient's right side, and the left index finger for the left side, the examiner invaginates the loose scrotal skin, starting at a low point on the scrotum (Fig. 13.10). The spermatic cord is followed upward to the external ring. With the finger either at the external ring or within the canal, the patient is asked to turn his face to one side, strain down, and cough. The examiner notes any palpable herniating mass as it touches the finger. An indirect hernia will touch the finger tip. In the presence of a direct hernia, the bulge will strike the side of the finger when the patient is straining, since it comes directly through the abdominal wall instead of down the inguinal canal.

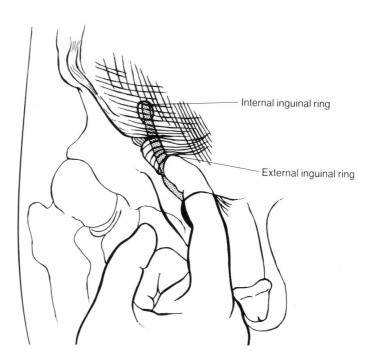

Internal inguinal ring

External inguinal ring

FIGURE 13.10. Examining for inguinal hernias.

The location of the femoral canal is estimated by placing the right index finger on the patient's right femoral artery. The middle finger will then lie over the femoral vein and the ring finger will lie over the femoral canal. If a femoral hernia is present, a soft mass will be felt which becomes larger as the patient strains or coughs.

The inguinal and femoral nodes are inspected and palpated at this time (Fig. 13.11).

Examination of the Rectum and Prostate

In Caucasians, cancer of the prostate is the third most common cause of death in men over the age of 55 and the main cause after the age of 75.[1] Cancer of the prostate is less common in other racial groups.[2] The rectum and prostate gland should be examined yearly on every man, and more frequently if the patient has a problem or a family history of cancer of the prostate. Examination of the rectum is not routinely done with children, unless the history indicates a problem.

The patient is given instructions to empty his bladder prior to beginning the rectal and prostate examination, because a full bladder causes loss of definition of the base of the prostate gland. To begin the examination, the examiner has the adult patient turn around and lean on the examining table with his toes pointed toward each other. If the patient is debilitated, a lateral Sims' position may be used. The young child should be in the supine position with his knees and hips flexed towards the abdomen. The anus of the adult is observed for fissures, hemorrhoids, and bleeding. In children, the examiner observes for a foreign body, fissure, skin tags, pilonidal dimple, bleeding, and signs of scratching (possibly due to the presence of pinworms).

Next, the examining hand should be gloved and the index finger well lubricated. The examiner places the index finger (the fifth finger may be used with children) at the anus and waits a few seconds to relax the sphincter. She then gently inserts the finger, noting muscle tone, sphincter tone, and tenderness. The lateral and posterior walls are systematically palpated for tumors, polyps, and stool. The prostate gland of the adult patient is felt on the anterior wall of the rectum. Each lobe is palpated, starting from the median furrow and moving out to the lateral aspects. Every portion of the gland is covered, noting its symmetry, consistency, size and tenderness (Fig. 13.12).

Both sides of the prostate should be symmetric and have a smooth, firm, rubbery consistency. A boggy prostate is abnormal and could be indicative of an infectious process. Any stony, hard nodules should make the examiner suspicious of cancer. The initial cancerous lesion usually involves the posterior portion of the prostate, which is readily palpable. Size of the prostate is not as important in detecting cancer as symmetry and consistency. Benign prostatic hypertrophy is extremely common in men older than 50 years. The prostate may bulge more than 1 cm into the rectal lumen. The hypertrophied tissue tends to obliterate the median furrow. The prostate is tender when inflammation is present. Cancerous lesions are usually nontender.

Finally, an attempt is made to palpate the seminal vesicles above the prostate. They are normally not palpable, but if they are involved in an inflammatory reaction, they may be dilated and extremely tender. At the completion of the examination, the

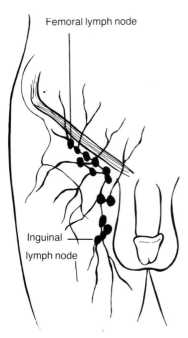

Femoral lymph node

Inguinal
lymph node

FIGURE 13.11. Inguinal and femoral lymph nodes.

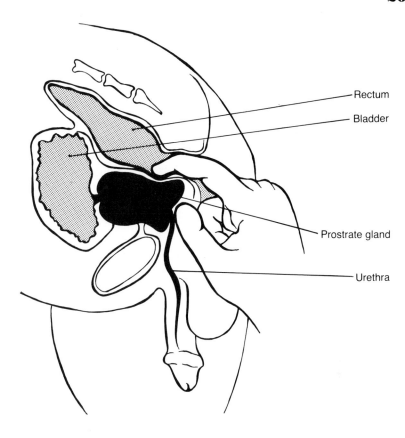

FIGURE 13.12. Palpating the prostate.

examiner should inspect the stool left on the glove for the presence of blood. The stool should be routinely tested for the presence of blood.

REFERENCES

1. Shortridge, L. M. & McLain, B. R. Primary care and prostate cancer. *Nurse Practitioner*, 1979, *4*, 25–27.
2. Rhodes, G., Glober, G., & Stemmermann, G. A review of some tumors of interest for demographic study in Hawaii. *Hawaii Medical Journal*, 1974, *33*, 283–284.

EXAMPLE OF A RECORDED HISTORY AND PHYSICAL

Subjective:

Chief Complaint (Reason for Visit): "I have had pain when urinating since yesterday."

HPI: This 19-year-old white college male considers himself to be in good health. Last night he had a sudden onset of urgency and painful urination. This morning he noticed a small amount of yellowish discharge from his penis. He has casual sexual relationships with three women. His last sexual contact was 3 days ago. He is not aware of having been exposed to venereal disease. He has never experienced these symptoms in the past. He denies hematuria, backache, lethargy, chills, fever, rashes in the genital area, genital lesions, past history of urinary tract infection, and past history of venereal disease. There is no family history of kidney disease. He is very concerned that he may have the "clap."

OBJECTIVE:

Penis: Circumcized. No lesions or rash; normal size; no masses; small amount of yellow discharge from the urethra with milking.

Scrotum: No rash, lesions, masses, or swelling; testes descended. No tenderness of epididymis or spermatic cord.

Prostate: Firm, no masses or tenderness.

Lymph nodes: Inguinal and femoral nodes not palpable or tender.

Abdomen: No tenderness over general abdomen or suprapubic or CVA areas. No masses palpated.

14

The Musculoskeletal System

The musculoskeletal system is highly complex and rarely evaluated independently. Because of the interrelationship of this system to the neurologic and cardiovascular systems, these systems would ordinarily be assessed together. This is particularly true of the extremities. For the purposes of this chapter, however, the specifics of history taking for and examination of the musculoskeletal system will be dealt with separately. Essential material relating to the pediatric population will be incorporated throughout the chapter. The musculoskeletal system in children is usually thoroughly assessed at each well child check. Adults, however, rarely need as complete an assessment as is described in this chapter, unless specific complaints are presented. Then the importance of being thorough cannot be overemphasized. An adult screening examination of the musculoskeletal system would consist primarily of joint inspection and determination of active range of motion and strength on resistance. Any difficulties would then be investigated more thoroughly, including assessment of the degrees of range of motion.

The examiner should develop the habit of establishing a baseline of data for each patient. This will allow for comparison of data, especially important for older patients so that true changes in function can be quickly established.

HISTORY

A careful history, especially if a particular problem exists, is absolutely vital. Frequently what may appear superficially to be a musculoskeletal disorder can be, in fact, the result of changes in the cardiovascular, respiratory, neurologic, or other organ systems.

Because pain and loss of function are the most common presenting complaints, a thorough history of present illness (HPI) relevant to that pain is mandatory, including answers to the following questions.

Onset: How did you feel before the pain started? When did the pain start (exact time and date, if at all possible)?

Setting: How did it start? What were you doing when it started (vacuuming, football, etc.)?

Location: Where exactly is the pain and does it radiate?

Character: Describe how the pain feels (aching, burning, sharp, stabbing, throbbing, etc.). How does the pain feel now as compared to when it started?

Sequence and chronology: Does the pain come and go or is it steady?

Associated phenomena: Headache? Fever? Weakness? Numbness and tingling? Nausea, vomiting and/or diarrhea, weight loss? Cough? Redness and swelling of joints?

Aggravating factors: What makes the pain worse (motion, etc.)?

Alleviating factors: What makes the pain better (medication, rest, etc.)?

Relevant personal history: Previous history of musculoskeletal problems (dates, diagnostic studies, treatment)? The examiner should be sure to elicit a trauma history in children and adolescents.

Relevant family history: Arthritis (type), gout, congenital defects, cardiovascular or neurologic disorders, cancer?

Disability: Changes in activity at home, work, and school? The type of outside work and current family or work stresses are also important, as they can have a bearing on continued disability.

The examiner should try to have the client be as specific as possible, because pain alone is a subjective experience and cannot be observed, except indirectly through facial expressions and, in severe instances, changes in vital signs.

Particular problems parents might notice that are relevant to the musculoskeletal system are flat feet, toeing in or out, poor posture, and limitation of movement when playing with others. A new mother might notice difficulty diapering the baby because one hip is tight. Even if parents do not notice or complain of the above problems, the examiner should ask about them specifically.

Sports injuries are all too common in the adolescent age group, particularly if height and weight are inadequate for the sport or class—i.e., football and wrestling. The adolescent may not complain about pain if he or (more recently) she knows this will result in activity limitation or ridicule by teammates. Sensitivity to this aspect of development will aide the examiner in gathering complete data.

Much of the history will be elicited during other sections of the health history or in the HPI. This information is generally gathered in relation to the ability to perform activities of daily living. The presence of loss of function without pain in a patient under the age of 40 unquestionably requires an in-depth evaluation.

ANATOMY

The skeletal system provides structure and support for the body and its 206 bones. This system is also involved in blood cell formation and acts as a protective structure for underlying organs (i.e., the brain and lungs). Individual bones are generally classified in four categories:

1. Irregular (i.e., vertebra)
2. Short (i.e., hand)
3. Long (i.e., leg)
4. Flat (i.e., pelvis)

Groups of bones are classified into two categories:

1. The axial skeleton (bones of the head, vertebral column, and ribs).
2. The appendicular skeleton (shoulder, pelvis, and extremities).

Voluntary or striated muscles, of which there are over 600, comprise approximately 40 percent of the body's muscle mass and attach themselves to various points on the bony skeleton. Involuntary or smooth muscles are found in parts of the body which act automatically or without effort on the part of the individual (i.e., blood vessels and the stomach). The heart is usually listed separately, for though it consists of striated muscle, it is not under voluntary control.

The articular system consists of various joints throughout the body and is generally broken down into three functional categories:

1. *Synovial joints*
2. *Fibrous joints*
3. *Cartilaginous joints*

The synovial joint consists of a *joint space,* a *joint capsule,* a *synovial membrane,* and an *articular cartilage* which forms over the ends of two adjoining bones (Fig. 14.1).

The *articular cartilage* acts as a cushion between two joint bones. The loose synovial membrane lines the joint space and secretes synovial fluid; both the membrane and the fluid allow for freedom of movement within the joint capsule. The knee and hip are examples of synovial joints.

Fibrous joints consist of two bones bound by fibrous material and are found where little, if any, movement is needed—i.e., the suture lines of the skull.

Cartilaginous joints allow for only limited motion. The *hyaline type* is found where the first rib joins the sternum. The *fibrocartilaginous type* is found in the vertebral column.

Tendons are tough fibers which are part of the muscle and join muscle to bone. *Ligaments* are fibers which join bone to bone. These are connective tissues which are also assessed in the physical examination.

Various joints of the body will be discussed at length in terms of their anatomy and range of motion. There are many differences among individuals in these joints due to age, general health, and amount of exercise undertaken. Degrees of motion given are averages. The table at the end of the assessment section can act as a guide during the nurse's assessment. Only major bony and muscle structures will be discussed (for greater depth the reader is referred to the reference section at the end of the chapter).

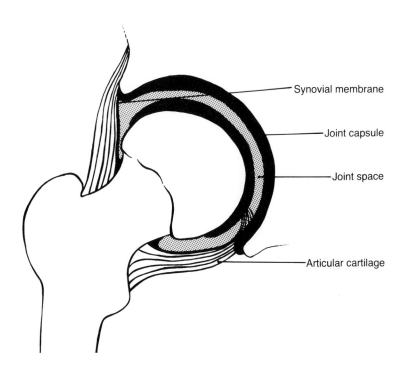

Synovial membrane

Joint capsule

Joint space

Articular cartilage

FIGURE 14.1. The anatomic structure of the joint capsule.

The Temporomandibular Joint

This joint is the point of articulation of the mandible with the skull and is the only movable joint in this portion of the axial skeleton (Fig. 14.2). It is also one of the most used joints in the body and is subject to great stress in the course of a lifetime. The hinge and glide motion is usually symmetrical and can be felt by placing an index finger in the anterior external auditory canal, or directly over the joint, while the patient opens and closes his mouth.

The Shoulder

Many of the structures of the shoulder can be easily identified (Fig. 14.3):

1. The *clavicle* articulates with the manubrium sternum at the *sternoclavicular joint* and the *acromioclavicular joint* in the shoulder. This is the only bone joining the shoulder girdle to the axial skeleton.
2. The *greater and lesser tubercle of the humerus* on the anterior aspect of the shoulder.
3. The *groove* for the biceps tendon.
4. The *deltoid muscle* which overlies the shoulder.
5. The *scapula*.
6. The *glenohumeral joint* between the scapula and the humerus.
7. The *biceps*.
8. The *triceps*.

The subacromial bursa, which lies between the deltoid and supraspinatus muscles, is not normally identifiable.

The Spine

From the posterior view the spinal column is normally straight from the base of the skull (Fig. 14.4). There are 7 *cervical*, 12 *thoracic*, 5 *lumbar*, 5 *sacral*, and 4 *coccygeal vertebrae*. The spinous processes may be seen easily if the patient is not obese, particularly the prominent processes of C_7 and T_1 on a plane with the superior tip of the scapular. L_4 can be identified by drawing a line between the right and left iliac crests. From the lateral view the cervical concave curves can be seen easily.

Major muscle bodies which can be identified in the neck include the *sternocleidomastoid*, which extends from behind the ear to the sternoclavicular junction, and the *trapezius*, which extends posteriorly from the base of the skull to the shoulder and to the mid-thoracic region in a triangle. Motions of both the neck and the rest of the spine include flexion, extension, rotation, and lateral bending.

The Elbow

The bony structures of the elbow are readily identified, as follows (Fig. 14.5).

1. The *olecranon* (the most visible point posteriorly).
2. The *olecranon fossa* (just superior to the olecranon).
3. The *medial* (closest to the body) and *lateral epicondyles* of the *humerus*.
4. The groove for the ulnar nerve just inferior to the medial epicondyle (frequently referred to by the patient as the "funny bone"); the *medial collateral ligament* overlies this groove and is not normally palpable.

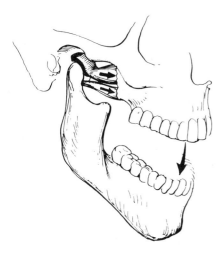

FIGURE 14.2. The external pterygoid muscle's two heads act asynchronously to open the temporomandibular joint. (From Hoppenfeld, S. *Physical examination of the spine and extremities.* New York: Appleton–Century–Crofts, 1976, p. 129)

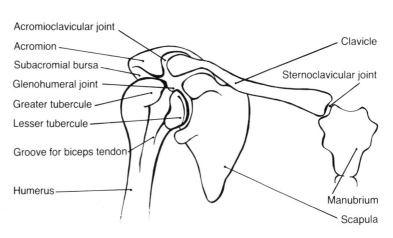

FIGURE 14.3. Bony structures of the shoulder.

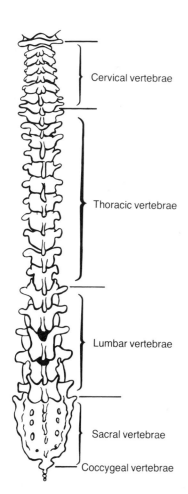

FIGURE 14.4. Posterior view of the spine.

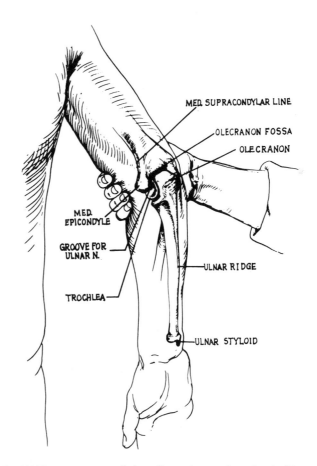

FIGURE 14.5. Anatomy of the elbow (posterior view). (From Hoppenfeld, S. *Physical examination of the spine and extremities.* New York: Appleton–Century–Crofts, 1976, p. 38)

The wrist flexors are palpable along the anterolateral portion of the forearm and the extensors are palpable on the anterior medial aspect. Of the latter, the *brachioradialis* can be easily identified by flexing the elbow to 90° and applying pressure against resistance at the wrist. The motions of the elbow include flexion, extension, hyperextension, supination, and pronation.

The Wrist, Hand, and Fingers

The bones of the forearm, the *radius* and *ulna*, meet at the wrist in the *radiocarpal joint*. In the hand there are 8 *carpal bones*, 5 *metacarpals*, and 12 *phalanges* (Fig. 14.6). The first joints of the hand below the wrist are called the *metacarpophalangeal joints*, or knuckles. With the exception of the thumb, which lacks the middle phalanx, the next joint is called the *proximal interphalangeal* and the third is called the *distal interphalangeal* joint. The thumb is considered the first finger, the index the second finger, and so on. Each of the bones and joints, with the exception of several of the carpal bones, can be easily identified.

Particularly prominent landmarks include the *ulnar styloid process*, the *pisiform bone*, and the *radial styloid*. The *anatomic snuff box* just distal and dorsal to the radial styloid can be seen when the thumb is extended. It is bordered by the *extensor pollicis longus* and *abductor pollicis longus*. The size of the *palmaris longus* muscle, the tendon of which lies superficially near the center of the flexor surface of the wrist, is variable among populations. It cannot be detected in 15 to 25 percent of patients of European descent, but is generally observable in Oriental and Black patients.[1] Many muscles and tendons are involved in performing the complex actions of the fingers, hands, and wrist.

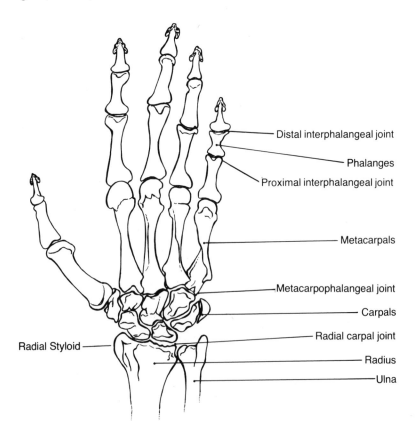

Distal interphalangeal joint

Phalanges

Proximal interphalangeal joint

Metacarpals

Metacarpophalangeal joint

Carpals

Radial carpal joint

Radius

Ulna

Radial Styloid

FIGURE 14.6. The anatomic structure of the wrist, hand, and fingers.

The motions of the wrist include flexion, extension, radial deviation, and ulnar deviation. At the metacarpophalangeal joints, motion includes flexion, extension, abduction, and adduction. At the proximal and distal interphalangeal joints, motion includes flexion and extension. Motions of the thumb include flexion, extension (radial abduction, palmar abduction/adduction), and opposition.

The Hip

Only a small portion of the hip and pelvis can be directly identified. Palpable landmarks include the *iliac crests*, the *anterior superior spines*, the *symphysis pubis*, and the *ischial tuberosities* (Fig. 14.7). If the examiner places her fingertips on the iliac crest and has her hand resting laterally, her palm will rest on the *greater trochanter* of the *femur*. There are three joints within the pelvic girdle: (1) the *symphysis pubis*, (2) the *sacroiliac*, and (3) the *hip joint*.

The first two are nearly immobile, with the hip joint providing nearly all mobility needed. The major muscle groups assist in movement of the hip and are easily identifiable. They include the *sartorius*, the *adductor longus*, the *gluteus medius*, the *gluteus maximus*, and the *quadriceps* (Fig. 14.8). Motions of the hip include flexion, extension, abduction, adduction, internal rotation, and external rotation.

The Knee

The knee areas in Figure 14.9 are easily identifiable. Ordinarily the *synovium*, the *medial* and *lateral collateral ligaments*, and the *menisci* are not palpable. The *anterior* and *posterior cruciate ligaments* are located behind the *patella* near the center of the knee joint. They provide stability to the knee and prevent dislocation of the *tibia* and femur anteriorly and posteriorly. The motions of the knee include flexion, occasionally hyperextension, and internal and external rotation.

The Ankle and Foot

The ankle is composed of more than one joint, but the major one is called the *tibiotarsal joint*. The major landmarks are the *Achilles*

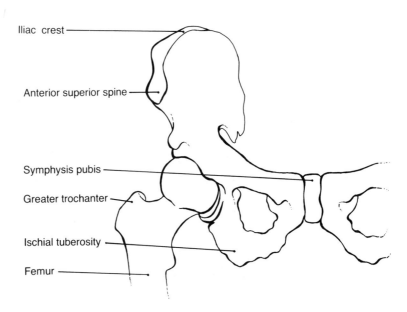

FIGURE 14.7. The hip joint (anterior view).

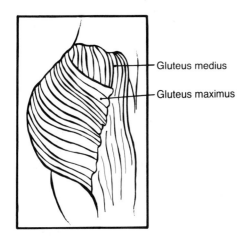

FIGURE 14.8. Muscles of the hip and thigh.

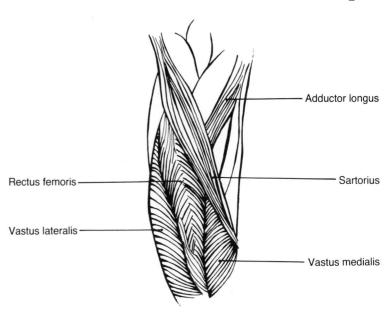

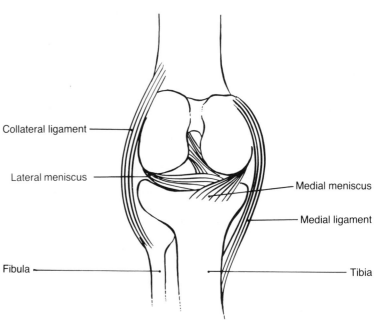

FIGURE 14.9. Anterior view of the knee.

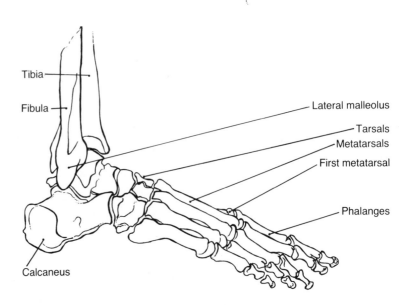

FIGURE 14.10. Lateral view of the ankle and foot.

tendon, the *medial malleolus* of the *fibula*, and the *first metatarsal phalange* (Fig. 14.10). The peroneus tertius muscle assists in dorsiflexion of the foot at the ankle and in elevation of the lateral border of the foot. Its tendon can be felt running from the region of the lateral malleolus at the ankle to the base of the fifth metatarsal. This muscle may be reduced or absent in some populations; absence is more frequent in Black and American Indian populations than in European or Oriental patients. Interestingly, this muscle may be present asymmetrically (in one leg only).[2]

There are 7 *tarsal* bones, 5 *metatarsals*, 14 *phalanges*, and 2 *sesamoid* bones. The great toe lacks a middle phalange and so the foot corresponds approximately in composition to the hand. There are many muscles, ligaments, and tendons in the ankle and foot. The major muscles supplying action to the foot are the *soleus* and *gastrocnemius*, the so-called calf muscles. The motions of the ankle include extension (dorsiflexion), flexion (plantar flexion), inversion and eversion, and adduction and abduction.

PHYSICAL ASSESSMENT

The examination should proceed in an orderly fashion, with a general inspection first and then a separate examination for each part, from the temporomandibular joint down. Inspection should always come first; palpation and measurement should come last. A flexible protractor or a measuring tool called a *goniometer* is helpful in accurately assessing range of motion in degrees. A comfortably warm room is a must because the patient must be undressed to do an adequate examination. Standing, sitting, supine, and prone positions are used throughout the examination.

General Inspection

The examiner should have the patient walk away from her in a straight line and then return, to assess his gait. The assessment actually begins when the patient first walks into the examining room, because he is then least apt to be aware that the examiner has already begun an early assessment. In addition the examiner should have the patient walk away from her in a straight line and then return to assess his gait.

Gait assessment is broken into the *stance* phase and *swing* phase. The stance phase has three parts: (1) *the heel strike*, (2) *midstance*, and (3) *push-off*. The swing phase also has three parts: (1) *acceleration*, (2) *swing-through*, and (3) *deceleration*. There should be minimal shifting of the pelvis and trunk during the gait, and the normal distance between the heels while walking is 2 to 4 inches. A wider gait is indicative of pathology. The examiner should watch for foot dragging, shuffling, or limping and record abnormalities in relation to the phase of the gait. She should also note the position of the trunk in relation to the legs while the client is walking. Active range of motion of the trunk should be within the following range (Figs. 14.11–14.14, Chart 14.1).

Flexion: 70–90°
Extension: 30° standing; 20° prone
Rotation: 30–45°
Lateral bending: 35°

A person with *acute low back pain* due to strain or disc problems will favor the side of greatest pain, the trunk will be tilted forward

CHART 14.1.

Range of Motion*

Joint	Motion	Approximate Measurement
Temporomandibular	Open wide (active)	Able to insert three fingers
	Mandible forward	Top teeth behind lower teeth
Neck	Flexion	45°
	Extension	55°
	Rotation	70°
Trunk	Flexion	70–90°
	Extension	30° standing
		20° prone
	Rotation	30–45°
	Lateral bending	35°
Shoulder	Forward flexion (arm straight)	180°
	Backward extension (arm straight)	50–60°
	Horizontal extension (arm straight)	130°
	Horizontal flexion (arm straight)	40°
	Abduction (arm straight)	180°
	Adduction (arm straight)	45–50°
	Abduction†	90°
	Adduction†	90°
Elbow	Flexion	150°
	Extension	150°
	Hyperextension	0–15°
	Supination	90°
	Pronation	90°
Wrist	Flexion	80–90°
	Extension	70° ±
	Radial deviation	20°
	Ulnar deviation	30°–50°
Fingers		
Metacarpophalangeal joints	Flexion	90°
	Extension	30–45°
	Abduction	20° between fingers
	Adduction	Fingers should touch
Proximal interphalangeal joints	Flexion	100–200°
	Extension	0°
Distal interphalangeal joints	Flexion	80–90°
	Extension	20°

(continued on p. 279)

CHART 14.1. (continued)

Range of Motion*

Joint	Motion	Approximate Measurement
Thumb	Flexion	Transpalmar abduction
	Extension	Able to touch tip of thumb to base of little finger and then extend away from the palm 50° between thumb and index finger
Metacarpophalangeal joint	Flexion	50°
	Extension	
Interphalangeal joint	Flexion	90°
	Extension	20°
Palmar	Abduction	70°
	Adduction	70°
Opposition	Able to touch each fingertip with tip of thumb	
Hip	Flexion	
	Knee flexed	110–120°
	Knee straight	90° or less
	Extension (prone)	30° or less
	Abduction	45–50°
	Adduction	20–30°
	Internal rotation	35–40°
	External rotation	45°
Knee	Flexion	120–130°
	Extension (hyper)	10–15°
	Internal rotation	10°
	External rotation	10°
Ankle and foot	Extension (dorsiflexion)	20°
	Flexion (plantar flexion)	45–50°
	Inversion (passive), hind foot	5°
	Eversion (passive), hind foot	5°
	Abduction, forefoot	10°
	Adduction, forefoot	20°
Toes		
First metatarso-phalangeal joint	Flexion (active)	45°
	Extension (active)	70–90°
Interphalangeal joints	Distal	
	Flexion	60°
	Extension	30°
	Proximal	
	Flexion	35°
	Extension	0°
Metatarsophalangeal joints	Flexion	40°
	Extension	40°
Toe spread	Abduction/adduction	Degrees vary

*Active unless otherwise stated.

†Elbow held at side and flexed.

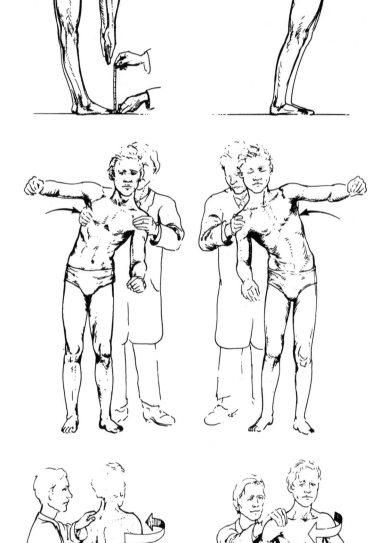

FIGURE 14.11. Left: Range of flexion in the lumbar spine. Right: Range of extension in the lumbar spine. (From Hoppenfeld, S. *Physical examination of the spine and extremities*. New York: Appleton–Century–Crofts, 1976, p. 248)

FIGURE 14.12. The range of lateral bending in the lumbar spine should be equal on both sides. (From Hoppenfeld, S. *Physical examination of the spine and extremities*. New York: Appleton–Century–Crofts, 1976, p. 248)

FIGURE 14.13. Range of rotation in the lumbar spine. (From Hoppenfeld, S. *Physical examination of the spine and extremities*. New York: Appleton–Century–Crofts, 1976, p. 249)

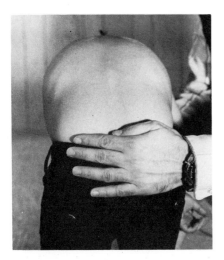

FIGURE 14.14. Testing forward flexion of the trunk and checking for curvature of the spine.

The Spinal Column

slightly or over the painful side, the lumbar curve will be absent or nearly absent, the gait will be hesitant and more widely spaced, and occasionally a marked pelvic tilt will be present. If an *unstable hip* or weak musculature is present, the pelvis will fall on the side of the uninvolved hip rather than as it usually does during normal gait or weight-bearing. As a general rule, gait is an excellent indicator of problems within the musculoskeletal and neurologic systems. The examiner should look at the patient's posture from the anterior and posterior views. She should check the spinal curves looking for any displacement—i.e., *scoliosis*, which is a lateral curve seen on the posterior view, usually of the thoracic spine, or *kyphosis*, an increased convexity of the thoracic spine on the lateral view. *Lordosis* is an increased concavity of the lumbar spine (Fig. 14.15). Lumbar lordosis is normally present in small children who have protuberant abdomens. This normal curvature is more pronounced in Black children. The examiner should also look for any gross deformities or asymmetry.

While the client is still standing, the examiner should have him bend over as far as he can. The spinal column should then have a smooth convex curve. A *functional scoliotic curve* due to poor posture will disappear. True scoliosis will be accentuated when the patient bends over. This test is quickly and easily done, but children are frequently not checked. The importance of checking for scoliosis in children cannot be too highly stressed. Early referral of even borderline scoliosis may prevent a worsened curvature, extensive surgery, and emotional trauma for the child. The spinal column will spread up to 4 inches in length and, depending on the patient's age and general condition, the examiner should be able to record forward flexion of between 70° and 90°. Next, the examiner should palpate the spinal processes and paravertebral muscles to assess for points of tenderness or swelling and record the level where pain occurs. She should observe how the patient gets onto the examining table and record any difficulties and need for assistance.

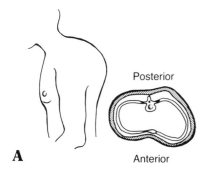

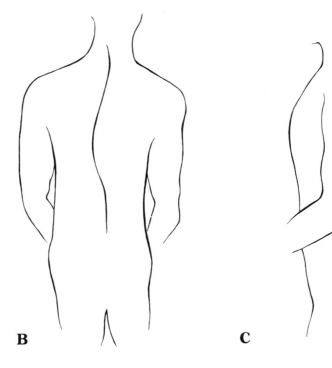

FIGURE 14.15. Abnormal curvatures of the spine: (A) kyphosis, (B) scoliosis, (C) lordosis.

The Temporomandibular Joint

The examiner should observe the patient's face and note any asymmetry, swelling, or evidence of trauma. She should have the patient open his mouth and note the smoothness of motion and any hesitancy of that movement. There should not be any shift of the mandible to the right or left and the examiner should be able to insert three fingers vertically into the patient's fully opened mouth.

To check the ease of joint function, the examiner should place the tips of the little fingers in both ear canals and press gently on the anterior portion of the canals. She should have the patient open his mouth, noting any marked click (possibly a *damaged meniscus*) or a grating sensation (*arthritis*). Poor dentition or poor occlusion may also cause trauma to the temporomandibular (TM) joint, in which case external palpation will elicit tenderness. If there is *spasm of the external pterygoid muscles*, pressure on the maxillary buccal mucosa posterior to the molars will cause tenderness. Occasionally opening the mouth wide into hyperextension, as in a big yawn, will cause the mandibular condyles to slip out of the glenoid fossa, creating an inability to close the mouth. The *dislocation* may be unilateral, as might occur with a blow to the chin or bilateral. In either case immediate referral to the physician for reduction of the dislocation is imperative.

The Cervical Spine

The examiner should observe the neck in the anterior, lateral, and posterior positions. She should check the cervical curvature for any abnormalities. Loss of curvature may result from severe muscle spasm after a *whiplash* accident. The examiner should compare the size and symmetry of the neck muscles, particularly the sternocleidomastoid and trapezius, and note any deviations or masses. She should palpate along the spinous process and also along the supraclavicular fossa for any points of tenderness, swelling, or nodules. Active range of motion (ROM) should be within the following range from the 0° position (Figs. 14.16–14.18, Chart 14.1):

Flexion: 45°
Extension: 55°
Rotation: 70° or chin in line with the shoulder
Lateral bending: 40–45°

The nurse should attempt to find a passive range of motion if the patient has difficulty with ROM on his own. She should test the strength of the neck muscles by providing resistance during active range of motion and compare sides. If there is a complaint of neck, shoulder, or arm pain, the *Adson test* should be performed to determine whether pressure is being exerted on the subclavian artery by the scalenus anticus muscle or a cervical rib (Fig. 14.19). The examiner should palpate the left radial artery and then have the patient extend his chin upward slightly, rotate his head to the left, and take a deep breath. If the pulse diminishes or disappears, the test is positive. This should be repeated on the opposite side for comparison.

The Shoulder

The examiner should inspect and compare both shoulders in terms of bony and muscular symmetry. She should note the presence of atrophy of the muscles, deformity, and/or masses involving elevation

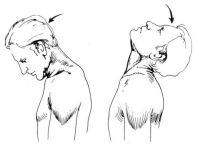

FIGURE 14.16

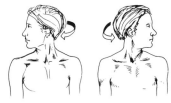

FIGURE 14.17

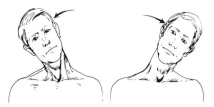

FIGURE 14.18

FIGURES 14.16–14.18. (14.16) Left. Normal range of neck flexion. Right. Normal range of neck extension. (14.17) Normal range of neck rotation. (14.18) Normal range of lateral bending. (From Hoppenfeld, S. *Physical examination of the spine and extremities.* New York: Appleton–Century–Crofts, 1976, p. 115)

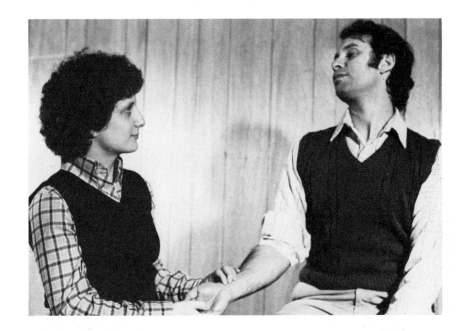

FIGURE 14.19. The Adson test.

or depression of the shoulder. She should identify the bony landmarks as indicated in the anatomy section and note any point tenderness or crepitation and its location. She should palpate the muscular structure and note any tenderness or spasm. The patient should be asked to attempt active range of motion, as follows (Figs. 14.20–14.27, Chart 14.1).

Forward flexion: 180°
Backward extension: 50–60°
Horizontal extension: 130°
Horizontal flexion: 40°
Abduction: 180°
Adduction: 45–50°
Abduction:* 90°
Adduction:* 90°

*Elbow at side and flexed 90°

The examiner should note any motions which elicit pain and record at what angle the pain and/or loss of function occurred. If difficulty

FIGURE 14.20. Example of the Apley scratch test: external rotation and abduction. (From Hoppenfeld, S. *Physical examination of the spine and extremities*. New York: Appleton–Century–Crofts, 1976, p. 21)

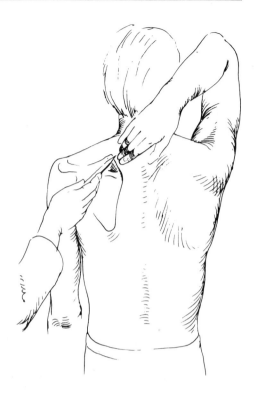

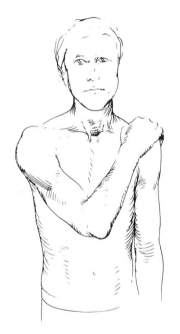

FIGURE 14.21. Test for internal rotation and adduction. (From Hoppenfeld, S. *Physical examination of the spine and extremities*. New York: Appleton–Century–Crofts, 1976, p. 21)

is encountered, the examiner should do passive ROM to see if shoulder mobility can be increased. She should also note the angle at which the scapula begins to move or elevate as the extended arm is abducted from the body. She should test muscle strength bilaterally by providing resistance against the arm in each motion. She should also have the client shrug his shoulders against resistance.

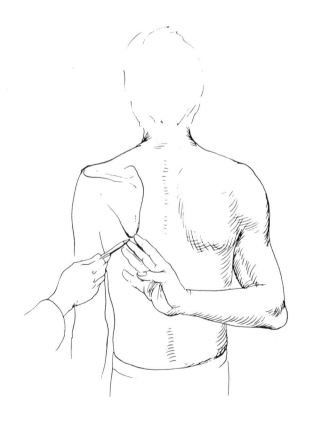

FIGURE 14.22. Internal rotation and adduction. (From Hoppenfeld, S. *Physical examination of the spine and extremities*. New York: Appleton–Century–Crofts, 1976, p. 21)

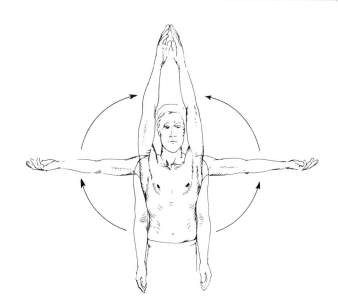

FIGURE 14.23. Range of motion. (From Hoppenfeld, S. *Physical examination of the spine and extremities.* New York: Appleton–Century–Crofts, 1976, p. 22)

The stability of the scapula should be tested by having the patient face a wall and push his hands against it. If there is weakness in the serratus anterior muscle, the scapula will become mobile and prominent, giving a "winged" effect.

Tears in the Rotator Cuff. The four muscles that guard and stabilize the shoulder joint can be assessed by passively abducting the extended arm to a 90° angle. The patient should be asked to slowly lower his arm. If a tear is present, he will be unable to do so; the arm will fall abruptly.

A common sports injury, aside from dislocation, is *subluxation* of the acromioclavicular joint. The patient will support his arm with the opposite hand and be reluctant to flex or abduct the shoulder. The nurse should have him place the hand of the affected side on the opposite shoulder and lean forward. Pressure on the distal end of the clavicle will cause pain and the clavicle will be mobile. Subluxation may also be encountered in the stroke patient when the paralyzed shoulder and arm are inadequately supported.

If *fracture* of the upper arm, particularly of the neck of the humerus, is suspected, the examiner should be sure to determine if pulses are present in the lower arm.

FIGURE 14.24. Test for abduction: motion occurs at the glenohumeral and scapulothoracic articulation in a 2:1 ratio. (From Hoppenfeld, S. *Physical examination of the spine and extremities.* New York: Appleton–Century–Crofts, 1976, p. 23)

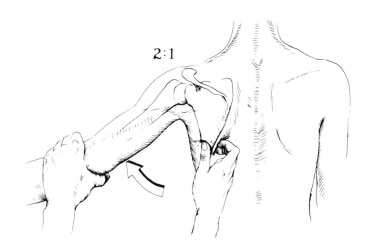

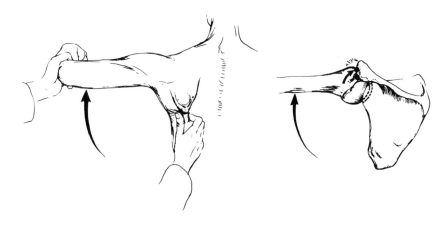

FIGURE 14.25. Abduction continues to approximately 120°, where the surgical neck of the humerus strikes the acromion. (From Hoppenfeld, S. *Physical examination of the spine and extremities.* New York: Appleton–Century–Crofts, 1976, p. 24)

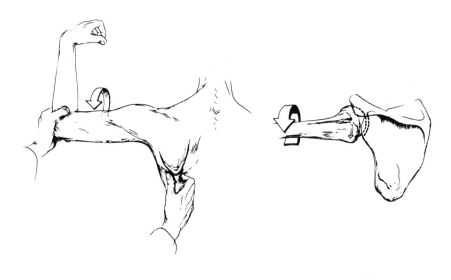

FIGURE 14.26. Full abduction is possible only when the humerus is externally rotated. (From Hoppenfeld, S. *Physical examination of the spine and extremities.* New York: Appleton–Century–Crofts, 1976, p. 24)

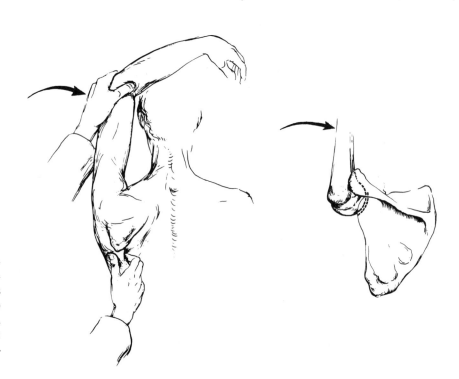

FIGURE 14.27. External rotation increases the articulating surface of the humeral head and turns the surgical neck away from the tip of the acromiom. (From Hoppenfeld, S. *Physical examination of the spine and extremities.* New York: Appleton–Century–Crofts, 1976, p. 24)

The Elbow

The examiner should inspect the elbow while it is in 90° of flexion, noting any redness, swelling, nodules, or deformities. A soft swelling over the olecranon process may be indicative of *olecranon bursitis*. The examiner should note the muscle structure in the forearm and upper arm and compare it with that of the opposite arm. She should palpate the elbow in a position of flexion and extension, determine the bony landmarks, and note any point tenderness, bogginess, or crepitation around the joint itself. The muscle bodies should be palpated to determine if tenderness or spasm is present. The examiner should then have the patient put his elbow through active range of motion (Figs. 14.28 and 14.29, Chart 14.1):

Flexion: 150°
Extension: 150°
Hyperextension: 0–15°
Supination: 90°
Pronation: 90°

If *tennis elbow* is present, palpation at or near the lateral epicondyle will elicit point tenderness.

The Wrist

The examiner should inspect the wrist for shape, deformity, swelling, lumps, or redness. She should palpate the prominent bony landmarks, the muscles, and the tendons, comparing the two wrists and determining whether any point tenderness exists. This part of the body is susceptible to dysfunction in *rheumatoid arthritis* and the *migratory arthritis* of rheumatic fever in children.

The examiner should have the patient move the wrist through active range of motion (Figs. 14.30 and 14.31, Chart 14.1):

Flexion: 80–90°
Extension: 70°
Radial deviation: 20°
Ulnar deviation: 30–50°

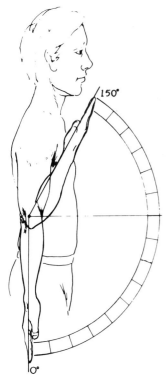

FIGURE 14.28. The elbow range of motion in flexion and extension. (From Hoppenfeld, S. *Physical examination of the spine and extremities.* New York: Appleton–Century–Crofts, 1976, p. 50)

If the patient has complained of difficulty flexing and extending his thumb and if tenderness is present in the tendons bordering the anatomic snuffbox, he may have *De Quervain's disease*, or *chronic stenosing tenosynovitis*. To test for this, the patient is asked to clench his fingers over his thumb and then put his wrist sharply into ulnar deviation. This is called *Finkelstein's test* and is positive if the patient experiences sudden pain from the snuffbox into his thumb. *Ganglions* are not uncommon on the posterior or dorsal surface of the wrist. These are soft, round, discrete lumps that are not attached to underlying structures and rarely cause pain or inhibit function in the wrist. If the patient has complained of pain and weakness in his thumb and index and middle fingers, there may be *compression of the median nerve* by the carpal tunnel ligament. Tapping the wrist on a ligament over the median nerve will cause pain in the fingers supplied by this nerve. This is called a positive *Tinel's sign*. The most common deformity in the wrist due to fracture is the silver fork deformity of a *Colles' fracture*. This is a fracture within 2–3 cm of the distal end of the radius, including, in some, fracture of the ulnar styloid process with dorsal displacement. When the wrist and hand are placed on a flat surface, the displacement looks like a fork

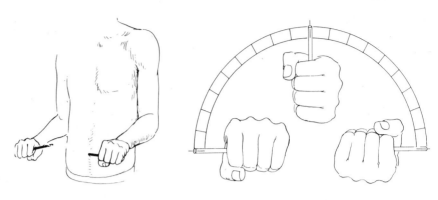

FIGURE 14.29. The elbow range of motion in supination and pronation. (From Hoppenfeld, S. *Physical examination of the spine and extremities.* New York: Appleton–Century–Crofts, 1976, p. 51)

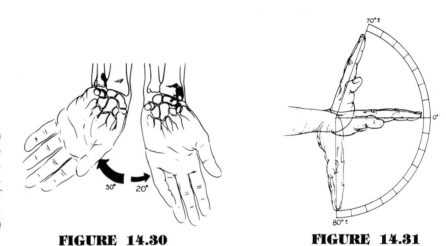

FIGURES 14.30 – 14.31. (14.30) Ulnar and radial deviation of the wrist. (14.31) Wrist flexion and extension range of motion. (From Hoppenfeld, S., *Physical examination of the spine and extremities.* New York: Appleton–Century–Crofts, 1976, p. 89)

FIGURE 14.30   **FIGURE 14.31**

turned with the tines pointing down on the surface. This is usually caused by a fall on an outstretched hand.

The Hand and Fingers

The examiner should inspect and compare the hands in terms of bony and muscular structure, looking for signs of swelling, redness, nodules, deformities, extra fingers (*polydactyly*), very short fingers (*brachydactyly*), or webbing between the fingers (*syndactyly*). The thenar eminence (the muscle body below the thumb) should be compared with the hypothenar eminence (the heel of the hand or palm). The examiner may be able to delight the patient by telling him which hand he used for the majority of activities simply by noting that the muscles are more prominent in the thenar and hypothenar areas in the dominant hand. In addition, the hand creases are deeper and more noticeable in that hand. In dark-skinned individuals, the palmar surfaces of the hands and plantar surfaces of the feet may normally show darkly pigmented creases. The presence of *palmar muscle atrophy* should also be noted. If pronounced, the palm (or volnar surface) will have a hollowed out appearance.

The examiner should palpate the body landmarks of the hand, paying particular attention to the joints. She should note the presence of tenderness, bogginess, or nodules. *Heberden's nodules,* which occur in osteoarthritis, may be present at the distal interphalangeal joints (Fig. 14.32).

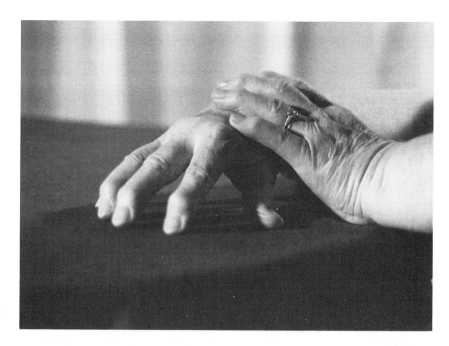

FIGURE 14.32. Example of Heberden's nodules.

The patient should be asked to perform active range of motion of the thumb and fingers. Independent movement of the distal phalanges is usually not possible without the examiner stabilizing the proximal interphalangeal joints in zero position—i.e., with the fingers extended in straight line position from the palm.

Further ranges of motion are listed below (Figs. 14.33–14.40, Chart 14.1).

1. Fingers
    a. Metacarpophalangeal joints
       (1) Flexion: 90°
       (2) Extension: 30–45°
       (3) Abduction: 20° between fingers
       (4) Adduction: Fingers should touch
    b. Proximal interphalangeal joints
       (1) Flexion: 100–120°
       (2) Extension: 0°
    c. Distal interphalangeal joints
       (1) Flexion: 80–90°
       (2) Extension: 20°
2. Thumb
    a. Flexion and extension: transpalmar abduction; able to touch tip of thumb to base of little finger and then extend away from palm 50° between thumb and index finger
    b. Metacarpophalangeal joint
       (1) Flexion: 50°
       (2) Extension: 50°
    c. Interphalangeal joint
       (1) Flexion: 90°
       (2) Extension: 20°
    d. Palmar
       (1) Abduction: 70°
       (2) Adduction: 70°
    e. Apposition: Able to touch each fingertip with tip of thumb

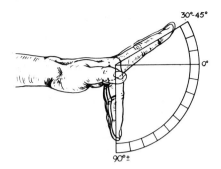

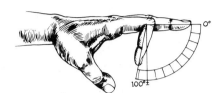

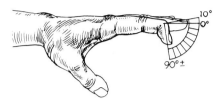

FIGURE   14.33   **FIGURE   14.34.**   **FIGURE   14.35.**

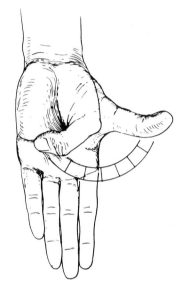

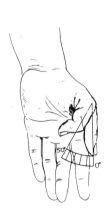

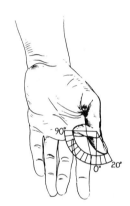

FIGURE   14.36.   **FIGURE   14.37.**   **FIGURE   14.38.**

FIGURES 14.33 – 14.40. (14.33) Metacarpophalangeal joint range of motion: flexion–extension. (14.34) Proximal interphalangeal joint range of motion: flexion–extension. (14.35) Distal interphalangeal joint range of motion: flexion–extension. (14.36) Thumb flexion and extension. (14.37) Thumb flexion and extension: metacarpophalangeal joint. (14.38) Thumb flexion and extension: interphalangeal joint. (14.39) Palmar abduction/adduction of the thumb. (14.40) Opposition of the thumb and fingertips. (From Hoppenfeld, S. *Physical examination of the spine and extremities.* New York: Appleton-Century-Crofts, 1976, p. 89–91)

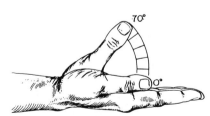

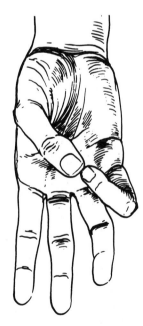

FIGURE   14.39   **FIGURE   14.40.**

The examiner should note any difficulty performing active or passive range of motion and where the difficulty occurs. A *contracture* of one of the fingers due to adherence of the tendon to the tendon sheath from tenosynovitis may prevent full extension of the fingers away from the palm. This is called *Dupuytren's contracture*.

Because *rheumatoid arthritis* most commonly affects the proximal interphalangeal and metacarpophalangeal joints, the examiner may note tenderness and swelling of those joints. With advanced disease a *swan's neck* or *boutonnière* deformity may be present (Figs. 14.41 and 14.42).

The Hip and Pelvis

The pelvis should be inspected with the patient in the sitting position. The level of the iliac crests should be level or parallel to the floor. The examiner should look for signs of trauma—i.e., bruising, abrasion, or swelling. She should palpate the crests, the anterior spines, the symphysis, and, when the client is lying down, the ischial tuberosities. If pressure exerted on any of these areas elicits a pain response from the patient and there is a history of body or pelvic trauma, *pelvic fracture* must be considered. The examiner should palpate along the spine for tenderness, swelling, or nodules.

The fingertips are placed over the anterior spines and the palm over the lateral hip. The greater trochanter of the femur will lie just under the palm. The area is palpated for tenderness and deformity. The muscles of the hip, thigh, and buttocks are palpated for tenderness. The examiner should have the patient perform active range of motion. He may need passive assistance to complete ROM (Figs. 14.43–14.48, Chart 14.1):

Flexion: knee flexed, 110–120°; knee straight, 90°
Extension(prone): 30° or less
Abduction: 45–50°
Adduction: 20–30°
Internal rotation: 35–40°
External rotation: 45°

The examiner should test for strength of the muscles by providing resistance during active range of motion. A *flexion contracture* of the hip may be demonstrated by having the patient, while in supine position, flex his leg against his chest. Ordinarily, the opposite leg barely rises during this motion. If contracture is present, the straight leg will begin to flex and this is measured in degrees. This is considered a positive Thomas test for hip flexion contracture. Pain precipitated in the lumbar spine by straight leg raising is called a positive Lasègue's sign. The degree at which pain occurs is then recorded.

In infants an *Ortolani click* may be heard in congenital dislocation of the hip(s) (Figs. 14.49 and 14.50). The knees of the infant are flexed to 90° and the hips are abducted and externally rotated so that the legs are flat on the table. If dislocation is present, a click will be heard as the head of the femur slips back into the acetabulum. A positive *Allis' sign* in congenital hip dislocation is present if one leg appears shorter than the other when the knees are flexed in the supine position and viewed anteriorly.

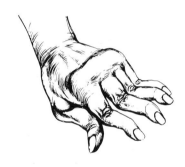

FIGURE 14.41. Swan's neck deformity. (From Hoppenfeld, S. *Physical examination of the spine and extremities.* New York: Appleton–Century–Crofts, 1976, p. 87)

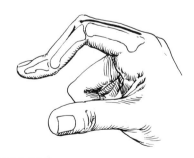

FIGURE 14.42. A boutonnière deformity. (From Hoppenfeld, S. *Physical examination of the spine and extremities.* New York: Appleton–Century–Crofts, 1976, p. 87)

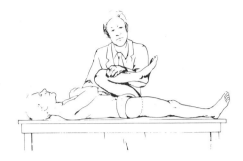

FIGURE   14.43.

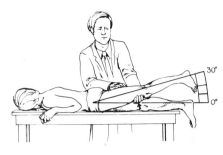

FIGURE 14.44.

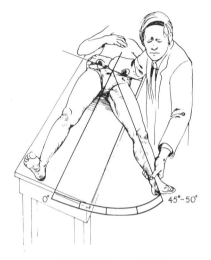

FIGURE   14.45.

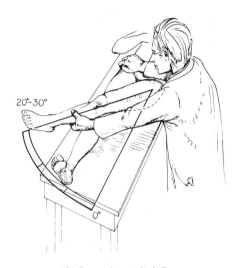

FIGURE   14.46.

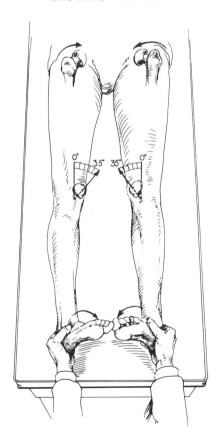

FIGURE   14.47.

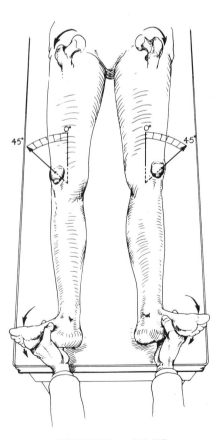

FIGURE   14.48.

FIGURES 14.43–14.48. (14.43) The normal limit for hip flexion is approximately 135°. (14.44) Test for hip extension. (14.45) The normal limits for hip abduction are 45° to 50°. (14.46) The normal limits for hip adduction are 20° to 30°. (14.47) The normal limit for internal rotation is 35°. (14.48) The normal limit for external rotation is 45°. (From Hoppenfeld, S. *Physical examination of the spine and extremities.* New York: Appleton–Century–Crofts, 1976, pp. 156–8.)

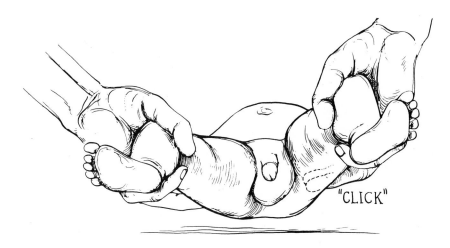

FIGURE 14.49. A diagnosis of a congenital dislocation of the hip. This may be confirmed by the Ortolani "click" test. The involved hip is not able to be abducted as far as the opposite one, and there is a "click" as the hip reduces. (From Hoppenfeld, S. *Physical examination of the spine and extremities.* New York: Appleton–Century–Crofts, 1976, p. 168)

FIGURE 14.50. In the newborn, both hips can be equally flexed, abducted, and externally rotated without producing a "click." (From Hoppenfeld, S. *Physical examination of the spine and extremities.* New York: Appleton–Century–Crofts, 1976, p. 168)

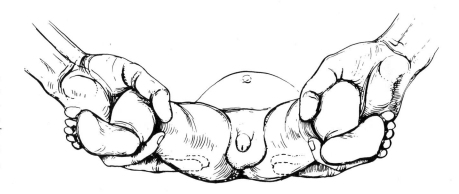

At this point the examiner should measure the leg lengths. This is done in two ways:

1. Apparent leg length: The examiner picks a nonfixed point, such as the umbilicus, and measures from that point to the medial malleolus. This is repeated on the opposite side.
2. True leg length: The examiner measures from the anterior spine of the pelvis to the medial malleolus. This is repeated on the opposite side.

These maneuvers determine if one leg is actually shorter than the other or if the pelvis is tilted.

Since the low back and hip are sites for referred pain from disease in the pelvis, the examiner may want to return after the musculoskeletal exam is completed and consider a pelvic exam on a female or a prostate exam on a male.

The Knee

The knees should be inspected while the patient is in the sitting position. Any deformities, redness, swelling, or nodules should be noted. *Tibial torsion* may be present if a plumb line dropped from the center of the patella does not intersect the toes in children. Tibial torsion may result from prolonged sitting in front of a television in a position called the "TV squat" (Fig. 14.51). The examiner should have the child stand and note the position of the legs. "Bow-

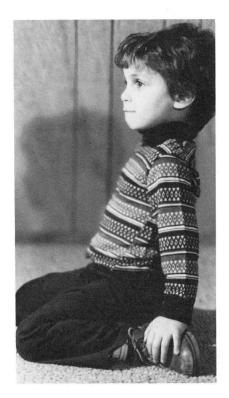

FIGURE 14.51. The "TV squat."

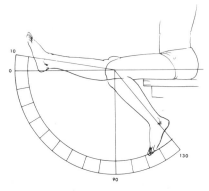

FIGURE 14.52. The range of knee motion in flexion and extension. (From Hoppenfeld, S. *Physical examination of the spine and extremities.* New York: Appleton–Century–Crofts, 1976, p. 187)

leggedness," or *genu valgum*, may be present if the medial malleoli are touching and the knees are more than 1 inch apart. Conversely, *genu varum* may be present if the knees are touching and the medial malleoli are more than 2–3 cm apart.

The examiner should palpate the bony and muscular structures and note any points of tenderness in the joint, muscles, or tendons and compare sides. The patella should move freely without discomfort. In adolescents, *Osgood–Schlatter* disease may be present if tenderness and swelling are found at the insertion of the infrapatellar tendon onto the tibial tubercle. *Chondromalacia* may be present if pain is produced as the patella is moved while pressing it against the femur.

Next, the examiner should have the patient move the knee through active range of motion and assist as necessary (Fig. 14.52, Chart 14.1).

> Flexion: 120–130°
> Extension (hyper): 10–15°
> Internal rotation: 10°
> External rotation: 10°

The nurse should test the strength of the muscles by providing resistance during active range of motion and perform a neurologic check of the lower extremities (see Chap. 15).

There are a number of tests the examiner can perform to check for stability and obstruction in the knee. The following are among the major tests.

McMurray's Test (for Mensical Tears). If the test is positive, a click is heard when the knee is lowered from a flexed and externally rotated position while pressure is applied to the knee (Figs. 14.53–14.56).

Test for Integrity of the Collateral Ligaments. The examiner holds the knee stable with one hand on the medial side of the femur and pushes laterally against the tibia. If there is a tear in the medial collateral ligament, the tibia will slide medially. If the hands are changed to the opposite sides and the maneuver is repeated, the tibia will slide laterally if there is a tear or weakness in the lateral collateral ligament (Figs. 14.57 and 14.58).

Test for Integrity of the Anterior and Posterior Cruciate Ligaments (Draw Sign). The examiner has the patient assume the supine position with his knees flexed to 90°. She then stands at the end of the table and applies pressure to the tibia with her hands, pushing toward the patient. If a tear or weakness of the posterior cruciate ligament is present, the tibia will slide posteriorly. The examiner then pulls the tibia toward her. If there is a tear or weakness of the anterior cruciate ligament, the tibia will slide forward (Figs. 14.59 and 14.60).

Test for Mechanical Obstruction. The examiner flexes the patient's knee and raises the leg off the table. She then holds the ankle in her hand and passively lowers the leg. The leg should "bounce" into a fully extended position. If it doesn't, some type of obstruction exists in the joint (Figs. 14.61–14.63).

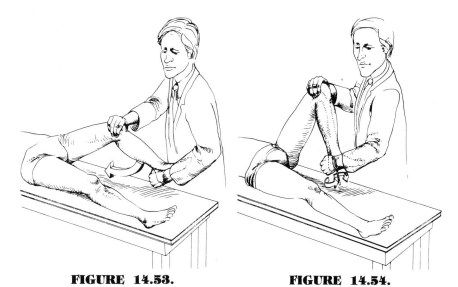

FIGURE 14.53.   **FIGURE 14.54.**

FIGURES 14.53 – 14.56. (14.53) The McMurray text for meniscal tears. The knee is flexed. (14.54) With the knee flexed, the examiner internally and externally rotates the tibia on the femur. (14.55) With the leg externally rotated, the examiner places a valgus stress on the knee. (14.56) With the leg externally rotated and in valgus, the examiner slowly extends the knee. If a click is palpable or audible, the text is considered positive for a torn medial meniscus, usually in the posterior position. (From Hoppenfeld, S. *Physical examination of the spine and extremities.* New York: Appleton–Century–Crofts, 1976, p. 192)

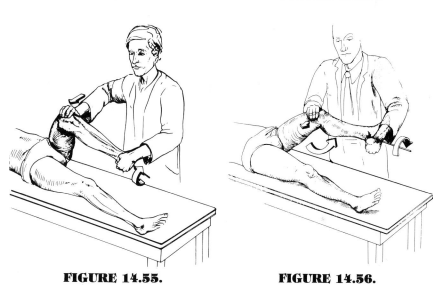

FIGURE 14.55.   **FIGURE 14.56.**

FIGURES 14.57 – 14.58. (14.57) To test the medial collateral ligament, the examiner applies valgus stress to open the knee joint on the medial side. (14.58) To test the lateral knee for stability, the examiner applies varus stress to open the knee joint on the lateral side. (From Hoppenfeld, S. *Physical examination of the spine and extremities.* New York: Appleton–Century–Crofts, 1976, p. 185)

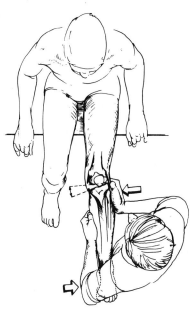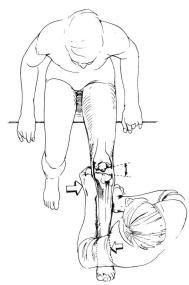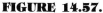

FIGURE 14.57.   **FIGURE 14.58.**

FIGURES 14.59 – 14.60. (14.59) A positive anterior draw sign: torn anterior cruciate ligament. (14.60) A positive posterior draw sign: torn posterior cruciate ligament. (From Hoppenfeld, S. *Physical examination of the spine and extremities.* New York: Appleton–Century–Crofts, 1976, p. 186.)

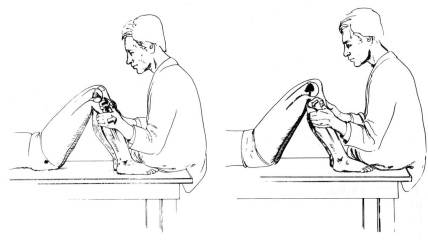

FIGURE 14.59.   **FIGURE 14.60.**

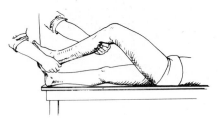 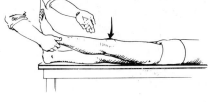 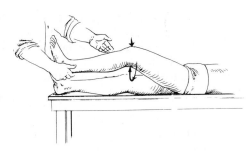

FIGURE 14.61.   **FIGURE 14.62.**   **FIGURE 14.63.**

FIGURE 14.61 – 14.63. (14.61) The "bounce-home" test. The examiner flexes the knee. (14.62) The knee is allowed to passively extend. It should fully "bounce home" into extension. (14.63) Fluid in the knee joint prevents the knee from "bouncing home;" instead it may rebound. (From Hoppenfeld, S. *Physical examination of the spine and extremities.* New York: Appleton–Century–Crofts, 1976, p. 194)

FIGURE 14.64. Test for minor effusion. (From Hoppenfeld, S. *Physical examination of the spine and extremities.* New York: Appleton–Century–Crofts, 1976, p. 196)

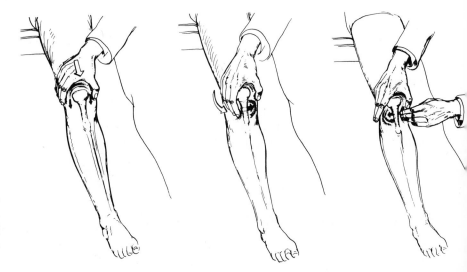

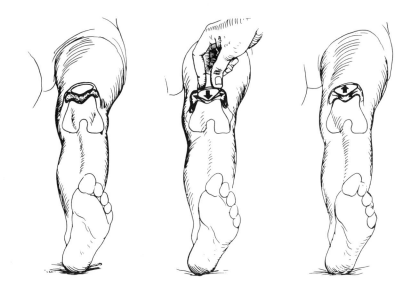

FIGURE 14.65. Test for major effusion: a ballottable patella. (From Hoppenfeld, S. *Physical examination of the spine and extremities.* New York: Appleton-Century-Crofts, 1976, p. 195)

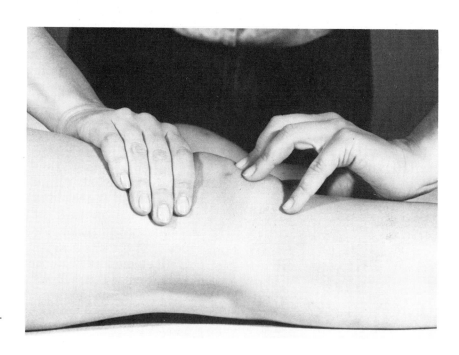

FIGURE 14.66. Testing for ballottement of the patella.

Test for Minor Swelling Beneath the Patella. The examiner milks the joint capsule downward and then applies pressure to the medial or lateral side. A bulge will appear on the side opposite the pressure if fluid is present (Fig. 14.64).

Test for Major Swelling Beneath the Patella. The examiner presses the patella sharply against the femur. If fluid is present, the patella will rebound or bounce back quickly. Another name for this test is *ballottement of the patella* (Figs. 14.65 and 14.66).

The Ankle, Foot, and Toes   The ankle is inspected for swelling, redness, nodules, and deformity. Swelling, redness, and marked tenderness to the lightest of palpation in either of the great toes may be indicative of *gout*. The examiner should note the presence or absence of the longitudinal arch of the foot, as well as any deformities of the toes (such as a *hammer toe*, or flexion contracture) and any calluses or warts. She should look for the presence of *hallux valgus*, which occurs when the great toe is laterally deviated toward and occasionally overlaps the second toe. Continuous trauma due in part to ill-fitting shoes may result in a bursa over the metatarsophalangeal joint, resulting in the so called painful *bunion*. The nurse should note the position of the ankle: the position is valgus if the medial malleolus angulates inward and varus if the lateral malleolus angulates outward. Inspecting the shoes for points of wear is often helpful in determining ankle and foot stress points.

In children it is important to note whether the entire foot toes out *(pes valgus)* or toes in *(pes varus)*. *Metatarsus valgus* describes the condition in which only the forefoot turns in. If attempts to passively correct these conditions fail, then referral for correction is necessary.

The sole of the foot should be inspected for any abnormalities—i.e., excessive callus formation, flattened arches, or wart formation. The nurse should palpate the bony and muscular structures of the foot for any points of tenderness and record any findings. The patient should be asked to perform active range of motion of the ankle, foot, and toes. Several of the maneuvers will have to be done passively, as listed below (Figs. 14.67–14.73, Chart 14.1).

1. Ankle and foot
   a. Extension (dorsiflexion): 20°
   b. Flexion (plantar flexion): 45–50°
   c. Inversion (passive), hind foot: 5°
   d. Eversion (passive), hind foot: 5°
   e. Abduction, forefoot: 10°
   f. Adduction, forefoot: 20°
2. Toes
   a. First metatarsophalangeal joint
      (1) Flexion (active): 45°
      (2) Extension (active): 70–90°
   b. Interphalangeal joints
      (1) Distal
         (a) Flexion: 60°
         (b) Extension: 30°
      (2) Proximal
         (a) Flexion: 35°
         (b) Extension: 0°
   c. Metatarsophalangeal joints
      (1) Flexion: 40°
      (2) Extension: 40°
   d. toe spread (abduction/adduction): degrees vary

Strength of muscle groups is tested by providing resistance during active range of motion (Chart 14.2). A test for strength of the gastrocnemius and soleus muscles in the posterior lower leg can be conducted by having the patient hop on the ball of his foot. If the muscles are weak the foot will land flat on the floor. He will not be

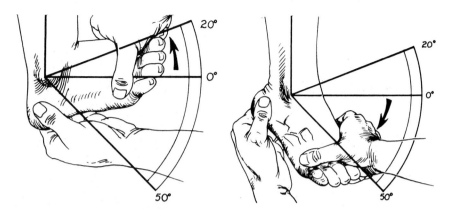

FIGURE 14.67.   **FIGURE 14.68.**

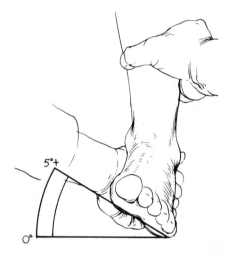

FIGURE 14.69.

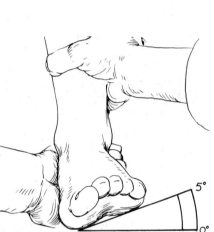

FIGURE 14.70.

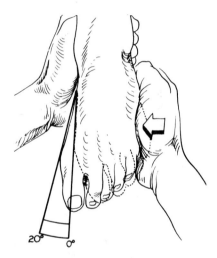

FIGURE 14.71.

FIGURES 14.67 – 14.73. (14.67) Range of ankle dorsiflexion. (14.68) Range of ankle plantar flexion. (14.69) Foot inversion test. (14.70) Foot eversion test. (14.71) Forefoot adduction test. (14.72) Forefoot abduction test. (14.73) The normal flexion/extension range of the first metatarsophalangeal joint. (From Hoppenfeld, S. *Physical examination of the spine and extremities.* New York: Appleton–Century–Crofts, 1976, pp. 223, 225, 226)

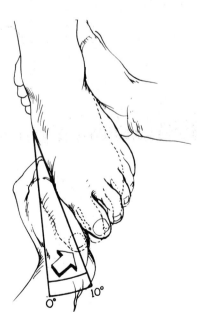

FIGURE 14.72.

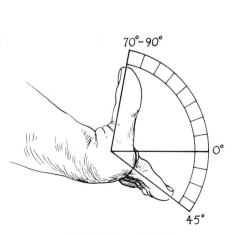

FIGURE   14.73.

CHART 14.2.

Muscle Grading Chart

Muscle Gradations	Description
5—Normal	Complete ROM against gravity, with full resistance
4—Good	Complete ROM against gravity, with some resistance
3—Fair	Complete ROM against gravity
2—Poor	Complete ROM, with gravity eliminated
1—Trace	Evidence of slight contractility; no joint motion
0—None	No evidence of contractility

able to hold himself on the ball of his foot. This test should be done in accordance with the age and general condition of the patient.

REFERENCES

1. Barnicot, N. Biological variation in modern populations. In G. Harrison, et al. (Eds.), *Human biology.* 1977, pp. 181–300.
2. Spuhler, J. Genetics of three normal morphological variations: Patterns of superficial veins of the anterior thorax, peroneus tertius muscle, and number of villate papillae. *Cold Spring Harbour Symposia on Quantitative Biology*, 1950, *15*, 175–189.

EXAMPLE OF A RECORDED HISTORY AND PHYSICAL

Subjective:

Chief Complaint: ". . . rheumatism in my hip for 10 hours."

HPI: This 54-year-old truckdriver was admitted to Memorial Hospital for "control of my diabetes." He considered himself to be in "pretty good" health prior to admission. Because of extreme lethargy he was placed on bedrest for the first 24 hours after admission. On the second day he began to complain of "rheumatism in my right hip. I knew this was going to happen if I stayed in bed too long. I do O.K. if I keep moving—even when I drive my truck, I have to stop every 2 hours or so and walk around. My doctor told me I had rheumatism—I guess he called it arthritis—about 5 years ago." He describes the "rheumatism" as "a steady deep aching in my right hip" that started about 10 hours ago. He stated it "feels real stiff, too; I can hardly move my leg." He denies low back pain or radiation to his (R) leg; aching increases with initial activity and eases if he continues the activity—i.e., walking. He usually takes 2 or 3 plain aspirin tablets "when I feel the aching begin" and gets "good" relief. There is no regular pattern of medication use. No known allergies. Denies fever, redness, or swelling in (R) hip. Denies history of trauma to either hip, pelvis, or lower extremities. Both parents had "rheumatism real bad when they got older."

States "I usually just keep right on truckin" as they say; can't let it get me down. I just try not to do a whole lot of stair climbing or lifting heavy boxes any more."

OBJECTIVE: T.98.4°F orally; P. 88 (radial); R. 18; B.P. 160/88 (sitting)

General: Patient presents as an alert, cooperative, 54-year-old man sitting on the edge of his bed. He grimaces occasionally when he tries to change his position. Needs assistance to ambulate three steps. Avoids putting full weight on (R) leg.

Face: Temporomandibular joint → crepitations felt bilaterally; able to open mouth 3 cm.

Neck: Full active ROM without complaints of pain or stiffness. No muscle atrophy, deformities, or masses noted.

Shoulders: Symmetrical; full active ROM without complaints of pain or stiffness. No muscle atrophy, deformities, masses, redness, or swelling noted.

Elbows: As for shoulders above.

Wrists: As for shoulders above.

Fingers: Deformities noted in distal interphalangeal joints of the second and third fingers, bilateral—flexion limited to 45° in these joints and 0° extension. All other joints have full active and passive ROM. No redness, swelling, or muscle atrophy seen.
Some 2 to 3 mm nodules noted below nailbed; one on second finger, 1 on third finger of right hand.

Spine: In sitting position appears straight in posterior view. Accentuated curve at cervical/thoracic junction in lateral view. No redness, swelling, tenderness or deformities seen.

Pelvis: In sitting position → iliac crests appear level. No tenderness to palpation or pressure.

Hips: Tender to pressure over (R) hip joint. No redness or swelling seen; no visible deformity. In lying position: full active/passive ROM in (L) hip.

> With knee straight < 45° before ↑ pain.
> With knee flexed < 60° before ↑ pain.
> Extension: Unable to extend right leg in prone position; 10° on left.
> Abduction: 25° to 30°
> Adduction: < 10°
> Internal rotation: < 20°
> External rotation: < 20°

Knees/Ankles/Toes: Full active/passive ROM without complaints of pain or stiffness. No redness, swelling, tenderness, muscle atrophy, or masses found.

15

The Neurologic Examination

The nervous system is the "integrator" of all the other systems in the body. Without its "intactness," many homeostatic controls will not function. The nervous system, which begins to develop in early embryonic life, starts its role as integrator even then.

By the time a baby is born, this system has already been very active. Because of the nervous system's major role in growth and development, it is vital that accurate assessments be made from birth. Throughout life the nervous system needs to be evaluated routinely.

In the neonatal period there are obvious neurologic signs that can be evaluated. If there is any clue of dysfunction, consultation should be sought. The earlier a problem can be recognized and the more quickly intervention takes place, the better the chances are for a more positive outcome.

With the infant and toddler, evaluations are done at well baby exams by taking a thorough history, doing a complete physical (including an appropriate neurologic exam), and administering a Denver Developmental Screening Test. With these three tools, most developmental abnormalities can be picked up.

For the school-age child and the adolescent, school is a good screening facility for many of the neurologic problems typical to this age group. Because health care at this age deals primarily with acute treatment and periodic physicals, it is important that thorough neurologic screening be done during the annual physical exam.

In the young adult and middle adult, neurologic problems are not common. However, there are some disorders that are typical to these age groups and will manifest with very vague complaints.

In the geriatric patient special concerns exist. When a patient notices decreasing mobility, loss of memory, and other similar problems, it is terrifically frightening to him. With a gradual decrease in neurologic functioning, his whole independent existence is threatened, and this has many implications. Not only is independence an issue, but the patient's self-image may be threatened as well. If the nurse is astute and includes anticipatory guidance in her care, the potential for a situational crisis may be decreased.

These examples illustrate the importance of the neurologic assessment. Because a thorough exam takes up to 45 minutes to perform, there are some screening tests that should be done routinely. If the results of any screening tests are questionable, a more detailed evaluation can be made. When choosing an appropriate level of depth for this exam, there are other considerations. The condition of the patient makes a great deal of difference—not only in his level of consciousness, but also in his ability to ambulate. Many portions of the exam require his being able to move and coordinate his extremities. Another factor in determining how much detail is required in the exam is the chief complaint of the patient. If his chief complaint relates to the neurologic system, as with "headaches," a most thorough assessment is essential. However, if the complaint is an injured knee, a screening level might be more appropriate. The last but none the less important consideration is the cooperation and participation of the patient.

The neurologic assessment is divided up into the history and the physical exam. The portions of the physical exam that this chapter will address are: (1) mental status (which includes speech, language, and intellectual functioning), (2) the cranial nerves, (3) the motor system, (4) the sensory system, (5) the reflexes, and (6) the Denver Developmental Screening Test (DDST).

HISTORY

The neurologic history is important for two reasons: (1) to get the patient's description of the functioning or malfunctioning of his nervous system and (2) to establish the mental status of the patient. Although assessment of mental status is part of the physical, much can be checked while eliciting the history, including the patient's orientation, intellectual abilities, language, and speech.

To say that there is one method or one format for the neurologic history would be incorrect. It has already been stated that the level of consciousness, the chief complaint, and the cooperation of the patient must be considered. Additional criteria include the developmental age and stage of the patient. Obviously, there are certain questions relevant to infant development that are not pertinent to the adolescent. However, there are some questions that are important to ask at any age. These concern any history of loss of consciousness, fainting, convulsions, trauma, tingling or numbness, tremors or tics, limping, paralysis, speech disorders, loss of memory, disorientation, mood swings, anxiety, depression, or phobias.

If the answer to any of these questions is "yes," further inquiry regarding circumstances is necessary—when they occur, the cause, treatment, and course of recovery.

A complaint of pain does not typically arise in relation to this system. If pain from a neurologic disorder is mentioned, it will probably come up during the system review for the head, back, or extremities.

Other complaints that may arise in this discussion are anxiety, nervousness, moodiness, and clumsiness. The patient should be queried about all these complaints, which should then be listed as pertinent negatives if the patient denies their occurrence.

Discussion concerning problems with smell, vision, taste, etc. is not necessarily included here. Although these senses are related to the cranial nerves, they are more appropriately covered under the system review of the eyes, nose, and oral cavity (see history within the appropriate chapters).

To approach the specific developmental areas of the system review, it is easiest to begin with infancy and work through the various stages of life.

In *infancy,* special attention is paid to the presence of certain reflexes. Not only can the nurse elicit the reflex response during the physical, but she can also question the parents about certain movements they should notice. This also gives the nurse information on the parent's observation of their child. Do they notice that if they touch the baby's cheek, he turns his head toward the side touched *(rooting reflex)*? Does the baby have difficulty with sucking or swallowing? Does he gag? When a loud noise is made or the crib is jarred, does the baby seem to be startled *(Moro's reflex)*? When an object or finger is placed in the baby's palm, does he grasp it *(palmar grasp reflex)*? When they hold the baby in a "standing" position with his feet on a flat surface, does he appear to be dancing *(dancing reflex)*? All these reflexes and others can be assessed as part of the Denver Developmental Screening Test. There are certain times specific reflexes are expected to disappear. This disappearance is as important as their presence (see the section on description of infant reflexes). However, even these reflexes may vary among population groups. In reporting on ethnic differences in infants, Freedman found that American Indian and Chinese babies showed a reduced Moro's reflex and "defense reaction" (turning away or swiping at a cloth held over the nose) when compared with Caucasian and Black babies.[1]

As the neonate progresses through infancy, certain growth and developmental tasks must be accomplished, such as rolling over, sitting, pulling himself up, and walking. All of these are milestones; the dates of occurrence can be elicited during the history and documentation can be done during the physical and the DDST. Although racial variation has been reported in the rate of motor development (black infants reportedly sit, stand, and walk at earlier ages than their Caucasian counterparts), no standardized developmental scales have used cross-racial subjects. Consequently, the examiner must also rely on family reports when assessing the developmental level of ethnic children of color.[1-3]

Parents of children in this age group should also be questioned about inappropriate movement or obvious problems with balance that may have been observed in the child. A balance problem may not be noticeable until late infancy, when the baby begins to walk. If there is a concern, most parents will observe inappropriate falling. It is important for the nurse to remember that normalcy in growth and development depends on the accomplishmnent of developmental tasks appropriate to that age and stage. If any discrepancies are found, evaluation of past accomplishment is necessary.

The last area of investigation in the neurologic review concerns any history of seizures. Seizures in this age group occur for one of two reasons: high fever or a neurologic disease. If elevated temperature is suspected as the reason, it is important to record the description of the seizure, including body temperature, body movement, loss of consciousness (for how long?), loss of urine or feces, number of occurrences within that illness, length of time they lasted, previous history of seizures, other members of the family who have had a seizure, and treatments implemented. If neurologic dysfunction is suspected, the same types of questions should be asked. However, the examiner will probably discover that an acute illness is not present.

The *toddler* has many developmental milestones, too. Most of these were reviewed in Chapter 1 (see Chart 1.2). Questioning the parents about the approximate dates of accomplishment of these milestones is worthwhile. Any inappropriate movements, falling, tics, tremors, head nodding, or head banging should be recorded, Seizing with an elevated temperature is not atypical in this age group. In fact, this response to a high fever may exist late into the school-age years. The nurse should always inquire about this, especially if it has occurred at other times in the past. It is also important to assess exposure to lead, particularly with children from poor families. The greatest incidence of lead poisoning occurs in children living in old houses in the inner city. Frequent exposure to lead may produce symptoms of "dullness." The child may thus be viewed as developmentally retarded when he is actually the victim of a poverty-perpetuated disease.[3]

During the *preschool, school-age, adolescent,* and *young adult* years, the nurse should inquire about the completion of developmental tasks (see Chart 1.2). Successful accomplishment of these and a negative general history (see neurologic general review of system) will take care of this system review. However, if any of the general questions asked get a positive response, further investigation is necessary. Applying the "eight areas of investigation" to a positive response will help the nurse gather the appropriate data.

Generally, the *middle-aged* patient has few neurologic complaints. He may notice some gradual changes, such as problems with presbyopia. Other neurologic changes are minimal during these years if the person is in reasonably good health. There are, however, specific diseases (such as multiple sclerosis) that are likely to occur in the middle years. Thus the nurse must always follow up on complaints with even the most vague resemblance to neurologic disturbances.

With the patient in the *later years,* the nurse must pay special attention to neurologic changes. Very often this patient may not be aware of the gradual neurologic changes that take place, as in hearing, tasting, and touching. There may be a decrease in memory and an overall weakening of the muscles. The patient should be asked about vision and hearing. Does he notice any change? Is there any weakening or paralysis of the extremities? The nurse should inquire about such sensory symptoms as paresthesias, numbness, and tingling. In terms of motor function, any falling, dizziness, uncontrolled muscle movements, tics, tremors, or speech disturbances should be noted. It is often difficult to get the patient to be specific about complaints along this line. The more concrete the data, the more helpful they will be. For this reason, the nurse may find herself using more direct questioning and guiding the patient to specific points.

ANATOMY

The study of the anatomy and physiology of the nervous system is difficult for two reasons; (1) the complexity of its structure, function, and effect on the human body and (2) the many varied theories and explanations of its structure, function, and effect, which have so much contradictory content.

For all practical purposes, the nervous system can be separated into the central nervous system and the peripheral nervous system. The *brain* and *spinal cord* make up the *central nervous system.* The spinal nerves and the *cranial nerves* compose the *peripheral nervous system.*

The Central Nervous System

The Brain. The brain can be divided up in several different ways. The simplest division includes the *forebrain,* the *brainstem,* and the *cerebellum* (Fig. 15.1). The forebrain includes the cerebrum (telencephalon) and diencephalon (thalamus and hypothalamus) and the brainstem includes the midbrain, pons, and medulla.

The Forebrain. The *cerebrum* is the largest portion of the brain center. In addition to its sensory and motor functions, it is said to be the place of the highest mental function. It stores all knowledge.

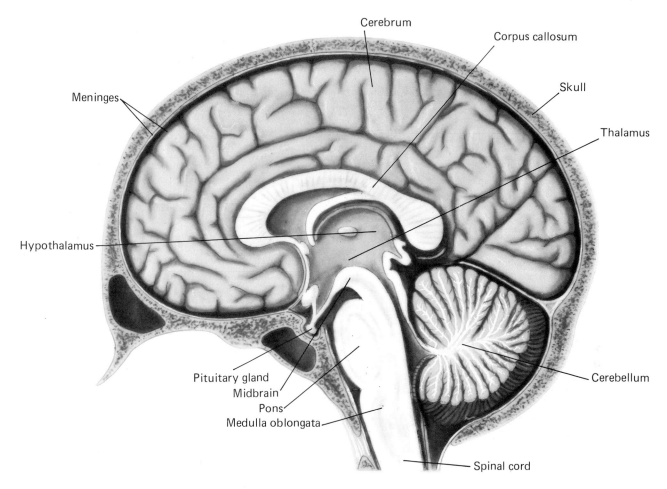

FIGURE 15.1. The brain: major structures. (From Heagarty, M., Glass, G., King, H., & Manly, M. *Child health: Basics for primary care.* New York: Appleton–Century–Crofts, 1980, p. 169).

The *diencephalon* is composed of the *thalamus* and the *hypothalamus*. The thalamus is the largest part of the diencephalon. It works along with the hypothalamus to affect hormones, smooth muscles, and glands. The hypothalamus is known as the regulator of the internal environment. It integrates and correlates autonomic, somatic, and hormonal operations. The hypothalamus also plays a part in emotion and satiation.

The Brainstem. All the *afferent and efferent tracks* between the spinal cord and the brain go through the brainstem. Many cranial nerves come from there and all the cell bodies of the efferent section of the cranial nerves are in the brainstem. The overall function includes the control of subconscious and reflex activity. The *midbrain* is involved in motor coordination. The *medulla* contains the autonomic control centers for breathing, arterial blood pressure, and vomiting. Not much is known about the pons and its separate function. It contains many fiber tracks between the spinal cord and the brain. It does seem to be a "relay center," with most messages going to the *cerebellum*.

The Cerebellum. The cerebellum is located in the occipital region of the head. It attaches to both the cerebrum and the brainstem. Functionally, the cerebellum deals with balance, posture, and equilibrium.

The Peripheral Nervous System

The Spinal Nerves. There are 31 pairs of spinal nerves: 8 cervical, 12 thoracic, 5 lumbar, 5 sacral, and 1 coccygeal. Each spinal nerve has an afferent and efferent component as well as a *dorsal* and *ventral branch* (Fig. 15.2). The ventral portion serves the limbs as well as the front and lateral aspects of the trunk. The spinal nerves that innervate specific areas of the skin are called *dermatomes* (Fig. 15.3). It is important to note that each spinal nerve may have a very large dermatome to serve.

The Cranial Nerves. There are 12 pairs of cranial nerves. In this case, each pair does not necessarily have an afferent and efferent component. These 12 cranial nerves are: *olfactory* (CN I), *optic* (CN II), *oculomotor* (CN III), *trochlear* (CN IV), *trigeminal* (CN V), *abducens* (CN VI), *facial* (CN VII), *acoustic* (CN VIII), *glossopharyngeal* (CN IX), *vagus* (CN X), *spinal accessory* (CN XI), and *hypoglossal* (CN XII). Each nerve has specific functions and is either sensory, motor, or both (Chart 15.1).

The peripheral nervous system can be further divided into afferent and efferent sections because most of the cranial nerves and all of the spinal nerves have both components.

The efferent segment is divided again into the *somatic* and *autonomic systems.* The somatic efferent motor nerves innervate skeletal muscle and the autonomic nerves stimulate smooth muscle, cardiac muscle, and the glands.

Autonomic Nervous System. What a misnomer! The nervous system is confusing enough without this misleading term. The au-

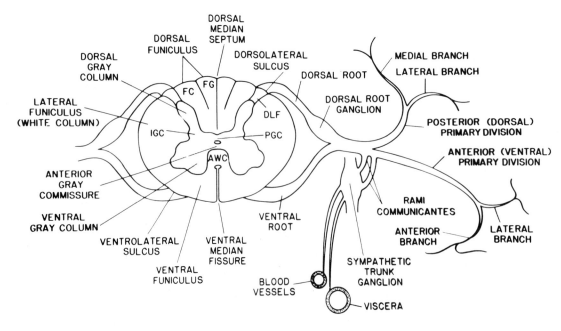

FIGURE 15.2. The spinal nerve: dorsal and ventral branches. (From Jensen, D. *The Human Nervous System.* New York: Appleton–Century–Crofts, 1980, p. 41).

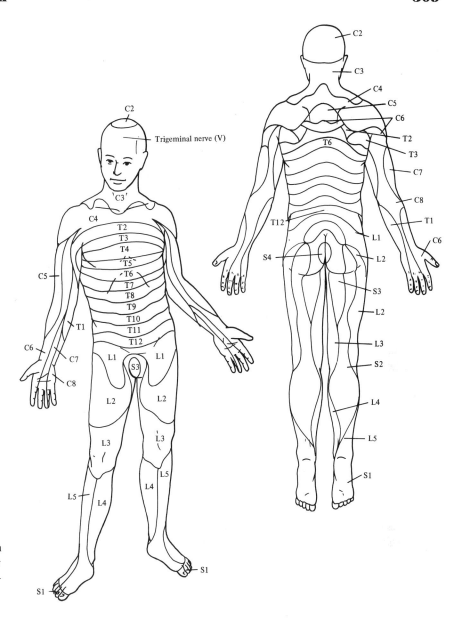

FIGURE 15.3. Dermatomes. (From Brill, E. & Kilts, D. *Foundations for nursing.* New York: Appleton–Century–Crofts, 1980, p. 225).

tonomic nervous system is not another nervous system. It is, in fact, one of the efferent portions of the peripheral nervous system. This innervation further breaks down into the *sympathetic and parasympathetic sections.*

The feature unit of this system involves the *ganglia,* which are groups of cells that lie outside the central nervous system (Fig. 15.4). The synapse of neural transmission occurs along this pathway. One difference in the sympathetic and parasympathetic divisions depends on the location of these ganglia. For the most part the ganglia in the sympathetic system lie close to the spinal cord. In the parasympathetic system the ganglia lie closer to the organ receiving the stimulation. The fibers on either side of the ganglia are called either *preganglionic* or *postganglionic.*

At the junction of the preganglionic and postganglionic neurons, where the synapse occurs, a chemical transmitter is released. This must happen prior to the synapse. The chemical released depends on the site of the ganglia. *Acetylcholine* is released between *preganglionic* and *postganglionic fibers* in both the sympathetic and

CHART 15.1.

The Cranial Nerves

Cranial Nerve	Motor (M) or Sensory (S) Origin	Function
CN I (olfactory)	S	Smell
CN II (optic)	S	Vision
CN III (oculomotor)	M Autonomic Somatic	Pupillary constriction Extraocular muscles: superior rectus, medial rectus, inferior rectus, inferior oblique
CN IV (trochlear)	M	Extraocular muscles: superior oblique
CN V (trigeminal)	S	Face and scalp; three divisions: ophthalamic, maxillary, mandibular
	M	Mandibular muscles: masseter, temporal, pterygoid
CN VI (abducens)	M	Internal deviation of eye
CN VII (facial)	S	Taste: anterior ⅔ of the tongue
	M	Facial muscles: face, scalp and outer ear Submandibular and sublingual salivary glands, lacrimal glands, and glands of nasal and palatine mucosa
CN VIII (acoustic)	S	Hearing, balance
CN IX (glossopharyngeal)	S	Taste: posterior ⅓ of the tongue
	M	Pharynx: swallowing, gagging, parotid gland
CN X (vagus)	S	Larynx; pharynx; esophagus; heart, abdominal organs
	M	Pharynx, larynx
CN XI (spinal accessory)	M	Muscles: sternocleidomastoid, trapezius
CN XII (hypoglossal)	M	Tongue

parasympathetic systems. The nerve fibers that release acetylcholine are *cholinergic* fibers. Acetylcholine is also released between the parasympathetic postganglionic fiber and the effector cell (Fig. 15.4). At the synapse of the sympathetic postganglionic fiber and effector cell, *adrenergic* (adrenalin) fibers release *norepinephrine*.[4] Whereas, in the parasympathetic response acetylcholine is again released between the postganglionic fiber and the effector cell.[1]

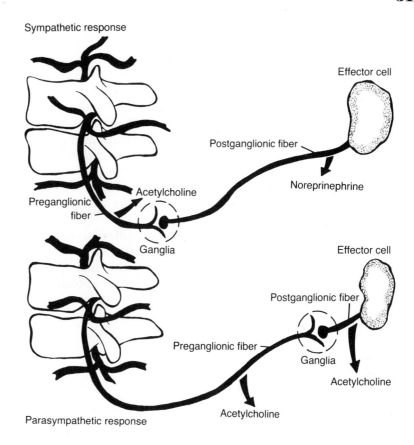

Sympathetic response

Effector cell

Postganglionic fiber

Noreprinephrine

Acetylcholine

Preganglionic fiber

Ganglia

Effector cell

Postganglionic fiber

Preganglionic fiber

Ganglia

Acetylcholine

Acetylcholine

Parasympathetic response

FIGURE 15.4. Autonomic nervous system.

The function of the autonomic nervous system is to provide a homeostatic environment for the body by controlling the activities of specific organs—primarily the smooth muscles, cardiac muscles, and glands. For the most part, this function is accomplished by involuntary controls.

Most organs that the autonomic nervous system affects receive dual innervation. This means that the organs have both sympathetic and parasympathetic stimulation. These systems work antagonistically against one another. The sympathetic deals with "fight or flight;" the parasympathetic effect is most easily evidenced at rest or recovery from sympathetic stimulation.

The Motor System. In order for the motor system to function appropriately, the following organs must be intact: the *cerebral cortex*, the *basal ganglia*, the *cerebellum*, the *brainstem*, and the *spinal cord nuclei*.

The cerebral cortex has an important role in motor function. The area of the cortex most involved is the posterior portion of the frontal lobe. This is known as the *motor cortex*.

The basal ganglia act as relays in the motor system. They receive messages from the cortex to stimulate purposeful control of fine, coordinated, rapid and slow movement. The mechanism of postural control lies here also. The brainstem, spinal cord nuclei, and *reticular formation* are portions of the descending tract that act in conjunction with the basal ganglia.

The cerebellum houses both afferent and efferent nerve fibers. Every motor stimulus must pass through the cerebellum. Motor stimulation is not initiated here, but all the integration of information from the basal ganglia and motor cortex takes place in the cerebellum.

If damage occurs in the cerebellum, not only does movement become uncontrolled and uncoordinated, but vestibular function is affected. Thus balance and posture are involved in the function of the cerebellar region.

The descending pathways which influence motor function and are an intricate part of this system are the *corticospinal* (pyramidal tract) and the *multineuronal* pathways (Fig. 15.5). Two-thirds of the nerve fibers in the corticospinal pathways cross over in the medulla before reaching the spinal cord. Thus if right-sided symptoms appear, damage will have most likely occurred on the left side of the brain.

The multineuronal pathway is not a separate descending pathway. It is the first connecting point for some motor neurons that synapse in the nuclei of the brainstem and cerebrum. Although the synapse occurs outside the motor cortex, the integration of all this electric activity is what allows for coordinated movement of the skeletal muscles.

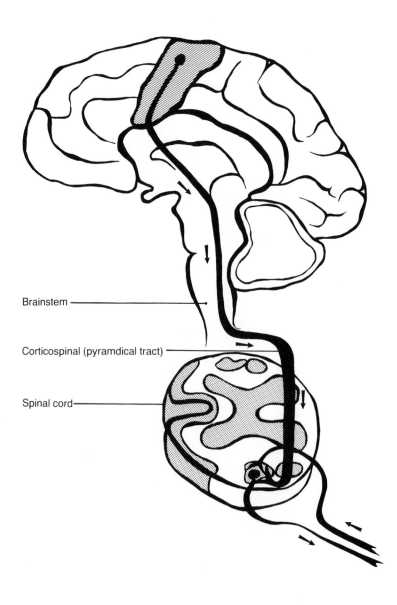

Brainstem

Corticospinal (pyramdical tract)

Spinal cord

FIGURE 15.5. Corticospinal pathways.

The Reflex Arc. The reflex arc is a homeostatic mechanism of the motor system. This is the basis for the *muscle stretch reflex.* The muscle stretch reflex is a *monosynaptic reflex.* This means that there is only one synapse between the receptor and the effector.

Deep tendon reflexes are examples of the monosynaptic reflex arc. This simple reflex arc can be described most easily by imagining what occurs between the moment a tendon is tapped by a reflex hammer and the contraction of the muscle (Fig. 15.6).

The *tendon* is tapped. The *muscle spindle* is activated and the impulse travels along an afferent nerve fiber along the peripheral nerve to the spinal nerve. Further along the pathway and just outside the spinal cord is the *posterior root.* When the stimulus enters the cord, the synapse takes place. The *anterior root* picks up the stimulus and it travels along efferent pathways, including the spinal nerve and the peripheral nerve. Ultimately, the impulse reaches the muscle and the contraction occurs. This illustrates *lower motor neuron function.*

The Sensory System. The *sensory system* is made up of *sensory receptors, afferent neurons, ascending pathways,* and the *primary sensory areas* of the cerebral cortex.

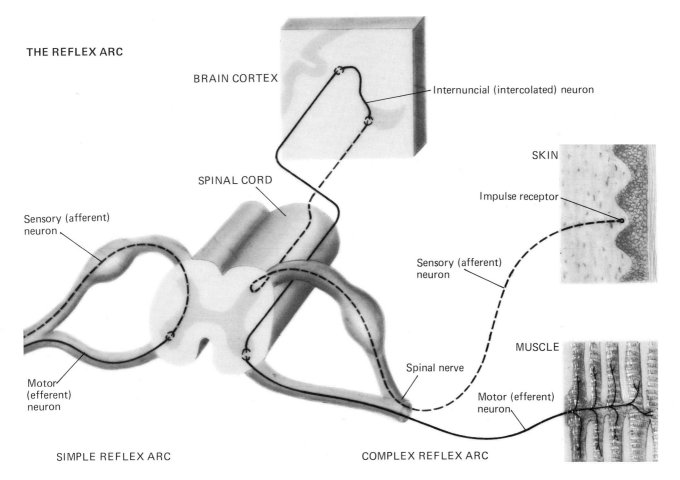

THE REFLEX ARC

BRAIN CORTEX

Internuncial (intercolated) neuron

SKIN

Impulse receptor

SPINAL CORD

Sensory (afferent) neuron

Sensory (afferent) neuron

MUSCLE

Spinal nerve

Motor (efferent) neuron

Motor (efferent) neuron

SIMPLE REFLEX ARC   COMPLEX REFLEX ARC

FIGURE 15.6. Nervous reflex: the reflex arc. (From Heagarty, M., Glass, G., King, H., & Manly, M. *Child health: Basics for primary care.* New York: Appleton–Century–Crofts, 1980, p. 170).

There are many different kinds of sensory receptors. These vary according to the types of stimuli they receive. The receptors are classified according to position; movement; and the sensations of heat, cold, pain, and touch. There are other types for muscle, joint, and tendon sense. There are also receptors in the viscera and blood vessels—these are not necessarily conscious receptors.

Two ascending pathways known to scientists at present are the *lateral spinothalamic* and the *posterior* columns. The lateral spinothalamic is responsible for pain and temperature. The posterior column is the tract that deals with position and movement.

Like all the other divisions within the nervous system, all the units must be intact and functioning for an appropriate response to occur, regardless of the orientation of the stimulus. If there is any interruption along the way, symptoms will appear. The physical assessment of the nervous system will help pinpoint the location of that interruption.

PHYSICAL ASSESSMENT

The physical assessment of the neurologic system involves two different approaches, depending on the reason for the examination. If the patient is undergoing a routine health assessment, a screening level exam is appropriate. If the chief complaint relates to the neurologic system, as with headaches, numbness, or weakness of an extremity, then a much more detailed assessment is required.

The screening examination includes a brief assessment of mental status and developmental level in children; assessment of specific cranial nerves (II, III, IV, V (motor), VI (motor), VII (motor), VIII, IX (motor), XI, and XII—most of these are unavoidably tested in examination of the head, ears, eyes, nose, and throat) assessment of motor function, including walking, knee bends, hopping, and walking on heels and toes (the examiner should test only those tasks appropriate to age and ability); evaluation of sensory function, including pain and/or vibration in the hands and feet; and assessment of deep tendon reflexes.

The equipment needed for the neurologic screening exam includes an ophthalmoscope, a tuning fork, a safety pin (sharp and blunt end), and a reflex hammer. For a more detailed exam the examiner needs two test tubes (one filled with warm water and one with cold), a wisp of cotton, a quarter, a paper clip, and two distinct substances with odors (alcohol swab, coffee grounds, or a peppermint).

Mental Status

Much of the mental status exam can be done during the interview. This is especially true for testing orientation to time, person, and place, and is also true for testing recall. The patient's responses to questions about his past health history reflect his memory for events that occurred earlier in his life. Elicitation of data about a recent complaint illustrates his recall for more recent events. Obviously, if he knows who he is, where he is, and the time of day, his time, person, and place orientation is intact. Although the nurse elicits subjective data, her observations of the patient's responses are objective data. Again, only a screening level exam is done, unless otherwise indicated.

The additional components of the mental status examination include:

1. General apperance: It is important to notice not only hygiene and grooming, but also whether the patient's clothing is appropriate for the place and weather.
2. Posture: The patient's sitting or standing position may be either upright or slouched. This can point out a mechanical problem or reflect his self-image.
3. Facial expression.
4. Mood: This is often evidenced in the posture and facial expression. The nurse should be careful to document this with her observational skills and not just give her opinon.
5. Speech: This includes tone and verbalization as well as the quality of what is being stated. The nurse must be sure that there are no educational or language barriers while making this observation.
6. Level of awareness and state of consciousness: This includes orientation to time, person, and place; ability to concentrate; and the level of consciousness (Chart 15.2).
7. Intellectual functioning: This includes memory (both recent and remote), basic knowledge (understanding and ability to learn), abstract thinking (the ability to explain abstract statements, such as "A rolling stone gathers no moss."), similarity association (the ability to take similar concepts and make an association—i.e., a chair is to a table as a pencil is to paper), and judgement (the ability to make decisions with common sense and appropriate thought processes).

All these observations are invalid if the nurse is testing at a level at which the patient cannot understand or participate. The nurse should be subtle in her approach in gathering this information and scatter the tests throughout the interview.

CHART 15.2.

Altered States of Consciousness

Term	Characteristics
Full consciousness	Alert, awake; aware of self and environment
Confusion	Disorientation in time; irritability and/or drowsiness; misjudgment of sensory input; shortened attention span; decrease in memory
Delirium	Disorientation, fear, misperception of sensory stimuli; may be out of contact with environment
Stupor	Unresponsive, but can be aroused back to a near normal state
Coma	Unresponsive to external stimuli

From McGehee–Harvey, A., et al. *The principles and practice of medicine* (19th ed.). New York: Appleton–Century–Crofts, 1976, p. 1510.

The Cranial Nerves

The decision as to whether or not to test all or some of the cranial nerves for screening purposes is a moot point. Because it takes so little time to test their intactness and because so many of them are tested within the head, ear, eye, nose, and throat exams, it is just as easy to test all the cranial nerves.

Cranial Nerve I (Olfactory). This nerve controls the sense of olfaction. The patient is told that he will be asked to smell a particular substance and identify it. For this he will have to close his eyes. After he closes his eyes, he is asked to place a finger over one nostril so he can only smell through one side at a time. The examiner should make sure the patient's nose is not obstructed from sinus drainage. She then places an odorous substance at the open nares—i.e., alcohol, coffee grounds, an orange, or a mint (especially good for children). The patient is asked to identify the scent, after which the other nostril is tested with a different substance. This is not done on the screening level.

Cranial Nerve II (Optic). The optic nerve is tested by evaluating visual acuity (with the Snellen chart and a funduscopic exam) and visual fields (with confrontation testing) (see Chap. 5).

Cranial Nerves III (Oculomotor), IV (Trochlear), and VI (Abducens). These are all tested together because of their related functions (see Chap. 5). These nerves are tested for appropriate extraocular movements, direct and indirect pupillary constriction, ptosis, lid lag, and nystagmus.

Cranial Nerve V (Trigeminal). This nerve has both a sensory and a motor component. The motor portion deals with the strength and symmetry of the masseter and temporal muscles. The patient is asked to clench his teeth. The examiner palpates the temporomandibular area and feels the strength of these muscles during the contraction. Unequal muscle contraction is significant and worthy of documentation and should be referred. The *sensory* division has three areas that need evaluation. The ophthalmic area is assessed by testing for the presence of the corneal reflex (see Chap. 5). The maxillary and mandibular divisions are tested for the sensations of pain or light touch. The patient is asked to close his eyes. The nurse explains to him that he will be feeling a sharp or dull sensation scattered around his face. He is to identify which he feels. The nurse uses an open safety pin and applies either the blunt or sharp end along the lateral aspect of the face, the forehead, the cheek, and chin. If there is any doubt after this test, the nurse asks the patient to identify the difference between hot and cold temperatures. For this the nurse has two test tubes filled with water—one hot, one cold. She applies the base of either tube in the same general area as she did the safety pin. The patient is asked to identify which is hot and which is cold. The nurse must remember to scatter the stimuli and alter the temperatures. The nurse can also stroke the patient's face at these selected areas with a wisp of cotton. The patient should be able to tell when the cotton is touching his face.

Cranial Nerve VII (Facial). The nurse initially observes for any tics, unusual movement, or asymmetry. The muscles of the face are tested by asking the patient to clench his teeth forcefully and smile,

(Fig. 15.7) blow out his cheeks with his mouth closed, frown or wrinkle his forehead, raise his eyebrows, and close his eyes tightly, not letting the examiner open them. The taste buds on the anterior two-thirds of the tongue are tested to evaluate the sensory component. The tongue can pick up the sensations of sweet (sugar), salty, sour (lemon), and bitter (aspirin). The patient should be able to differentiate among the tastes. The nurse should be sure to have him rinse his mouth between tastes to avoid overlap. The taste test is not done on the screening level.

Cranial Nerve VIII (Acoustic). Auditory acuity can be tested by audiometry and the Weber and Rinné tests (see Chap. 6). Testing vestibular function is beyond the scope of this book. The test involves injecting ice water into the external ear and observing nystagmus, vertigo, or falling. Anyone with intact vestibular function will have nystagmus. Patients find this test most uncomfortable.

Cranial Nerves IX (Glossopharyngeal) and X (Vagus). These two nerves are tested together. To test the glossopharyngeal nerve, the patient is asked to open his mouth and say "ah." The nurse should note the soft palate rising as well as the uvula. The nurse touches the uvula with a tongue depressor and elicits a gag reflex. This gag reflex tests the motor function of the vagus nerve. The nurse listens for any hoarseness of the voice. All this can be observed in taking the history and while examining the mouth.

Cranial Nerve XI (Spinal Accessory). The strength of the sternocleidomastoid and trapezius muscles is tested. The nurse places her hands on the patient's shoulders. The patient shrugs his shoulders and the nurse pushes down on them. The patient is asked to resist this pressure (Fig. 15.8A). For the other portion of this test, the examiner puts her hand on the side of the patient's face (Fig. 15.8B). She asks him to push against her hand while she applies pressure toward his face. The patient should be able to resist this pressure

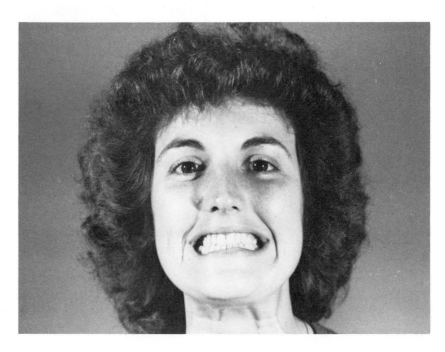

FIGURE 15.7. Testing cranial nerve VII.

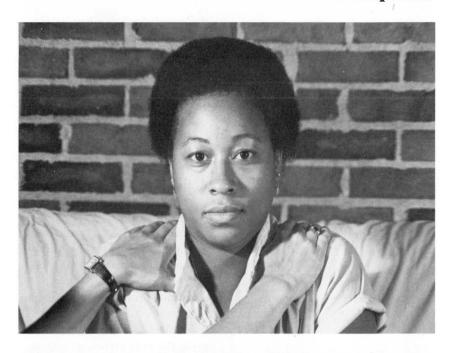

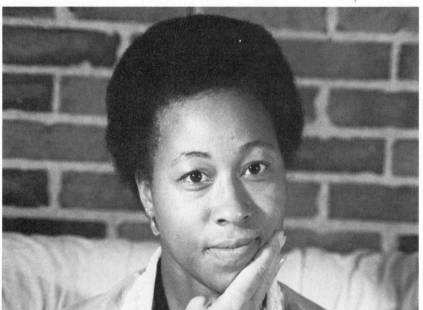

FIGURE 15.8. Testing cranial nerve XI.

with the strength in his facial muscles. The other side of the face is then tested.

Cranial Nerve XII (Hypoglossal). The patient's tongue is inspected while noting the mouth size and any irregular movement or asymmetry. The patient is then asked to stick out his tongue while the nurse looks for the same irregularities.

This completes the tests for the twelve cranial nerves.

The Motor System

Consistent with the other components of the neurologic examination, the testing of the motor system has a screening level and a more detailed approach. Some parts of the screening exam can be completed by watching the patient as he walks into the room and while he is sitting during the interview. The screening exam includes posture, swinging of the arms, movement of the legs, inspection of musculature of the body, the quality of muscle tone (especially in children and older people), and balance.

The more detailed version of the examination of motor system function is the same for both children and adults. The information elicited depends on the patient's ability and cooperation. This portion of the exam becomes necessary when abnormalities are suspected from the results of the screening exam. The evaluation at this point involves a further assessment of muscle tone, muscle strength, and coordination.

Posture and Muscle Tone. Posture can be evaluated by observing the patient's walk, his sitting position, and obvious deviation along the spinous process, back, or shoulders. Most people when they sit will have some degree of rounding of the shoulders. However, if this is exaggerated or corresponds with a portion of the chief complaint, further evaluation is necessary.

The posture and muscle tone of the newborn should be evaluated as well. In normal resting posture, the baby's legs are partially flexed and there is a slight abduction of the hips. Thorough inspection and palpation of muscle tone is essential, especially in infants and children (see Chap. 14). In the older patient muscle mass may atrophy and will appear to have less "substance."

Swinging of the arms in conjunction with movement of the legs can be observed easily when the patient walks into the room. Abnormalities in this movement are obvious.

Balance. Observing the patient's overall balance is the first step. Again, obvious abnormalities can be detected when he walks into the room.

The Romberg test, a test for cerebellar function, is a quick screening test for balance that should be done with all age groups, from toddlers to the elderly. For this test the patient is asked to stand up with his feet together. He is then asked to close his eyes. He is observed for swaying. The nurse should be close to the patient with her arms extended around him in case the patient starts to fall (Fig. 15.9). Some swaying is normal, especially in older patients.

Other cerebellar tests for balance, for the ambulatory patient who is able, include a shallow deep-knee bend, hopping in place (one foot at a time), heel to toe walking, walking on tip-toes and then on heels, and standing on one foot at a time with the eyes closed.

Inspection of the General Muscle Mass. The muscles of the body are inspected for atrophy, asymmetry, fasciculations (twitching) and involuntary movement. Further discussion of this examination can be found in Chapter 14.

The more detailed exam, when necessary, includes the following.

Muscle Tone. The patient should be lying in a supine position. The nurse should explain to him that the extremities of his body will be flexed and extended to test for pain, resistance, and flaccidity. Testing each side separately, the examiner supports the extremity being tested and takes it through a *passive range of motion*. On the

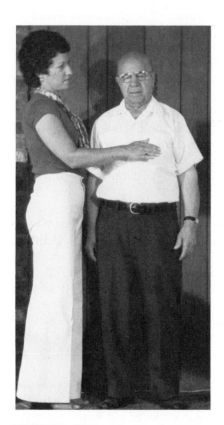

FIGURE 15.9. The Romberg test.

upper half of the body, the fingers, wrists, elbows, and shoulders are assessed. Then the toes, ankles, and knees are flexed, extended, abducted, adducted, and rotated for the same purpose.

Muscle Strength. Muscle strength is tested against the resistance of the examiner. Symmetrical responses are significant and permit the examiner to use the patient as his own control. Considerations should be given to the age and health of the patient as well as to the integrity of the skeletal muscles. The specific tests should be applied quickly and systematically, without fatiguing the patient. These include:

1. The finger-grip: The patient is asked to squeeze the examiner's first two fingers. The grip should be reasonably strong, but most important, it should be equal in both hands (Fig. 15.10).
2. Finger abduction: The patient is asked to separate his fingers. The examiner explains to him that she will try to push them together. The patient is to resist this pressure. The examiner notes any weakness or asymmetry in strength (Fig. 15.11).
3. Wrist dorsiflexion: The patient is asked to make a fist with both hands. The examiner tries to push them down while the patient resists. Any weakness is noted (Fig. 15.12).
4. Flexion and extension of the elbow: The patient is asked to push against the examiner's hands with his forearm (extension) (Fig. 15.13A). He is then asked to pull against the resistance of the examiner's hand at the forearm (flexion). Any pain or resistance is noted (Fig. 15.13B).
5. Shoulder and scapulae resistance: The patient is asked to extend both arms out in front of him for 20 seconds. He is told to resist the push about to be applied. The nurse then tries to push the arms down (Fig. 15.14). Any pain or weakness with this manuever is noted. This is a common site for sports injuries, arthritis, and bursitis. Next the patient is asked to raise both arms above his shoulders. The nurse tries to push his arms down to his sides. The patient is once again instructed to resist this maneuver.
6. Lateral bending, flexion, and extension of the trunk: The lower half of the body is assessed in a manner similar to that used for the upper half, with the patient lying down (see Chap. 14).
7. Hip flexion: The patient is asked to raise his leg against the examiner's hand, which is applying pressure on the thigh, trying to flatten the leg. Any pain with this movement is noted, especially in the geriatric client.
8. Hip abduction: The patient is asked to flex his knees so that his feet are flat on the table (or bed). The nurse places her hands over the lateral collateral ligaments. The patient then tries to push against the examiner's hands with his knees. The nurse resists the push (Fig. 15.15). There should be no pain or asymmetry in strength.
9. Hip adduction: The patient's legs are in the same position used with hip abduction, except that they are slightly spread apart. This time the nurse places her hands over the medial collateral ligaments. The patient is asked to bring his knees together against the nurse's resistance.

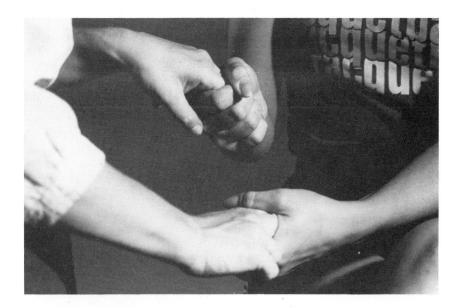

FIGURE 15.10. Symmetrical finger-grip strength.

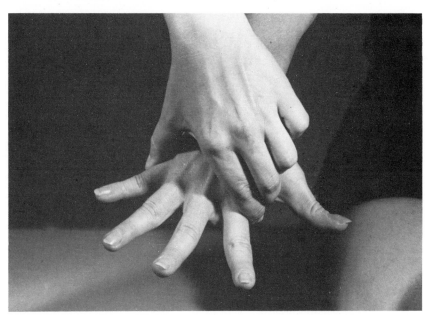

FIGURE 15.11. Finger abduction.

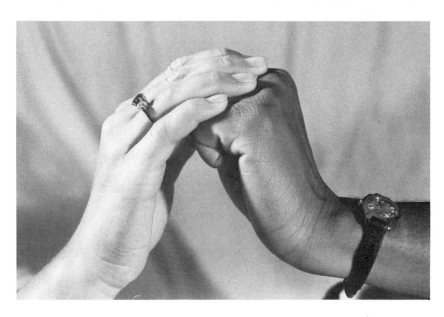

FIGURE 15.12. Wrist dorsiflexion.

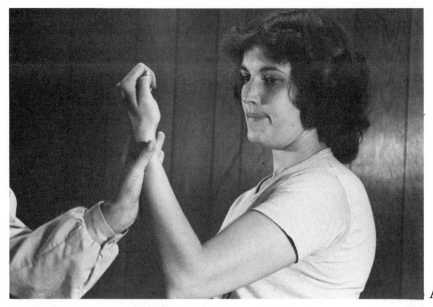

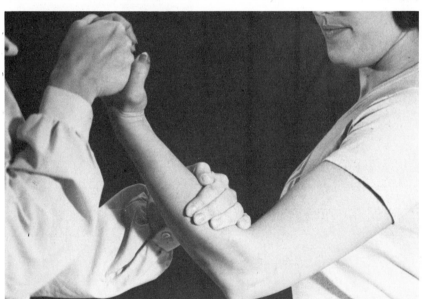

FIGURE 15.13. A: Extension of the elbow. B: Flexion of the elbow.

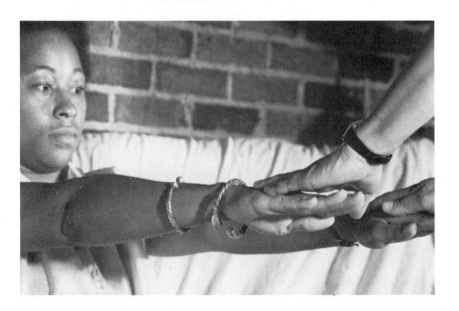

FIGURE 15.14. Shoulder and scapulae resistance.

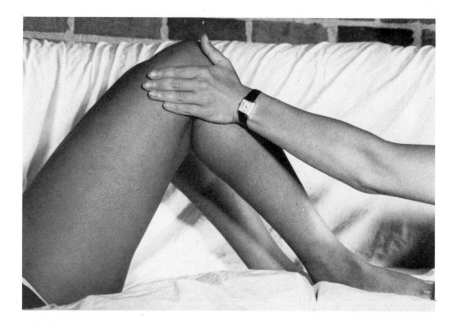

FIGURE 15.15. Hip abduction.

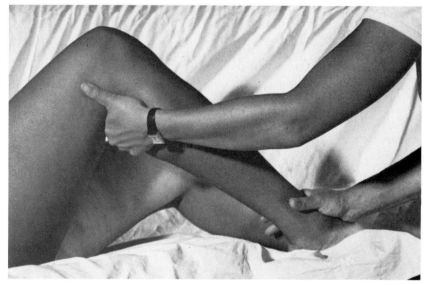

A

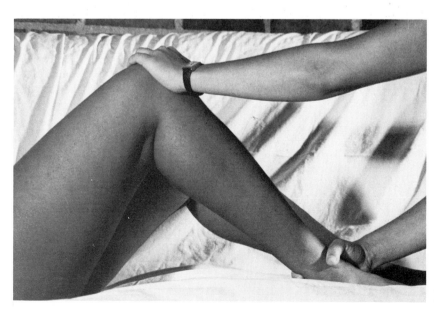

FIGURE 15.16. A: Knee extension. B: Knee flexion.

B

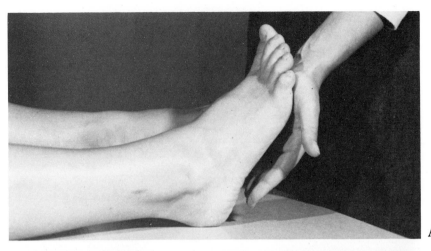

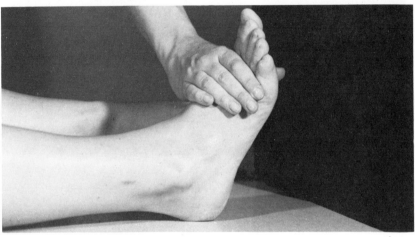

FIGURE 15.17. A: Plantar flexion of the ankle. B: Dorsiflexion of the ankle.

10. Knee extension and flexion: Again the patient's legs are flexed at the knees with his feet flat on the bed. To test extension of the knee, the nurse places one of her hands behind the patient's knee and the other on the ankle. The patient is asked to straighten his leg against the nurse's hand, which is on his ankle (Fig. 15.16A). Then the nurse's hand at the knee is taken from behind and placed on top of the knee. The patient is asked to keep his foot flat on the bed as the nurse tries to extend his leg and straighten it. (Fig. 15.16B)

11. Plantar flexion and dorsiflexion of the ankle: This test is commonly used to help locate the origin of back and leg pain. The patient is still supine with his legs flat on the bed. The nurse puts her hand on the ball of the patient's foot. The patient is asked to push against the nurse's hand while the nurse applies resistance to the patient's push (Fig. 15.17A). Then the patient is asked to pull against the nurse's hand, which is cupped around the superior aspect of each foot (dorsiflexion) (Fig. 15.17B). In specific back injuries, pain will be elicited with this test.

12. Abdominal muscle strength: While the patient is in the supine position, he is asked to raise himself at the waist or sit up. A child is asked to look at his "belly button." Pain with this maneuver may be indicative of meningeal irritation.

Coordination. This portion of motor system function, which in fact tests for intact cerebellar function, evaluates fine, purposeful movement and coordination of the upper and lower extremities. The tests are not complicated, but the instructions may be confusing. In order to be sure that the patient understands the directions, it is wise for the nurse to demonstrate to the patient what she expects him to do. Assessing rapid rhythm movement is the first test. There are two phases in this evaluation. First the patient, who is sitting up, is asked to pat the superior aspects of his thighs as rapidly as possible. He is then asked to turn his hands back and forth with the same rapid motion (palm to dorsum of hand) (Fig. 15.18). This is observed for 30 seconds. Speed and symmetry are noted.

For the second test, the patient is asked to take his thumb and touch all his fingers consecutively, repeating this several times. Each hand is tested separately. The examiner notes problems with consecutive touching or missing the fingers completely.

Next, the nurse asks the patient to touch his nose with his index finger and then put that finger on the examiner's finger. The nurse holds her finger 2 feet in front of the patient's face. The patient is asked to touch the examiner's finger with his index finger and then touch his nose with his index finger. He must move his finger back and forth several times from the nurse's finger to his nose. The patient is then asked to close his eyes, first looking at the nurse's finger. Again he is to touch his nose and then her finger—this time with the eyes closed. The nurse should not move her finger during this part of the test.

Testing fine coordination of the lower extremities is simple. The patient should be in a supine position. He is instructed to close his eyes and place the heel of his foot on the opposite knee. Next he is asked to slide his heel down his shin to his foot. The nurse observes the smoothness of this maneuver. This test is repeated on the other extremity.

This detailed exam can take a reasonably long time to perform. The nurse should be alert for patient fatigue during this extensive testing. Accuracy and validity are essential.

With children, many of these tests are made into games. It is important to remember that geriatric patients tire more easily and that some decrease in their abilities is within normal limits.

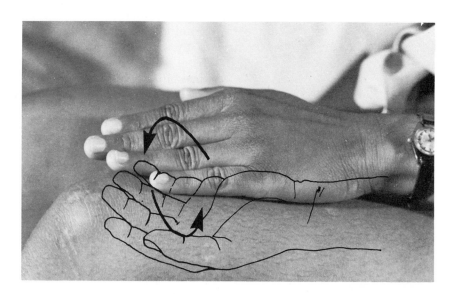

FIGURE 15.18. Hand coordination.

The Sensory System

The screening examination for the sensory system includes assessment of pain, vibration, and light touch. Where a more detailed evaluation is required, the nurse adds temperature sensation, position sense, discriminative sensation (stereognosis and two-point discrimination), point localization, and extinction.

The sensory examination can be done quickly and efficiently, without fatiguing the patient if an organized approach is used. There are certain rules that should be applied consistently throughout the exam. First, stimuli should be scattered and applied symmetrically wherever possible, so that all the dermatomes and peripheral areas are covered. Second, the more distal areas should always be tested first. If they are undamaged, the more proximal areas will be intact. Third, if any areas are suspect, the boundaries of the sensory changes need to be clearly mapped out.

The equipment used is a wisp of cotton, a safety pin, two straight pins, and a tuning fork. If the pain or light touch sensations are questionable, two test tubes with hot and cold water should be available.

The patient needs a careful explanation of the procedure because he will be asked to keep his eyes closed during the testing. Reassuring him that nothing will hurt him will help to gain his trust.

Screening For The Sensory System

Pain. A response to painful stimuli can be easily elicited with a safety pin. The patient is asked to close his eyes. Either the sharp or the dull end of the pin is placed at specific points on the body. The patient should be able to distinguish between sharp and dull. The nurse should start with the more distal areas (face, feet, and hands) and apply the pin in symmetrical positions, going from right to left or left to right. The sharp and dull stimuli should be varied irregularly so that the patient does not come to rely on a pattern.

Vibration. This testing is carried out in a manner similar to that used for sharp and dull testing. The patient is again asked to close his eyes. The nurse places the vibrating tuning fork on bony prominences, such as the wrist, ankles, and forehead. The patient should be able to say when he feels the vibration on his body. A lower pitched (larger) tuning fork will give stronger sensations. An alternate method involves placing the vibrating fork on a bony prominence and stopping the vibrations suddenly. The patient is asked to say when the sensation stops. If there is any doubt after testing the distal areas, little time is needed to evaluate the elbows, shoulders, knees, iliac crests, and spine. If these are found to be normal, the distal places should be retested to confirm findings.

Light Touch. Using the wisp of cotton, the nurse strokes the patient, while his eyes are closed, on different parts of his body. He is asked to state where he is being touched. Symmetrical testing is important here.

Detailed Examination of the Sensory System. These tests are used when there are complaints of numbness, tingling or loss of sensation, loss of motor function, areas of tissue breakdown, and/or muscle atrophy. Obviously, these tests can also be used to expand on information elicited during the screening test.

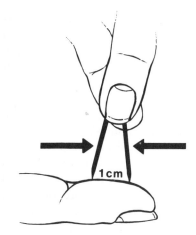

FIGURE 15.19. Two-point discrimination.

Temperature. This is applied when the patient is unable to distinguish between sharp and dull stimuli. The two test tubes, filled with hot and cold water, are placed on various parts of the body. The patient is asked to distinguish between hot and cold.

Position. The patient is asked to close his eyes. He is told that his big toe will be moved either up or down. He is to say when the toe is up and when it is down. This is repeated with the other foot and then with each hand.

Discriminative Sensation

Stereognosis. For this test a familiar object, such as a key, coin, or paper clip, is used. The patient is asked to open his hand and close his eyes. The nurse places the object in one hand and the patient is allowed to feel it with that hand. He is asked to identify the object. Another variation of this test is to write a number familiar to the patient in his palm. The blunt end of the reflex hammer or the nurse's finger will do. The patient should be able to identify the number. Both hands are tested.

Two-point Discrimination. The heads of two straight pins are placed on the patient's fingertip about 3 cm apart. The points are brought closer and closer together until he can only distinguish one point. The pins should not be more than 2 or 3 mm apart. One finger is tested on each hand (Fig. 15.19).

Point Localization. This test is relatively simple. The patient, with his eyes closed, is touched by the nurse somewhere on his body. She removes her hand. After that he opens his eyes and points to where he has been touched. This test is repeated on various parts of the patient's body.

Extinction. The patient's eyes are closed and the nurse touches him on corresponding parts of his body at the same time (upper arms, knees, etc.). He is asked to state where he has been touched.

If discrepancies are found after completing the above tests, a referral is usually necessary. However, several factors may skew the results: fatigue on the part of the patient, poor instructions, or common skin abnormalities, such as callouses. Evaluating test results in children may be difficult. Making games out of all these tests will add to a child's cooperation.

If there is a degree of uncertainty, evaluation on a different day, in a different setting, or at a different time may prove worthwhile. It should be remembered that documenting the specific boundaries of areas under suspicion is essential. To record the information, it may be easier to draw an outline of a person on the chart and label the involved areas. If there is any question, prompt referral is in order.

Reflexes

The discussion of assessment of the reflexes will include *infant reflexes*, *superficial reflexes*, and *deep tendon reflexes*. In all three cases a reflex is a "reaction" to a provocation within the nervous system. It is not voluntary, learned, or conscious. However, with infant reflexes it is important to remember that the disappearance of specific reflexes at certain ages is appropriate and normal.

The quality of a reflex response to a stimuli will vary among individuals. In certain pathologic conditions (i.e., thyroid disorders), an abnormal reflex response may be a sign of the problem. Since the nervous system of the aging person may deteriorate gradually, it is possible that a patient's reflex responses will become less intense through the years.

Reflex Activity in the Newborn and Infant. The major reflexes in the newborn and infant are the *rooting, sucking, moro, palmar grasp, dancing, tonic neck,* and *Babinski's.* As previously discussed, the intensity of these responses may vary considerably among population groups.

The Rooting Reflex. When the baby's cheek is stroked, he will turn his head toward the side being stroked. This response should be present from birth to about 4 months (when awake).[5] If the upper lip on either side of the face is stroked, the baby will tip his head back, turn toward the stimulus, and open his mouth.

The Sucking Reflex. This reflex is also present at birth and can last to about 7 months. Putting something (a finger, nipple, etc.) in the baby's mouth will cause vigorous sucking. This is the action of the sucking reflex.

Moro Reflex. This is also known as the startle reflex. It can be elicited by creating a sudden noise, shaking the bed, or changing the baby's position suddenly. The first two of these stimuli will give a more accurate response. The loud noise can easily be supplied by clapping loudly over the baby's head. An alternate method of eliciting this response is to lift the baby by his hands from a supine position about 30°. He is then lowered slowly to the table. As soon as his head touches the table the nurse lets go of his hands (Fig. 15.20A). The response is an immediate extension of both arms and legs, with hands and fingers extending, too. The next portion of this response is the baby's bringing all the extended extremities closer to his body. The legs follow an elongating movement like the upper torso response, but not as exaggerated. This reflex is present at birth and lasts up to 3 months.

The Palmar Grasp Reflex. When a finger or another object is placed in the palmar aspect of the baby's hand (usually slid in on the ulnar side), the baby will surround the object with a strong grip for an extended period of time (Fig. 15.20B). This reflex is present at birth and lasts for 6 months.

The Dancing (Stepping) Reflex. This reflex can be elicited from birth to about 12 months (Fig. 15.20C). The baby is held in a standing position with support under the arms. When the baby's feet touch a flat surface, he will make dancing or stepping movements.

The Tonic Neck Reflex. This reflex does not develop until 2 months and only lasts until 6 months. The tonic neck reflex resembles the fencing position. When the baby is in the supine position and his head is turned in one direction, the arm and leg on the side he is facing will extend. The other arm and leg will flex. Special attention should be paid to the disappearance of this reflex. If it remains evident after 6 to 9 months, a referral is in order.

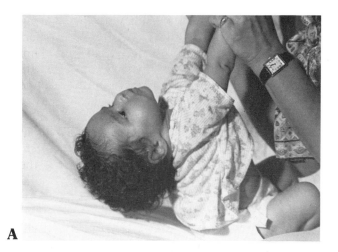
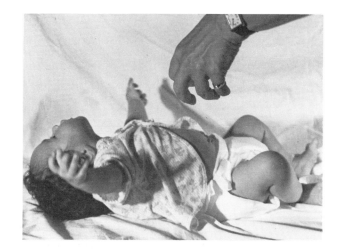

A

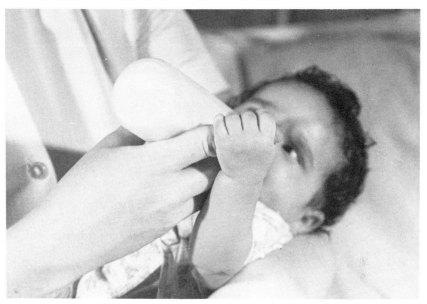

FIGURE 15.20. A. (left and right) Moro reflex. B. Finger grasp reflex. C. Dancing reflex.

B

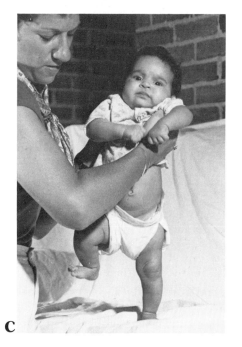

C

Babinski's Reflex. There is some controversy over the validity of this reflex in an infant. Because there are reflexes which cause extension and flexion of the toes, some authorities hesitate to trust its reliability. When the bottom of the baby's foot is stroked, the most likely response will be extension of the toes followed by the curling of the toes toward the sole of the foot (Fig. 15.21). This reaction is such in babies until approximately 18 months.

Deep Tendon Reflexes. Proper technique in eliciting deep tendon reflexes is essential for two reasons. First, it has already been stated that everyone will have a different quality of response to the stimulus. The nurse must know how to evaluate the boundaries of different ranges of "normal." Second, if technique is faulty, there is likely to be an asymmetrical response, which will result in false findings. A bilateral symmetrical reflex response is probably the most valid tool for ascertaining absence of disease. Thus, good dexterity with and knowledge of this skill is a must.

A reflex hammer is used to elicit a deep tendon reflex. The hammer is held loosely between the thumb and index finger. The wrist must also be very loose and the hammer is swung up and

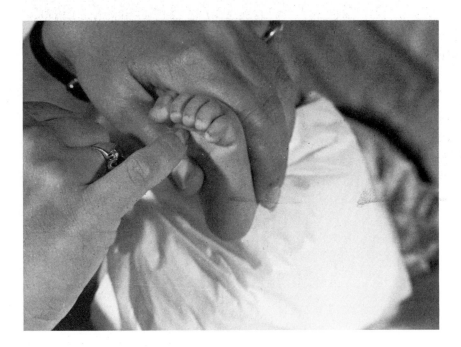

FIGURE 15.21. Babinski's reflex. Response in an infant.

down. The loose wrist motion is similar to the wrist motion used with percussion. Further detail on how to elicit each deep tendon reflex is presented below.

Appropriate elicitation of reflexes goes beyond the dexterity of the nurse. The patient must be relaxed or no response will occur. Therefore, the nurse must be sure that the patient understands the procedure, so that he can relax.

For measurement of the reflex response, a scale is available with a gradation from 0 to 4 (Chart 15.3). Because there is so much room for subjective interpretation of this scale, it is most reliable to evaluate the response in terms of symmetry. For this reason, the nurse should test each reflex bilaterally before moving down the body. This allows for immediate comparison of the response.

The deep tendon reflexes to be elicited are: the *biceps*, the *triceps*, the *brachioradialis* (supinator), *patellar*, and *Achilles tendon* reflexes. All of these are tested with a reflex hammer.

The Biceps Reflex (Spinal Cord Level: C_5, C_6). The patient's arm is flexed at the elbow and held by the nurse. The nurse places her thumb horizontally over the biceps tendon. A blow is delivered with the hammer to her thumb (Fig. 15.22). There will be slight flexion of the elbow, and the nurse will be able to feel the biceps's contraction through her thumb.

The Triceps Reflex (Spinal Cord Level: C_7, C_8). The patient's arm is again flexed at the elbow. The nurse palpates for the triceps tendon about 2–5 cm (1 or 2 inches) above the elbow. She then delivers the blow with the hammer directly to the tendon (Fig. 15.23). The patient is observed for contraction of the triceps's tendon and slight extension of the elbow.

The Brachioradialis Reflex (Spinal Cord Level: C_5, C_6). The patient's forearm can rest on the nurse's forearm or his own leg. The hammer strikes the radius 2–5 cm (1 or 2 inches) above the wrist. The

CHART 15.3.

Gradation of Reflex Responses

υ = No reflex response
+1 = Below normal
+2 = Average
+3 = Stronger than average
+4 = Very intense response (may resemble clonus)

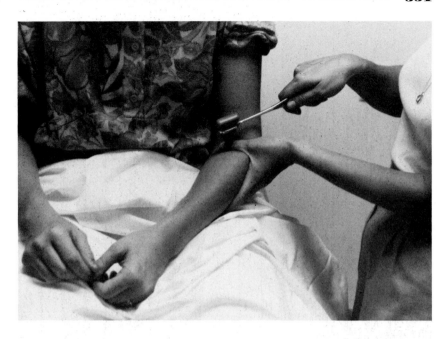

FIGURE 15.22. The biceps reflex.

patient is observed for flexion and supination of the forearm (Fig. 15.24). The fingers of the patient's hand may also extend slightly in this response.

The Patellar Knee Jerk (Spinal Cord Level: L_2, L_3, L_4). This can be more difficult to elicit if the patient is not relaxed completely. The patient should be sitting up if possible with his legs dangling over the side of the bed or table. If he is unable to sit up, the examiner slides her arm under the patient's knees as he flexes them. The patellar tendon is tapped with the hammer (Fig. 15.25). The tendon is usually found directly below the patella itself. When no response can be obtained, often the patient's legs are not relaxed enough. In this case he is asked to interlock his fingers and pull. This allows him to loosen up his legs so that the accuracy of the brisk response is not distorted.

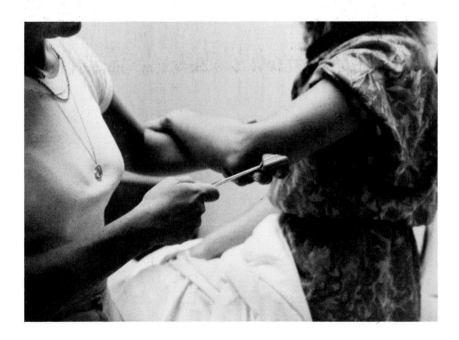

FIGURE 15.23. The triceps reflex.

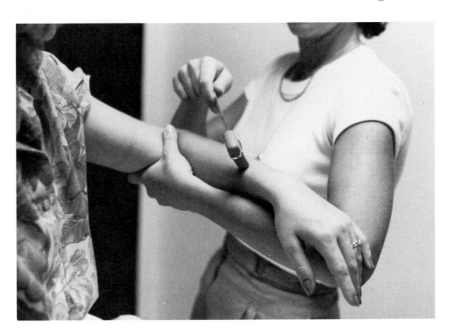

FIGURE 15.24. The brachioradialis reflex.

The Achilles Tendon Reflex (Spinal Cord Level: S_1, S_2). This should follow the patella reflex so that the patient can remain in the same position. To tap this reflex, the patient's ankle is dorsiflexed. With the foot held in this position, the examiner delivers the blow to the Achilles tendon just above the heel (Fig. 15.26). The reaction will be plantar flexion of the heel. The nurse will feel this in her hand as well as see it. If the patient is unable to sit up, the nurse can take the foot and place it on the opposite shin. This forces dorsiflexion as well. Another method to use if the patient is ambulatory is to ask him to kneel on the seat of the chair with his feet dangling over the edge (Fig. 15.27). This, too, forces dorsiflexion of the foot.

Clonus. This is not actually a reflex. However, it is an involuntary oscillation of a specific area which may be indicative of upper motor neuron disease. Ankle clonus is most frequently tested if the Achilles response is hyperactive.

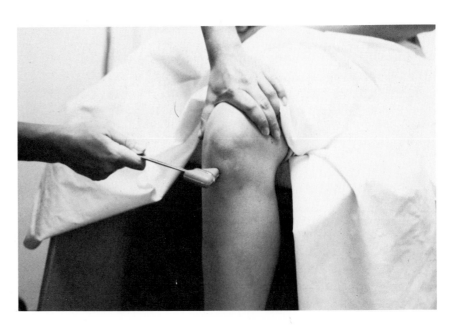

FIGURE 15.25. The knee-jerk reflex.

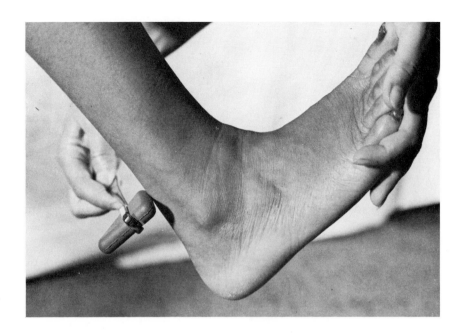

FIGURE 15.26. The Achilles tendon reflex (sitting).

To test for ankle clonus, the patient assumes the supine position. The nurse places one hand under the patient's knee, dorsiflexes the foot, and holds it in that position for a short period of time. The patient is observed for the oscillation while the foot is dorsiflexed.

Superficial Reflexes. The superficial reflexes include the *abdominal reflex*, the *cremasteric reflex*, the *corneal reflex*, and *Babinski's reflex*.

The Cremasteric Reflex (Spinal Cord Level: L₁, L₂). This can only be elicited in men. It is present by the age of 6 months. The inside of the patient's upper thigh is stroked upward with an object (a finger will do). The response to note is the rising of the testicle on the side being stroked.

The Corneal Reflex. See the section on the cranial nerves in this chapter; also see Chapter 5.

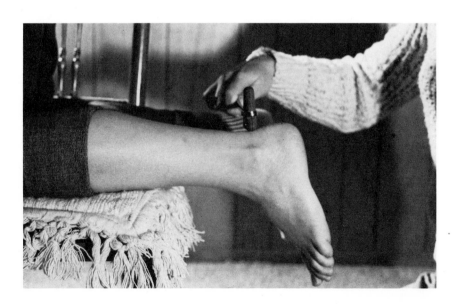

FIGURE 15.27. The Achilles tendon reflex (kneeling over a chair).

Babinski's Reflex (Spinal Cord Level: L_4, L_5, S_1, S_2). As stated earlier, this should not be positive in an adult. Performance of this test is the same for both infants and adults. All toes should flex if there is no disease. Extension of the toes indicates pathology (Fig. 15.28).

Meningeal Signs

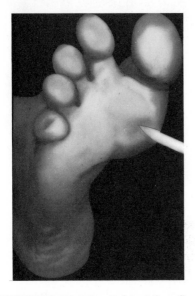

FIGURE 15.28. Babinski's reflex. Pathologic response in an adult. (From Heagarty, M., Glass, G., King, H., & Manly, M. *Child health: Basics for primary care.* New York: Appleton–Century–Crofts, 1980, p. 170).

Meningeal inflammation is not assessed for screening purposes. However, any time a child presents with symptoms of an upper respiratory infection, these tests should be done. In an adult any suspicion of intracranial dysfunction (due to infection, for instance), systemic problems, or trauma is an indication for this evaluation. Any positive findings justify immediate referral and further investigation. The signs tested for the presence of meningeal inflammation include Brudzinski's sign, Kernig's sign, and nuchal rigidity.

Brudzinski's Sign. The patient should be lying flat on his back. The nurse places her hand under patient's head (on the occiput) and raises his head toward his chest. A child may comply more readily if asked to look at his "belly button." The patient with a positive sign will resist this or have pain. Hip and knee flexion may also occur.

Kernig's Sign. The patient is still supine. One leg is flexed at the hip and then the knee at about 90°. The nurse attempts to straighten the knee (Fig. 15.29). Resistance or pain in the hamstrings is a positive sign for meningeal irritation.

Nuchal Rigidity. Any pain or resistance with flexion or rotation of the neck can be indicative of meningeal irritation. However, this may be the result of muscular problems. The nurse should be sure the history and other symptoms correlate with a neurologic problem as opposed to muscular injury or tension.

Developmental Assessment in Children

Assessment of the developmental level of a child is not only important in the neurologic examination, but also serves as major screening for all children. The developmental level is measured by

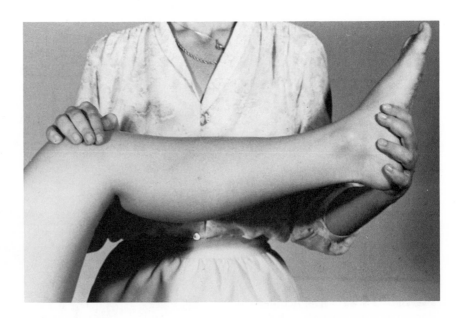

FIGURE 15.29. Kernig's sign.

testing certain abilities, including motor, communicative, and interactive skills. Special emphasis is placed on the population between birth and 6 years of age. After 6 years, one assumes that the school will take over a major portion of this testing. Even so, the examiner performing the annual health assessment should ask certain questions pertinent to the developmental tasks and test certain motor skills that are appropriate to each age group.

There are several standardized tests available to measure the accomplishment of these tasks. In selecting a particular test, it is important to consider its reliability, validity, standardization, simplicity of administration, expense, ease in scoring, and interpretation. As previously discussed, while racial developmental differences have been reported, no cross-racial standardized tests are yet available.

To exemplify the screening process, the most universally accepted test will be described: The Denver Developmental Screening Test (DDST). This test was developed at the University of Colorado in the late 1960s. Its widespread use is the result of extensive reliability and validity in testing as well as ease in administration.

The DDST evaluates four areas of development:

1. Gross motor, which involves an emphasis on the musculoskeletal and nervous systems.
2. Communication skills, including comprehension, expression, hearing, and speech.
3. Fine motor skills, which involve eye–hand coordination.
4. Personal, including social behavior, which relates to self-care and interaction with others.

The DDST is *not* a diagnostic test. It does test the developmental level in children from birth to age 6. Lack of achievement in certain areas warrants further investigation but does not label a child as "retarded," "handicapped," or "slow."

There are two ways to approach the DDST: the indirect and the direct methods. In the indirect method the examiner asks the parent about specific abilities and behaviors, while in the direct approach the examiner observes the child performing a task.

The direct method is much more valid. However, there are some tasks the child may refuse to perform, but which he is capable of doing. In this instance, the examiner should check with the parents and accept their word.

There are several factors to consider before testing the child:

1. The facility: The setting should be nonthreatening, well lit, and quiet.
2. Health of the child: The test should be deferred if the child has been ill or under stress or has experienced recent trauma.
3. Attention span: If the child is at a stage where his attention span is short, this should be taken into account.
4. Fatigue: If the child has spent a long day in school or it is late in the day, another time should be scheduled.
5. Eating: If an infant has just been fed, he is likely to want to sleep. In addition, some spitting up may occur just after feeding, especially during motor skill testing. Nor will a

hungry child be very cooperative. All these conditions are contradictory to a good testing environment.

6. Painful or frightening procedures: All testing should be done before any painful or frightening procedures are administered.

7. Explanation to parents: An explanation to the parents is essential. The nurse should emphasize that this is *not* an intelligence test, that the child will be asked to do certain things an levels he will not be expected to have achieved yet. Whether or not the parent should be present depends on the interaction between the parent, child, and examiner. If the child is more comfortable with the parent(s) present, then the parent(s) should be allowed to stay.

8. Rapport: This may be the most important uncontrollable item on this list. A sense of trust must exist between the examiner and the child or all the information elicited may be invalid.

The equipment needed for this test is available in an inexpensive kit. The kit's contents include red wool, raisins, a rattle with a narrow handle, eight 1-inch-square colored blocks (red, blue, yellow, green), a small glass bottle with an opening no bigger than 5/8 inch, a small bell, a tennis ball, and a pencil. Also needed are the test sheet and the instructions on its reverse side.

How To Administer The Test

1. The chronologic age of the child must be established (Fig. 15.30). This is done by subtracting the birthdate from the date of the test.

Date	Year	Month	Day
Date of test	80	7	15
Birthdate	75	3	10
Chronologic age	5	4	3

2. The nurse takes the test form and draws a line from the top to the bottom of the page at the corresponding age. The line should be drawn through all four areas of development. If the child was premature, the number of weeks premature should be subtracted from the chronologic age (Fig. 15.31). The line is drawn at the adjusted age.

3. The date the test is administered is written at the top of the age line. If an adjustment was made for prematurity, this should be indicated under the date.

4. Full instructions are on the back of the sheet.

5. At this point the child is tested. The tasks he should be asked to do are listed along the drawn line.

6. Each item is represented by a bar. The bar is placed on paper to show that 25, 50, 75, or 90 percent of all children (standardized population) can perform that task. The short slash shows the 50 percent cut-off, the left end of the shaded area represents the 75 percent group, and the right end of the shaded area shows the 90 percent performance level.

7. There is also a standardized method of scoring. If a child refuses to perform a particular item, the nurse should let the parent try. If still unsuccessful, *R* (refusal) should be

```
                                    DATE
                                    NAME
            DIRECTIONS              BIRTHDATE
                                    HOSP. NO.
```

1. Try to get child to smile by smiling, talking or waving to him. Do not touch him.
2. When child is playing with toy, pull it away from him. Pass if he resists.
3. Child does not have to be able to tie shoes or button in the back.
4. Move yarn slowly in an arc from one side to the other, about 6" above child's face. Pass if eyes follow 90° to midline. (Past midline; 180°)
5. Pass if child grasps rattle when it is touched to the backs or tips of fingers.
6. Pass if child continues to look where yarn disappeared or tries to see where it went. Yarn should be dropped quickly from sight from tester's hand without arm movement.
7. Pass if child picks up raisin with any part of thumb and a finger.
8. Pass if child picks up raisin with the ends of thumb and index finger using an over hand approach.

9. Pass any enclosed form. Fail continuous round motions.
10. Which line is longer? (Not bigger.) Turn paper upside down and repeat. (3/3 or 5/6)
11. Pass any crossing lines.
12. Have child copy first. If failed, demonstrate

When giving items 9, 11 and 12, do not name the forms. Do not demonstrate 9 and 11.

13. When scoring, each pair (2 arms, 2 legs, etc.) counts as one part.
14. Point to picture and have child name it. (No credit is given for sounds only.)

15. Tell child to: Give block to Mommie; put block on table; put block on floor. Pass 2 of 3. (Do not help child by pointing, moving head or eyes.)
16. Ask child: What do you do when you are cold? ..hungry? ..tired? Pass 2 of 3.
17. Tell child to: Put block on table; under table; in front of chair, behind chair. Pass 3 of 4. (Do not help child by pointing, moving head or eyes.)
18. Ask child: If fire is hot, ice is ?; Mother is a woman, Dad is a ?; a horse is big, a mouse is ?. Pass 2 of 3.
19. Ask child: What is a ball? ..lake? ..desk? ..house? ..banana? ..curtain? ..ceiling? ..hedge? ..pavement? Pass if defined in terms of use, shape, what it is made of or general category (such as banana is fruit, not just yellow). Pass 6 of 9.
20. Ask child: What is a spoon made of? ..a shoe made of? ..a door made of? (No other objects may be substituted.) Pass 3 of 3.
21. When placed on stomach, child lifts chest off table with support of forearms and/or hands.
22. When child is on back, grasp his hands and pull him to sitting. Pass if head does not hang back
23. Child may use wall or rail only, not person. May not crawl.
24. Child must throw ball overhand 3 feet to within arm's reach of tester.
25. Child must perform standing broad jump over width of test sheet. (8-1/2 inches)
26. Tell child to walk forward, ⌒⌒⌒⌒➤ heel within 1 inch of toe. Tester may demonstrate. Child must walk 4 consecutive steps, 2 out of 3 trials.
27. Bounce ball to child who should stand 3 feet away from tester. Child must catch ball with hands, not arms, 2 out of 3 trials.
28. Tell child to walk backward, ◄⌒⌒⌒⌒ toe within 1 inch of heel. Tester may demonstrate. Child must walk 4 consecutive steps, 2 out of 3 trials.

DATE AND BEHAVIORAL OBSERVATIONS (how child feels at time of test, relation to tester, attention span, verbal behavior, self-confidence, etc,):

FIGURE 15.30. Directions for the Denver Developmental Screening Test. (From Frankenburg, W. K. & Dodds, J. B., University of Colorado Medical Center, 1969).

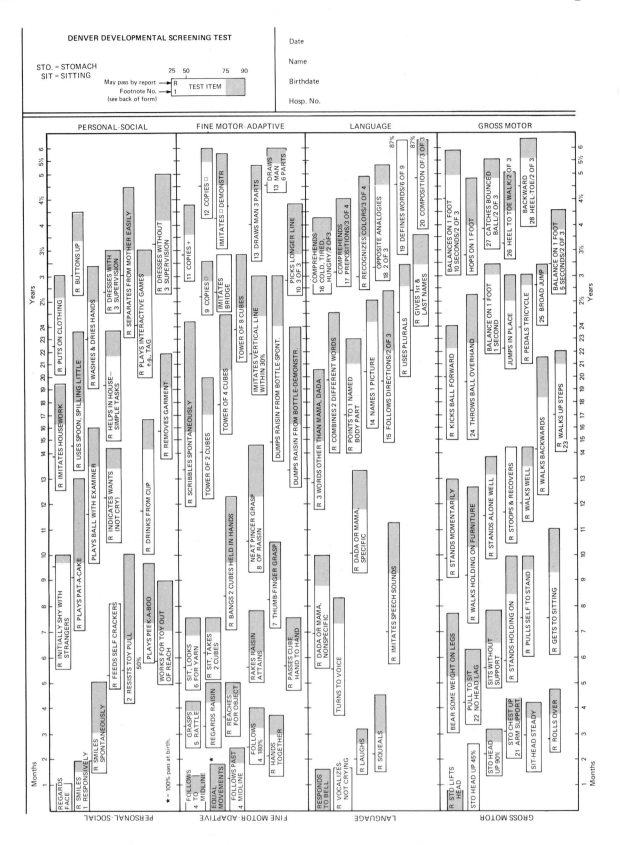

FIGURE 15.31. Form for the Denver Developmental Screening Test. (From Frankenburg, W. K. & Dodds, J. B., University of Colorado Medical Center, 1969).

recorded, as opposed to *F* (failure). *P* is the letter used to indicate a "pass." The last score option is *N.O.* (no opportunity). In some cases, a child may not have had the opportunity to learn certain skills, such as riding a tricycle. In other instances, cultural differences may interfere with performance. If this is the case, it is certainly not fair to fail the child in that area. Thus, the score "N.O." should not be used in the interpretation.

Before designating the score *F*, it is important to give the child at least three chances to perform the test. Administering the test on another day should be considered, too.

A "delay" is any item failed by the child which is completely to the left of the age line. In other words, the child may have failed an item which 90 percent of children normally pass at a younger age. This is documented on the form by coloring the right end of the bar of the delayed item. If the bar touches the age line, it should not be considered a delay.

The child should be tested on all items which pass through the age line. In addition, the child should be tested within each section for at least three expected failures and three expected passes. It helps build up the child's confidence to start with three items well below his age level.

At the completion of the test, the parents should be asked if the child's performance was typical of his activities at other times.

The results are classified within each sector as *normal, abnormal,* or *questionable.* The term *normal* is accepted when there is no doubt about the results. The term *abnormal* can be used under the following circumstances: (1) there are two or more delays in two or more sectors or (2) there are two or more delays in one sector, one delay in one or more sectors, and no passes intersecting the age line in the latter sector (s). The term *questionable* can be used when there are (1) two or more delays in one sector or (2) one delay in one or more sectors and no passes intersecting the age line in that (those) sector(s).

Children who are *abnormal* or *questionable* should be reevaluated within 2 or 3 weeks. If another *abnormal* score is obtained and the parent indicates that this is a typical performance level for the child, further evaluation is warranted.

The reliability of the test results depends a great deal on the sensitivity of the examiner to the child and the environment. Illness, fear, or the atmosphere of the testing area may distort the results. For this reason, it is important for the nurse to write down her observations of the child's behavior. The behavior observed includes attention span, nonverbal communication, and the relationship with the nurse or parent.

Observation of the parent–child interaction during the test may prove valuable to the nurse. Any signs of overdependency or hostility may manifest here. The nurse can also assess problems of emotional development during this entire process—for instance, lack of interest, lack of eye contact, preoccupation, withdrawal, or excessive shyness.

Above all, it is important to remember that this is a screening test, *not* a diagnostic tool. Its basic purpose is to alert the examiner to any need for further evaluation!

REFERENCES

1. Freedman, D. Ethnic differences in babies. *Human Nature*, 1979, *2*, pp. 36–44.
2. Freedman, D. & DeBoer, M. Biological and cultural differences in early child development. *Annual Review of Anthropology*, 1979, *8*, pp. 579–600.
3. Branch, M. & Paxton, P. *Providing safe nursing care for ethnic people of color.* New York: Appleton–Century–Crofts, 1976.
4. Luciano, D.S., Vander, A.J., Sherman, J.H., *Human Function and Structure.* New York: McGraw-Hill, 1978, p. 258.
5. Rudolph, A., Barnett, H., Einhorn, A. (Eds.) *Pediatrics* (16th ed.) New York: Appleton–Century–Crofts, 1977.
6. Thorpe. Developmental ser. of preschool children: A critical review of the interventions used in health and education programs. *Pediatrics*, 1974, *53*, p. 3.

EXAMPLE OF A RECORDED HISTORY AND PHYSICAL

Subjective:

Chief Complaint: "Headache and dizziness twice today."

HPI: This 75-year-old male considers himself to be in "fair" health. He has "severe arthritis" which has been a problem for "years." His day began as usual with no problems until 10:00 AM, when he suddenly noticed he had a dull ache behind his forehead. About 15 minutes later he felt dizzy, too. "The room began spinning around." He took two aspirins, laid down for an hour and "felt fine." About 2 hours ago, the same pain in his head began again, but was more "intense." About 1 hour ago his wife told him that his words were slurring. Half an hour ago his vision became blurry—only out of his left eye. He has no previous history of this type of episode, loss of consciousness, fainting, convulsions, trauma, tingling or numbness, tremors or tics, paralysis, or speech disorders. He takes Motrin 400 mg. t.i.d. for his arthritis. Does not take any other medications except an occasional aspirin. There is a family history of heart disease. Both parents died in their "mid-seventies" of a "stroke." His wife called their family doctor and he instructed her to take her husband to the emergency room. Patient feels he is "losing control of the situation."

Objective: T. 98.8°F axillary; P. 96 radial; R. 24; B.P. (R) 180/100 (lying), (L) 182/106.

MENTAL STATUS. Patient, when sitting in wheelchair, was somewhat slouched. He is frowning and his face reflects tension. His speech is slurred, but words can be understood. He is oriented to time, person, and place. He recalls recent and remote events. Abstract thinking and similarity association testing deferred.

CRANIAL NERVES

I: Right deferred at present.

II: Light—able to read paper 1 foot away. Left—not able to distinguish letters or words. Visual fields: right—within normal limits; Left—(?) < on periphery. Funduscopic: Right—unremarkable; Left—A–V ratio approximately 2:4, disc unremarkable; no A–V nicking, exudates, or hemorrhages.

III, IV, VI: Right—no ptosis, lid lag, PERRLA; no nystagmus; extraocular movements intact. Left—ptosis present, unable to hold glance at upper-left outer quadrant; no nystagmus, lid lag; consensual reaction to light slow.

V: *Sensory*—corneal reflexes present in both eyes. Able to distinguish light touch and sharp from dull on right side of face, chin, and right temporal area. Unable to feel stimulus from wisp of cotton on left temporal or left side of face. Can distinguish sharp from dull all over left side of face. Can also distinguish between hot and cold in the area where light touch is decreased. *Motor*—unable to clench teeth firmly. Temporomandibular contractions weaker on left side.

VII: No tics, tremors, unusual movement, or asymmetry. When asked to clench teeth, smile, unable to hold this position. Difficulty blowing out cheeks with mouth closed, more pronounced on left. Taste testing deferred at present.

VIII: Deferred at present.

IX, X: Uvula rises. No asymmetry of soft palate. Gag response elicited. No hoarseness.

XI: Left—weakness of shoulder when push applied to shrugged shoulders. Weakness also noted when patient pushes face against hand. Right—can resist shoulder shrug and push face against hand.

XII: No asymmetry, unusual movement or deviation of tongue.

MOTOR SYSTEM. Dragging left foot when walking from wheel chair to stretcher. Romberg—could not stand without falling with eyes closed.

	Right	*Left*
Finger grip	Strong	Very weak
Finger abduction	Unremarkable	Weaker than right
Wrist dorsiflexion	Unremarkable	Weaker than right
Flexion and extension of elbow	Unremarkable	Weaker than right
Shoulder and scapulae resistance	Unremarkable	Weaker than right
Hip flexion	Unremarkable	Weaker than right
Hip abduction	Unremarkable	Weaker than right
Hip adduction	Unremarkable	Weaker than right
Knee extension and flexion	Unremarkable	Weaker than right
Plantar flexion and dorsiflexion of ankle (no pain with testing)		

Sensory: Able to distinguish sharp from dull along the right side from shoulder to foot. On left side not able to do this on foot or shin, hand or forearm. Thigh, hip, abdomen, chest, and upper arm intact. Able to distinguish vibratory sensation along right side, wrist, knee, elbow, shoulder, hip, and foot. Unable to feel vibratory sensation on left wrist and left hip. Other areas distinguishable. Unable to distinguish position (up or down) of left big toe. Other areas intact. Rest of sensory exam deferred at present due to fatigue of patient.

Deep Tendon Reflexes: All intact; +2 and symmetrical. No right or left ankle clonus.

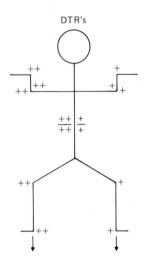

Chest: Respirations regular. Chest expansion symmetrical. Clear to ausucultation. No adventitious breath sounds.

Heart: Regular rate. No murmurs heard. Left carotid bruit present. Right carotid, no bruit.

Pulses:

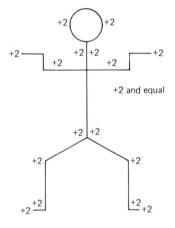

Appendix

EXAMPLE OF A RECORDED PHYSICAL EXAMINATION

Name:	L.R.		Age:	19		Sex:	Female

Height: 5'5''   **Weight:** 125 lbs.

Vital Signs: T. 98.2° F. orally   P. 60 radial   R. 15

B.P.: Arm   Standing: Right 98/68/64   Left 98/68/62

Sitting: 102/72/68   106/70/66

Supine: 108/70/66   106/68/64

Leg   120/80/74

GENERAL: Well developed, well nourished, young-looking adult. Articulate and pleasant. Ambulates without difficulty and is in no distress.

SKIN: Uniformly pinkish white in color, soft, warm, moist, elastic. No edema, masses, or lesions. Occasional lentigos over anterior and posterior trunk. Hair is thick, brown, straight, and shoulder-length. Nails are firm. No clubbing, biting, or discolorations.

HEAD: Cranium is normocephalic, with no tenderness. Scalp shows no lesions, lumps, scaling, or parasites. Face is symmetrical at rest and without edema. Alert and expressive.

EYES:

Visual Acuity: Snellen (no corrective lenses) R:20/20, L:20/25

Alignment: Corneal light reflex symmetrical; no strabismus.

Visual Fields: Full fields.

Extraocular Movements: Intact. No nystagmus.

Lids: No lid lag, edema, or crusting.

Lacrimal Apparatus: No tenderness, masses, or discharge.

Conjunctiva: Clear.

Cornea: No abrasions.

Sclera: White and without redness.

Anterior Chamber: No narrowing.

Irises: Uniformly blue.

Pupils: Equal and round. React to light and accommodation.

Lenses: No opacities.

Funduscopic: Red reflex elicited bilaterally. Disc margins sharp. A–V ratio 3:4. No A–V nicking, hemorrhages, exudate, or papilledema noted. Maculas unremarkable.

EARS:

Hearing: Hears whispered voice at 2 feet bilaterally. Weber—does not lateralize. Rinné—AC > BC bilaterally.

External Ear: No lesions, scaling or tenderness bilaterally.

Otoscopic: Canals clear. Tympanic membranes—pearly gray; shiny light reflex; no redness, bulging, or retraction. Landmarks visible.

NOSE and SINUSES: Nasal septum midline. No tenderness with palpation. Mucosa moist, red, and without inflammation or lesions. Turbinates visualized. No polyps. Frontal and maxillary sinuses are without tenderness.

ORAL CAVITY: No mouth odor. No lesions or bleeding of lips, gums, or tongue. Mucous membranes pink and moist. Teeth well aligned. No plaque or obvious decay. Tongue movement symmetrical. No swelling or lesions. Pharynx pink and without exudate. Tonsils present, without enlargement.

NECK: No edema, masses, or tenderness. Trachea midline. Thyroid nontender and not palpable. No lymphadenopathy.

CHEST: Abdominal breathing. Respirations regular. No signs of labored breathing. Excursion symmetrical. A–P diameter within normal limits. Tactile fremitus equal bilaterally. No masses or tenderness. Lung fields resonant. Diaphragmatic excursion 3 cm right side, 2 cm left. Posterior thorax—vesicular breath sounds throughout. Anterior thorax—bronchovesicular breath sounds over bronchial tree, otherwise vesicular. No adventitious breath sounds.

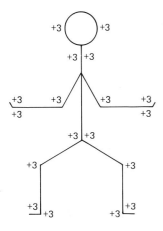

CARDIAC AND PERIPHERAL VASCULAR:

Pulses: +3 and equal; elastic; regular rate and rhythm; of normal contour. (see stick figure illustration)

Cardiac: Apical pulse 60 and of regular rate and rhythm. No visible or palpable masses, abnormal pulsations, lifts, or heaves. No palpable pulsations in the epigastric area. PMI 2 cm wide, palpable in the fifth ICS in the MCL and is a short sound synchronous with S_1. Percussion not done. S_1 is a single sound and is loudest at the apex; S_2 is loudest at the base and is split slightly with inspiration. No S_3, S_4, rubs, murmurs, or extra sounds heard.

Carotid Artery: No bruits auscultated.

Jugular Veins: External and internal jugular veins are elevated 2 cm above the sternal angle with the head of the bed elevated 45°. The *a* wave is synchronous with S_1, as the *v* wave is with S_2.

BREAST: Symetrical, small. No scars, lesions, dimpling, masses, or tenderness bilaterally. Nipples everted. No discharge or crusting.

ABDOMEN: Symmetrical. No protruberance. Strong muscle tone. No scars or striae. Bowel sounds audible in all four quadrants. No bruits over aorta or renal arteries. No masses or tenderness. Liver edge palpable, nontender. Span of 7 cm at MCL. Spleen nontender or palpable. Kidneys not palpable, no CVA tenderness. Bladder not distended or tender. No inguinal, femoral, or umbilical hernias. Inguinal and femoral lymph nodes not palpable or tender.

MALE GENITALIA: Not applicable.

FEMALE GENITALIA:

External: Female hair distribution, no lesions. Introitus pink. Bartholin's and Skene's glands not palpable; no discharge from urethra.

Vagina: Mucosa pink, without lesions. Well rugated. No discharge. No cystocele or rectocele. Strong muscle tone.

Cervix: Pink, nulliparous os. Anterior, firm, mobile. No erosions, cysts, or lesions.

Uterus: Small, pear-shaped, firm. Anteflexed. No mases or tenderness.

Adnexae: Ovaries and tubes not palpable or tender.

Rectum: No lesions, rashes, hemorrhoids. Strong sphincter tone. No masses.

MUSCULOSKETAL:

Neck: Full range of motion without pain. Temporomandibular joint—no slipping or crepitation.

Back: Sits without slouching. No tenderness of vertebral column or paravertebral muscles. No deformity or curvature. Full extension, lateral bending, and rotation. Heights of shoulders and scapulae equal. No pain or discomfort with full ROM.

Extremities: Arms and legs symmetrical. Full ROM of all joints without pain, tenderness, or crepitation. No redness, swelling varicosities, or edema. Epitrochlear nodes not palpable. No muscle atrophy.

NEUROLOGIC:

Mental Status: Alert and oriented to time, person, and place. Can recall recent and past events. Able to name nationally elected officials. Able to interpret abstract thought—i.e., "Don't change horses in the middle of the stream."

Motor Function: Even, regular gait. Able to perform heel to toe walking. No ataxia. Finger grip strong bilaterally. Romberg—able to stand with eyes closed without falling. Able to do hop, skip, and deep-knee bend. Rapid alternating movements of finger to nose and heel sliding down shin done without difficulty. No tremor, tic, or fasciculations.

Sensory: Able to distinguish sharp from dull on face and extremities. Position—able to distinguish up and down movement of toes and fingers bilaterally.

Deep Tendon Reflexes: All intact, +2, symmetrical. (see stick figure illustration)

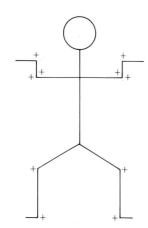

Cranial Nerves:
I: Not done.
II, III, IV, and VI: See *Eye*.
V: Jaws strong, lateral movement intact. Sensation of face intact. See *Sensory*.
VII: Smiles, wrinkles forehead, puffs cheeks, whistles. Symmetrical facial movements.
VIII: See *Ear*.
IX, X: Gag reflex present. Symmetrical rise of uvula and palate. Uvula midline.
XI: Shoulders rise symmetrically in shrug of shoulders and able to resist push.
XII: No asymmetry, fasciculations, or tremor of the tongue.

Bibliography

Alexander, M., & Brown, M. S. *Pediatric history taking and physical diagnosis for nurses* (2nd ed.). New York: McGraw–Hill, 1979.

Barrer, J., Stokes, L., Billings, D. Sensory interference with safety and security—vision. In *Adult and child care*. St. Louis: Mosby, 1973.

Basmajian, J. *Primary anatomy* (6th ed.). Baltimore: Williams & Wilkins, 1970.

Bates, B. *A guide to physical examination* (2nd ed.). Philadelphia: Lippincott, 1974.

Beeson, P. B., & McDermott, W. (Eds.). *Textbook of medicine* (14th ed.). Philadelphia: Saunders, 1975.

Chow, M., Durand, B. A., Feldman, M. N., & Mills, M. A. *Handbook of pediatric primary care*. New York: John Wiley and Sons, 1979.

DeAngelis, C. *Pediatric primary care* (2nd ed.). Boston: Little, Brown, 1979.

deCastro, F. Rolfe, U., & Drew, J. *The pediatric nurse practitioner: Guidelines for practice* (2nd ed.). St. Louis: Mosby, 1976.

DeGowin, E., & DeGowin, R. *Bedside diagnostic examination* (3rd ed.). New York: Macmillan, 1976.

Diekelmann, N. *Primary health care of the well adult*. New York: McGraw–Hill, 1977.

Duvall, E. *Family development* (4th ed.). Philadelphia: Lippincott, 1971.

Fowkes, W. Jr., & Hunn, V. *Clinical assessment for the nurse practitioner*. St. Louis: 1973.

Gallagher, J., Heald, F., & Garell, D. *Medical care of the adolescent*. New York: Appleton–Century–Crofts, 1976.

Ganong, W. *Review of medical physiology* (6th ed.). Los Altos: Lange Medical Publications, 1973.

Harmon, V., & Steele, S. *Nursing care of the skin: A developmental approach*. New York: Appleton–Century–Crofts, 1975.

Harvey, A. M., Johns, R. J., Owens, A. H., Jr., & Ross, R. S. *The principles and practices of medicine*. (19th ed.). New York: Appleton–Century–Crofts, 1976.

Hoppenfeld, S. *Physical examination of the spine and extremities*. New York: Appleton–Century–Crofts, 1976.

Hughes, J. G. *Synopsis of pediatrics* (3rd ed.). St. Louis: Mosby, 1971.

Jacob, S. W., & Francone, C. A. *Structure and function in man* (3rd ed.). Philadelphia: Saunders, 1974.

Judge, R. D., & Zuidema, G. D. (Eds.). *Methods of clinical examination: A physiologic approach*. Boston: Little, Brown, 1974.

Lewis, H. *The history and the physical examination*. New York: Appleton–Century–Crofts, 1979.

Luciano, D. S., Vander, A. J., & Sherman, J. H. *Human function and structure*. New York: McGraw–Hill, 1978.

Malasanos, L., Barkauskas, V., Moss, M., & Stoltenberg–Allen, K. *Health assessment*. St. Louis: Mosby, 1977.

Martin, L. *Health care of women*. Philadelphia: Lippincott, 1978.

Murray, R. B., & Zentner, J. P. *Nursing assessment and health promotion through the life span* (2nd ed.). Englewood Cliffs, N.J.: Prentice–Hall, 1979.

Office of Cancer Communications. *The breast cancer digest: A guide to medical care, emotional support, educational programs and resources.* DHEW Publication No. (NIH) 79–1691. Bethesda, Md.: National Cancer Institute, 1979.

Prior, J., & Siberstein, J. *Physical diagnosis: The history and examination of the patient* (4th ed.). St. Louis: Mosby, 1973.

Pritchard, J. A., & MacDonald, P. C. *Williams obstetrics* (15th ed.). New York: Appleton–Century–Crofts, 1976.

Rudolph, A., & Barnett, H. L. (Eds.). *Pediatrics* (16th ed.). New York: Appleton–Century–Crofts, 1977.

Schottelius, B., & Schottelius, D. D. *Textbook of physiology* (17th ed.). St. Louis: Mosby, 1973.

Selkurt, E. E. (ed.). *Basic physiology for the health sciences.* Boston: Little, Brown, 1975.

Sherman, J., & Fields, S. *Guide to patient evaluation.* Flushing, N.Y.: Medical Examination Publishing, 1974.

Slattery, J., Pearson, G., & Torre, C. (Eds.). *Maternal and child nutrition: Assessment and counseling.* New York: Appleton–Century–Crofts, 1979.

Vaughn, V., & McKay, R. J. (Eds.). *Nelson textbook of pediatrics* (10th ed.). Philadelphia: Saunders, 1975.

Zuidema, G. (Ed.). *The Johns Hopkins atlas of human functional anatomy.* Baltimore: Johns Hopkins University Press, 1977.

Index

f indicates figure legend; *c* indicates chart